Nutritional Management of Inflammatory Bowel Diseases

Ashwin N. Ananthakrishnan
Editor

Nutritional Management of Inflammatory Bowel Diseases

A Comprehensive Guide

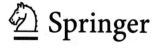 Springer

Editor
Ashwin N. Ananthakrishnan, M.D., M.P.H.
Harvard Medical School
Massachusetts General Hospital
Boston, MA, USA

ISBN 978-3-319-80035-6   ISBN 978-3-319-26890-3   (eBook)
DOI 10.1007/978-3-319-26890-3

Springer Cham Heidelberg New York Dordrecht London
© Springer International Publishing Switzerland 2016
Softcover reprint of the hardcover 1st edition 2016

Printed on acid-free paper

Springer International Publishing AG Switzerland is part of Springer Science+Business Media
(www.springer.com)

*I would like to dedicate this book to the
patients with inflammatory bowel diseases,
their family, healthcare professionals,
and researchers working to address
the challenges of these complex diseases*

Foreword

The management of a patient with inflammatory bowel disease (IBD) is complex and multilayered. Choosing appropriate effective yet safe therapy is utmost in the minds of most providers, but to the patient "Doctor what can I eat?" is the most important discussion that occurs in the office. While the science moves forward with understanding the intricate interplay of the microbial environment of the GI tract, it is apparent that what a patient consumes becomes part of that environment as well. For some, enteral nutrition is the treatment of choice for their Crohn's disease.

So the timeliness of this book cannot be understated. The authors here have broken down the different aspects of "nutrition" for providers so that they can have informed discussions with their patients regarding this important topic. Separating fact from fiction and science from speculation, this book will ultimately help patients make responsible choices and hopefully prevent even more complications that can result from elimination or fad diets meant to promote "health" or "healing."

I welcome the knowledge points brought forth in this book and hope that other readers use this information in formulating informed, evidence-based management plans for their patients with IBD.

Mayo Clinic   Sunanda Kane, M.D., M.S.P.H., F.A.C.G.
Rochester, MN, USA

Preface

Nutrition and Inflammatory Bowel Diseases: A Complex and Continuous Interface

Inflammatory bowel diseases (IBD), comprising Crohn's disease and ulcerative colitis, affect an estimated 1.5 million Americans, 2.2 million individuals in Europe, and several thousands more worldwide. They are complex in their origin, arising due to a dysregulated immune response to the microbiome in a genetically predisposed individual. The past two decades have witnessed an exponential increase in our understanding of the pathogenesis of these complex diseases, highlighting the role of innate and adaptive immune responses, integrity of the intestinal barrier function, as well as alterations in the diversity and composition of the intestinal microbiome. Yet, much remains unknown regarding the origin and natural history of these diseases. In particular, the role of modifiable environmental and behavioral factors, and in particular diet, remains poorly understood.

The effects of dietary influences on the onset of IBD as well as its potential effect on the natural history and maintenance of remission are among the most frequently voiced concerns by patients and family members. Indeed, despite the advances in therapeutic agents targeting the immune response that have revolutionized IBD care, safety and durability of such therapies over the long term remains an important concern. Most patients with IBD express an interest in active management of their disease and in particular through dietary modifications. Yet this is an area where there is limited data and consequently a dearth of resources to guide patients and providers. Additionally, by virtue of pan-gastrointestinal tract involvement in IBD and the effect of both disease and treatments on absorption and eating behavior, malnutrition and specific nutritional deficiencies are common in these patients.

This book was developed to serve as a comprehensive resource to healthcare providers involved in the management of IBD. Leading experts in the field summarize the state of the art in diet and nutritional management in IBD and provide useful practical tips for patient care.

Part I lays the ground for how dietary factors may influence the development and subsequent course of inflammatory bowel diseases. The first chapter on the influence of diet on the gut microbiome proposes mechanisms how dietary factors may alter the microbiome sufficiently to serve as a pro-inflammatory trigger for immune responses, while the second chapter examines the epidemiologic evidence supporting the association between various dietary patterns, micro- and macronutrient intake, and disease onset and relapse.

Part II of this book addresses the nutritional deficiencies that affect patients with IBD with specific chapters on iron and vitamin D, both of which are frequently deficient. The third chapter in this section provides a comprehensive A-to-zinc overview of other micronutrient deficiencies and guide to their management.

Part III provides insights on various dietary therapies for the management of established inflammatory bowel disease by first reviewing the most rigorously supported dietary intervention—enteral nutrition. Less well-supported but nevertheless widely popular interventions such as elimination diets, prebiotics, and probiotics are addressed in the next two chapters.

Part IV closes with a discussion of the most complex nutritional issues affecting patients with protracted and complicated courses of their IBD. The long-term outcomes and complications of total parenteral nutrition are discussed. The next two chapters summarize the pathophysiology, nutritional, and pharmacologic management of short bowel syndrome. Finally, the role of small bowel transplantation in those with refractory disease is discussed.

Contents

Contributors

Bincy P. Abraham, M.D., M.S., F.A.C.P. Division of Gastroenterology and Hepatology, Houston Methodist Hospital and Weill Cornell Medical College, Fondren Inflammatory Bowel Disease Program, Lynda K and David M Underwood Center for Digestive Disorders, Houston, TX, USA

Philip J. Allan, M.B.B.S., B.Sc., D.P.H.I.L., M.R.C.P. The Translational Gastroenterology Unit, Oxford University Hospitals NHS Trust, John Radcliffe Hospital, Oxford, UK

The Oxford Transplant Centre, Oxford University Hospitals NHS Trust, Churchill Hospital, Oxford, UK

The Intestinal Failure Unit, Salford Royal NHS Foundation Trust, Salford, UK

Alyce Anderson, B.S. Division of Gastroenterology, Hepatology and Nutrition, University of Pittsburgh School of Medicine, UPMC Presbyterian Hospital, Pittsburgh, PA, USA

David G. Binion, M.D. Division of Gastroenterology, Hepatology and Nutrition, University of Pittsburgh School of Medicine, UPMC Presbyterian Hospital, Pittsburgh, PA, USA

Athos Bousvaros, M.D., M.P.H. Division of Gastroenterology and Nutrition, Harvard Medical School, Boston Children's Hospital, Boston, MA, USA

Simon S.M. Chan, M.B. B.Chir., Ph.D., M.R.C.P. University of East Anglia, Norwich, Norfolk, UK

Department of Gastroenterology, Norfolk and Norwich University Hospital, NHS Foundation Trust, Norwich, Norfolk, UK

Athanasios P. Desalermos, M.D. Division of Gastroenterology, University of California, San Diego, USA

Francis A. Farraye, M.D., M.Sc. Section of Gastroenterology, Boston University Medical Center, Boston, MA, USA

Mahesh Gajendran, M.B.B.S. Department of Internal Medicine, University of Pittsburgh Medical Center, Pittsburgh, PA, USA

Thomas Greuter, M.D. Division of Gastroenterology and Hepatology, University Hospital Zurich, Zurich, Switzerland

Andrew R. Hart, M.B. Ch.B., M.D., F.R.C.P. University of East Anglia, Norwich, Norfolk, UK

Department of Gastroenterology, Norfolk and Norwich University Hospital, NHS Foundation Trust, Norwich, Norfolk, UK

Kurt Hong, M.D., Ph.D. Department of Medicine, Keck School of Medicine at University of Southern California (USC), Los Angeles, CA, USA

Department of Medicine, Center for Clinical Nutrition and Applied Health Research, Keck School of Medicine at University of Southern California (USC), Los Angeles, CA, USA

Jason K. Hou, M.D., M.S. Houston VA HSR&D Center of Excellence, Michael E. DeBakey Veterans Affairs Medical Center, Houston, TX, USA

Department of Gastroenterology and Hepatology, Baylor College of Medicine, Houston, TX, USA

Caroline Hwang, M.D. Department of Medicine, Keck School of Medicine at University of Southern California (USC), Los Angeles, CA, USA

Simon Lal, M.B.B.S., Ph.D., F.R.C.P. The Intestinal Failure Unit, Salford Royal NHS Foundation Trust, Salford, UK

Priya Loganathan, M.B.B.S. Division of Gastroenterology, Hepatology and Nutrition, University of Pittsburgh School of Medicine, UPMC Presbyterian Hospital, Pittsburgh, PA, USA

Renée M. Marchioni Beery, D.O. Department of Gastroenterology, Hepatology and Endoscopy, Brigham and Women's Hospital, Harvard Medical School, Boston, MA, USA

Hannah L. Miller, M.D. Connecticut Gastroenterology Consultants, New Haven, CT, USA

Eamonn M.M. Quigley, M.D., F.R.C.P., F.A.C.P., F.A.C.G., F.R.C.P.I. Division of Gastroenterology and Hepatology, Houston Methodist Hospital and Weill Cornell Medical College, Fondren Inflammatory Bowel Disease Program, Lynda K and David M Underwood Center for Digestive Disorders, Houston, TX, USA

Claudia Ramos Rivers, M.D. Division of Gastroenterology, Hepatology and Nutrition, University of Pittsburgh School of Medicine, UPMC Presbyterian Hospital, Pittsburgh, PA, USA

William Rivers, B.S. Division of Gastroenterology, Hepatology and Nutrition, University of Pittsburgh School of Medicine, UPMC Presbyterian Hospital, Pittsburgh, PA, USA

Jenny Sauk, M.D. Department of Gastroenterology, Massachusetts General Hospital, Boston, MA, USA

Anil Vaidya, M.D. The Oxford Transplant Centre, Oxford University Hospitals NHS Trust, Churchill Hospital, Oxford, UK

Stephan R. Vavricka, M.D. Division of Gastroenterology and Hepatology, University Hospital Zurich, Zurich, Switzerland

Division of Gastroenterology and Hepatology, Triemli Hospital Zurich, Zurich, Switzerland

Vijay Yajnik, M.D., Ph.D. Massachusetts General Hospital, Crohn's and Colitis Center, Boston, MA, USA

Part I
Diet and the Pathogenesis of Inflammatory Bowel Diseases

Chapter 1
Diet and Microbiome in Inflammatory Bowel Diseases

Jenny Sauk

Introduction

The pathogenesis of inflammatory bowel disease (IBD) remains elusive. As genetics accounts for only 30–40 % of disease penetrance, focus has shifted towards the contribution of environmental factors, such as antibiotics, smoking, and diet, on IBD disease risk and trajectory [1–7]. Alterations in the intestinal microbiota parallel changes in these environmental factors, with evidence suggesting a role of the intestinal microbiota in immune modulation [8–11]. Of all the exogenous factors, long-term diet has the largest effect in shaping the intestinal microbiome [12]. Therefore, understanding the effect of diet on the intestinal microbiome in IBD and in health can potentially identify new dietary therapeutic avenues to modulate disease course.

Intestinal Microbiome: Primer

Our gastrointestinal tract harbors a rich microbial community varying in composition and density based on anatomic site, host secretions, and intestinal transit time. Due to high acidity and rapid transit, the stomach and proximal small intestine hold relatively few microorganisms. However, the large intestine is home to roughly 10^{11} bacteria/g of luminal content in the colon, dominated mainly by obligate anaerobic bacteria that ferment non-digested dietary components [13].

J. Sauk, M.D. (✉)
Department of Gastroenterology, Massachusetts General Hospital,
165 Cambridge Street, 9th Floor, Boston, MA 02114, USA
e-mail: jsauk@mgh.harvard.edu

© Springer International Publishing Switzerland 2016   3
A.N. Ananthakrishnan (ed.), *Nutritional Management of Inflammatory Bowel Diseases*, DOI 10.1007/978-3-319-26890-3_1

Colonization of our intestinal tract begins at birth with fluctuations noted until age 2–3 years, after which the intestinal microbiota stabilizes and resembles that of the adult [14]. Early life factors, such as mode of delivery and breastfeeding, affect intestinal colonization of the infant, with *Lactobacillus* and other microbial communities resembling the mother's vaginal microbiota, more frequently colonizing the intestinal tract of infants born via vaginal delivery versus C-section. Once diet is introduced, there is frequently a shift in the dominant community, with *Bifidobacterium* species more consistently represented in breastfed infants versus formula-fed infants [15, 16].

With more sophisticated DNA-sequencing technologies and bioinformatics tools, our understanding of the intestinal microbiota has progressed rapidly. Both targeted 16S rRNA gene sequencing and whole-genome shotgun sequencing can be used to determine the microbial populations present and their abundance within a community. Whole genome shotgun sequencing has the added benefit of providing information on all genes, including bacterial sequences for which no reference sequence is available and sequences of eukaryotic, archaeal, and viral origin. Furthermore, as shotgun-sequencing samples the entire community gene content, genes associated with microbial function can also be determined [17].

Intestinal bacteria recovered from the stool belong to mainly two phyla, Bacteroides and Firmicutes. Bacteroides phylum breaks down further to two main genera, Bacteroides and Prevotella. Firmicutes include several species recognized as butyrate producers capable of breaking down indigestible polysaccharides. Other phyla, such as Actinobacteria and Proteobacteria are much less abundant in the healthy intestinal microbiota. These lesser abundant organisms can still play an important role in disease and health. As the intestinal microbiome includes 150-fold more genes than the human microbiota, it is likely that the intestinal microbiome plays a significant role in health and disease [18, 19].

IBD and the Microbiome: Overview

The dysbiosis described in IBD is characterized by lower microbial diversity and species richness, a greater prevalence of pro-inflammatory pathobionts, mainly described within the phylum, Proteobacteria, and a lower prevalence of commensal bacteria within the phylum, Firmicutes [20–23].

In ulcerative colitis, Firmicutes within the Clostridia cluster IV and XIVa, such as *Faecalibacterium prausnitzii* and *Roseburia hominis*, have been shown to have decreased representation in active UC than controls with an inverse correlation between disease activity and the presence of these organisms [24]. Furthermore, *Faecalibacterium prausnitzii* recovery after relapse also has been associated with maintenance of clinical remission in UC [25]. Reductions in bacteria involved in butyrate or proprionate metabolism, such as *Ruminococcus bromii*, *Eubacterium rectale*, and *Roseburia* sp. with increases in pathobionts such as *Fusobacterium* sp., *Campylobacter* sp., *Helicobacter* sp., *and Clostridium difficile* have been reported with UC [26]. A recent study also showed that the healthy sibling within a twin pairs discordant for IBD harbored the same microbial alterations as seen in the UC affected twin, suggesting that alterations in the gut microbiota may precede disease [27].

Similar sibling studies in CD have demonstrated a reduced microbial diversity, with lower abundance of *Faecalibacterium prausnitzii*, noted in the unaffected sibling of patients with CD [28]. *Faecalibacterium prausnitzii* has also featured prominently in other studies in CD that showed its decreased abundance is associated with a higher risk of postoperative recurrence in ileal CD. A lower proportion of *F. prausnitzii* in the resected ileal CD mucosal specimen was also associated with a higher risk of endoscopic recurrence at 6 months [29]. A recent, multicenter pediatric study in treatment-naive, newly diagnosed CD patients went further to show a decreased abundance of Erysipelotrichales, Bacteroidales, and Clostridiales with an increased abundance of Enterobacteriaceae, Pasteurellaceae, Veillonellaceae, and Fusobacteriaceae in both ileal and rectal biopsies [30]. Larger, longitudinal studies are necessary to determine the cause–effect relationship between the microbiome and disease onset. Cross-sectional studies at diagnosis and before diagnosis in higher risk individuals suggest that a microbial dysbiosis is present early in the course of disease.

Diet, IBD, and Microbiome: Overview

As the incidence of IBD has increased in developing nations such as East Asia, India, and Northern Africa, there is greater attention centered on the effects of the "Westernized" diet on IBD [1, 31, 32]. Supporting the role of the "Westernized" diet on intestinal inflammation, a study comparing the intestinal microbiome of European (EU) children with that of children from a rural African village of Burkina Faso (BF) revealed a higher representation of Enterobacteriaceae (*Shigella* and *Escherichia*) in EU children than BF children [33]. In parallel, there was a greater abundance of short-chain fatty acids (SCFA) seen in BF children than EU children thought to be related to high plant polysaccharide consumption in BF children and leading to the hypothesis that the SCFA-producing bacteria that figured prominently in BF children could help prevent the establishment of pathogenic bacteria. Other studies have supported a greater abundance of bile-tolerant organisms (*Alistipes*, *Bilophila*, *Bacteroides*) with decreased Firmicutes noted on an animal-based diet, which is prominently featured in a Westernized diet. One bile-tolerant organism represented with higher abundance on the animal-based diet, *Bilophila wadsworthia*, in particular, has been linked to IBD in animal studies [34, 35].

Long-term dietary habits influence an individual's final microbial composition. However, short-term microbiome changes can occur with brief dietary perturbations [19, 36]. Wu *et al.* performed a controlled feeding experiment on ten healthy subjects where subjects were given either a high-fat/low-fiber diet or low-fat/high-fiber diet and the stool samples were analyzed over 10 days. While changes were detectable within 24 h, the change was not significant enough to alter the major bacterial groups. Furthermore, the microbiome after intervention was still more similar to the individual before intervention than that of other subjects. A study by David *et al.* also demonstrated rapid alterations in microbial composition with dietary intervention (animal-based diet) will return to baseline within 2 days of the end of the intervention [34]. Long-term dietary interventions are likely necessary to lead to more significant and permanent shifts in microbial composition.

As these studies demonstrate the impact of diet on microbial composition in health and disease with dysbiosis prevailing in IBD, a greater effort to understand the effects of various components of our diet on the IBD microbiome may reveal mechanisms by which we can alter the course of the disease.

Fiber

Carbohydrates can be classified by their availability for metabolism in the small intestine. Carbohydrates (simple sugars/starch) are hydrolyzed and absorbed in the small intestine. Resistant starches, including inulin, pullan, fructooligosaccharides, and galactooligosaccharides, are carbohydrates that cannot be hydrolyzed in the small intestine but are fermented by the microbiota in the large intestine. Lastly, insoluble fiber, such as cellulose or bran, pass through the digestive tract intact but can have a laxative effect and add bulk to intestinal contents [37].

Higher dietary fiber, fruits and vegetable intake has been shown to have an inverse relationship to risk of Crohn's disease in pediatric and adult studies [38, 39]. In a large prospective study, soluble fiber from fruits and vegetables drove the strong inverse association between dietary fiber and CD risk [39]. Insoluble fiber, from whole grain and cereal, did not decrease this risk in CD or UC. However, intervention studies where fiber was used to affect disease course have had heterogeneous outcomes [6].

Microbial fermentation products from fiber, particularly short-chain fatty acids (SCFAs), can promote immune tolerance by increasing T regulatory (Treg) cell expression, via G-protein coupled receptor-mediated (GPR43) epigenetic modifications involving the inhibition of histone deacetylase [6, 10]. Supporting the importance of SCFAs, Erickson *et al.* demonstrated in twins discordant for CD that the affected twin experienced a decrease in microbial diversity along with a reduction in SCFA production [40]. Morgan *et al.* also revealed a decrease in SCFA pathways in CD patients compared to healthy controls [23]. A TNBS-induced colitis model suggested the role of roughly 17 bacterial strains from the Clostridia clusters IV, XIVa, and XVIII in expanding the colonic Treg population with a study by Smith *et al.* suggesting that SCFAs regulate the size and function of this colonic Treg pool [41, 42].

While specific fruits or vegetables have not been targeted as having particular health benefit in UC or CD, several small studies have evaluated immunologic and microbial changes with prebiotics, nondigestible fiber compounds that pass undigested through the upper part of the gastrointestinal tract and are meant to stimulate the growth of commensal bacteria, in CD and UC. Inulin, resistant starches, and fructo-oligosaccharides (FOS) have been studies as potential prebiotics.

The anti-inflammatory effects of FOS were explored in one small study of 10 CD patients receiving 15 g of FOS for 3 weeks revealing a significant reduction in the Harvey Bradshaw Index with an increase in *Bifidobacteria* concentrations [43]. Subsequently, FOS was studied in 103 CD patients receiving 15 g a day of FOS versus placebo for 4 weeks. While there was no significant clinical benefit seen in patients receiving FOS, there was a decrease in IL-6-positive lamina propria dendritic cells (DC) with increased DC IL-10 staining. No significant differences in *F. prausnitzii* or *Bifidobacteria* were noted in stool samples after the 4-week intervention [44].

In UC, a prospective, randomized, placebo-controlled trial of 19 patients treated with mesalamine showed that the group who received an oligofructose-enriched inulin supplementation for 2 weeks had a significantly lower fecal calprotectin level than controls (day 0: 4377; day 7: 1033; $p < 0.05$). No microbiome data were presented in this study [45]. Inulin supplementation was also explored in a study on pouchitis, where 24 g of inulin supplementation in 3 weeks lowered concentrations of *Bacteroides fragilis*, increased butyrate levels in the stool and decreased endoscopic inflammation [46].

In several UC studies, germinated barley food (GBF) has been explored, demonstrating induction of remission in patients with mild-to-moderate ulcerative colitis with one study revealing an increase in butyrate concentrations in the stool and another study finding increased levels of *Bifidobacteria* and *Eubacterium limosum* after GBF supplementation [47–49]. Larger, controlled clinical studies in well-phenotyped patients using prebiotic formulations linking microbial and metabolomic changes with disease outcome are needed to elucidate the patient population that would benefit most from these interventions.

Fat

The Western diet is characterized by higher fat and lower fiber. In mouse and human studies, high fat, in particular, high n-6 polyunsaturated fatty acid (PUFAs), consumption has been associated with increased risk of IBD and acceleration of inflammation [50–53].

A high-fat diet (HFD) is thought to propagate inflammation by changing the intestinal barrier function, activating various pro-inflammatory signaling pathways and altering the composition of the intestinal microbiota [54–57]. For example, a HFD was fed to wild-type mice and mice that overexpressed carcinoembryonic antigen-related cell adhesion molecules, CEACAMs, of which CEACAM6 is overexpressed in CD patients, leading to increases in *Ruminococcus torques* species that degrade mucus. Changes in intestinal permeability and goblet cell numbers, further promoted adherent-invasive *E. coli* (AIEC) invasion [56].

In another mouse model, a high milk fat diet accelerated the onset of colitis in IL-10-deficient mice, promoting taurine conjugation of bile acids, greater availability of luminal sulfur and subsequent expansion of a specific sulfite-reducing opportunistic pathogen, *Biophilia wadsworthia* [35]. To parallel these findings, humans placed on an animal-based diet showed an expansion of *B. wadsworthia* and other bile-tolerant microbes in the stool [34]. Decreases in microbes associated with plant polysaccharide metabolism, including *Eubacterium rectale, Roseburia* sp., and *Ruminococcus bromii* were also decreased in these human subjects on an animal-based HFD. Reduced microbial carbohydrate fermentation products, particularly short-chain fatty acids, were also witnessed in this group.

To expand on these observations, a mouse study further determined that parental HFD during gestation and lactation could impact immunity of the pups, leading to higher circulating bacterial LPS and lower bacterial diversity in the HFD pups. Therefore, the effects of parental high-fat diet consumption could potentially pass on to the subsequent generation [57, 58].

Enteral Nutrition

Enteral nutrition (EEN) is a complete liquid diet composed of one of the three formulas: elemental, comprised of partially or completely hydrolyzed nutrients; semi-elemental, comprised of peptides, simple sugars, glucose or starch polymers, and fats (as medium chain triglycerides); and polymeric, which includes intact fats, carbohydrates, and proteins [37]. These formula diets have been studied extensively for induction and maintenance of remission of CD with 4–12 weeks of the exclusive EEN typically required to induce remission and partial EEN required to maintain remission [19].

Mainly in pediatric studies, EEN is equivalent to corticosteroids in inducing remission with up to 80 % of active CD patients experiencing reductions in Pediatric Crohn's Disease Activity Index (PCDAI) scores and a decrease in inflammatory markers (C-reactive protein) following 8–12 weeks of EEN therapy [59–61, 92]. As adults struggle more with compliance, studies demonstrating efficacy of EEN have not been consistent in the adult population [62].

The mechanism by which EEN reduces inflammation in CD patients is largely unknown. Elemental formulas are absorbed in the proximal small intestine, eliminating any dietary components that reach the distal small bowel and colon [6]. Studies suggest that EEN work by improving intestinal barrier function, directly reducing proinflammatory cytokines and alterating the intestinal microbiota [63–65].

The microbial patterns with EEN treatment have not been consistent. Shiga and colleagues examined the microbiome of 33 active CD patients and 17 healthy subjects after elemental diet (8 patients) and total parental nutrition (TPN; 9 patients) via terminal restriction fragment length polymorphism (T-RFVPs) and revealed a significant decline in the *Bacteroides fragilis* population after elemental diet while maintaining overall diversity [65]. Leach et al. explored various microbial targets of interest and suggested that decreases in *C. leptum* correlated negatively with changes in the PCDAI, suggesting that *C. leptum* group stability was associated with reduced intestinal inflammation and disease activity [66].

Two studies have reported a decrease in microbial diversity with EEN therapy [60, 67]. Most recently, Kaakoush and colleagues used 16S rRNA and whole genome shotgun sequencing to determine changes in the fecal microbiota of 5 CD children before, during and after EEN therapy and compared these changes with 5 healthy controls to determine the effect of EEN on the intestinal microbiota. There was a reduced microbial diversity and reduced number of OTUs in CD patients, which correlated with disease remission [60]. It is likely that depletion of commensals by EEN therapy decreases the immune reactivity towards the CD microbiota. Larger studies are needed to further characterize the effects of EEN on the intestinal microbiota.

Aryl Hydrocarbon Receptor

Several studies in IBD have suggested a protective role of the aryl hydrocarbon receptor (AhR), a pathway involved in the detoxification of environmental substances with immunological functions. Compounds from cruciferous vegetables, such as broccoli, cauliflower, and cabbage, can activate the AhR pathway [10, 57]. AhR-deficient mice fail to produce IL-22 and are unable to mount a protective innate immune response to *Citrobacter rodentium* with severe colitis and high bacterial titers in the draining lymph nodes, liver, and feces [68]. In another study, the absence of AhR ligands increased the severity of colitis in mice, and when mice were placed on diets enriched in AhR ligands, alterations could be partially reversed [69]. IBD patients have decreased AhR expression in the intestinal tissue with activation of AhR signaling shown to decrease colitis [70].

Microbial metabolites or dietary factors may affect this pathway. For example, when availability of tryptophan, an essential amino acid, is high in the gastrointestinal tract, several species of microbes, predominantly *Lactobacilli acidophilus*, are able to utilize this amino acid, producing indole-3-aldehyde, activating AhR-driven IL-22 production by innate lymphoid cells to maintain mucosal homeostasis and confer colonization resistance to *Candida albicans* [71].

Another example of AhR modulation is with a microbial metabolite, 1,4-dihydroxy-2-naphthoic acid (DHNA), a precursor of Vitamin K2 made by *Propionibacterium freudenreichii* ET-3, found in cheese [10]. Via the AhR pathway, DHNA administration increased synthesis of antimicrobial peptides, RegIIIβ and γ, thus preventing the induction of DSS colitis [72]. Dietary or microbial factors that activate the AhR can affect expression of cytokines (such as IL-22) and production of antimicrobial peptides can influence intestinal homeostasis [57].

Micronutrients

Vitamin D deficiency has emerged as a key factor in the pathogenesis in IBD [73, 74]. An association between polymorphisms in the vitamin D receptor (VDR) and IBD suscepti-bility has been demonstrated [75, 76]. One study evaluated barrier function in polarized epithelial Caco-2bbe cells grown in medium with or without vitamin D and challenged with adherent invasive E. coli (AIEC) strain LF82. Caco-2bbe cells incubated with 1,25(OH)$_2$D$_3$ were protected against AIEC-induced disruption of transepithelial electri-cal resistance and tight junction protein redistribution. Mice were also fed vitamin D sufficient or deficient diets for 5 weeks and then were infected with AIEC, in the absence or presence of a low-dose Dextan Sodium Sulfate (DSS). Vitamin D-deficient mice given 2 % DSS exhibited pronounced epithelial barrier dysfunction and were more susceptible to AIEC colonization. Vitamin D-deficient mice also had significant increases in the rela-tive quantities of Bacteroidetes. Therefore, vitamin D was able to maintain epithelial barrier homeostasis, protecting against the effects of AIEC [77].

Iron

Iron is an essential nutrient in humans but also in nearly all bacterial species that coex-ist with humans. Animal and human studies have revealed an effect of oral iron on microbial composition [78–80]. In IBD, the role of oral iron is controversial. Mouse models of CD suggest ingested iron aggravates disease activity, whereas parenteral iron has no disease promoting effect [80]. Microbial composition parallels these trends with a decrease in *Desulfovibrio* sp. seen with luminal iron depletion [80]. However, conflicting results arise from human IBD studies evaluating disease-modi-fying effects of oral iron supplementation with one study showing an increase in dis-ease activity, but other studies showing no clear difference in disease activity between oral and intravenous iron treatment [81–83]. Studies have not explored the microbi-ome with respect to iron status in IBD patients, but dysbiosis has been described in anemic African children after oral iron fortification, resulting in an unfavorable ratio of fecal Enterobacteriaceae to *Bifidobacteria* and *Lactobacilli*, with an associated increase in fecal calprotectin correlating with the increase in fecal Enterobacteriaceae [84]. As most ingested iron is not absorbed but passes on to the terminal ileum and colon, iron can potentially create an inflammatory milieu by increasing local produc-tion of reactive oxygen species [85]. Further studies should be performed to under-stand the effects of parenteral versus oral iron in the IBD microbiome.

Food Additives

Polysaccharides, such as carrageenan, carboxymethyl cellulose, and maltodextrin, added to foods as emulsifiers, stabilizers, or bulking agents have been linked to bacteria-associated intestinal disorders [86–89]. The increasing consumption of polysaccharides in Western diets parallels the rise in CD [37]. Maltodextrin (MDX), in particular, has been shown to be linked to CD pathogenesis, with studies demonstrating an increased prevalence of bacteria for MDX metabolism in the ileal mucosa of CD patients. MDX also markedly enhanced AIEC LF82 strain-specific biofilm formation [90]. However, MDX alone was not sufficient to induce spontaneous intestinal inflammation in wild-type mice or full-term piglets [37, 91]. Dietary additives likely require the presence of concomitant risk factors to produce intestinal inflammation.

Conclusion

Modulating the intestinal microbiota remains an attractive therapeutic potential for IBD.

While the armamentarium of promising IBD medications continue to expand, many act as immunosuppressive agents and concern regarding adverse side effects prevail. As dietary interventions lack the side effect profile of immunosuppressive agents, patients frequently ask and desire a dietary prescription to treat IBD. Further understanding of the role of diet in IBD pathogenesis is needed and as diet affects the microbiome, it is only natural to explore how diet can modulate the course of IBD and affect the intestinal microbiome. While dietary modulation can alter the intestinal microbiota, the studies above demonstrate that these changes appear short-lived with relatively minor impact on the stable individual microbial composition.

Nevertheless, larger and longer studies have yet to be performed to assess if long-term dietary changes can create more durable changes with greater impact on the intestinal microbiome. Future studies should explore whether dietary interventions earlier in the course of disease could make more of an impact in disease course or if dietary interventions should be considered more as maintenance agents than induction therapies for IBD. Such considerations would influence future dietary intervention studies. Furthermore, understanding the individual variation in the microbiome and the unique immune response to an individual's microbiome may lead to the creation of a personalized microbial therapeutic prescription including dietary modulation that can provide a safe and durable treatment and maintenance option for patients with IBD in the future.

References

1. Ananthakrishnan AN. Epidemiology and risk factors for IBD. Nature Rev Gastroenterol Hepatol. 2015;12(4):205–17.
2. Bernstein CN. Antibiotics, probiotics and prebiotics in IBD. Nestle Nutr Inst Workshop Ser. 2014;79:83–100.
3. Frolkis A, Dieleman LA, Barkema HW, Panaccione R, Ghosh S, Fedorak RN, et al. Environment and the inflammatory bowel diseases. Can J Gastroenterol. 2013;27(3):e18–24.

4. Halmos EP, Gibson PR. Dietary management of IBD—insights and advice. Nat Rev Gastroenterol Hepatol. 2015;12(3):133–46.
5. Hou JK, Lee D, Lewis J. Diet and inflammatory bowel disease: review of patient-targeted recommendations. Clin Gastroenterol Hepatol. 2014;12(10):1592–600.
6. Lee D, Albenberg L, Compher C, Baldassano R, Piccoli D, Lewis JD, et al. Diet in the pathogenesis and treatment of inflammatory bowel diseases. Gastroenterology. 2015;148(6):1087–106.
7. Ungaro R, Bernstein CN, Gearry R, Hviid A, Kolho KL, Kronman MP, et al. Antibiotics associated with increased risk of new-onset Crohn's disease but not ulcerative colitis: a meta-analysis. Am J Gastroenterol. 2014;109(11):1728–38.
8. Biedermann L, Brulisauer K, Zeitz J, Frei P, Scharl M, Vavricka SR, et al. Smoking cessation alters intestinal microbiota: insights from quantitative investigations on human fecal samples using FISH. Inflamm Bowel Dis. 2014;20(9):1496–501.
9. Biedermann L, Zeitz J, Mwinyi J, Sutter-Minder E, Rehman A, Ott SJ, et al. Smoking cessation induces profound changes in the composition of the intestinal microbiota in humans. PLoS One. 2013;8(3):e59260.
10. Leone V, Chang EB, Devkota S. Diet, microbes, and host genetics: the perfect storm in inflammatory bowel diseases. J Gastroenterol. 2013;48(3):315–21.
11. Wu GD, Bushmanc FD, Lewis JD. Diet, the human gut microbiota, and IBD. Anaerobe. 2013;24:117–20.
12. Xu Z, Knight R. Dietary effects on human gut microbiome diversity. Br J Nutr. 2015;113(Suppl):S1–5.
13. Graf D, Di Cagno R, Fak F, Flint HJ, Nyman M, Saarela M, et al. Contribution of diet to the composition of the human gut microbiota. Microb Ecol Health Dis. 2015;26:26164.
14. Koenig JE, Spor A, Scalfone N, Fricker AD, Stombaugh J, Knight R, et al. Succession of microbial consortia in the developing infant gut microbiome. Proc Natl Acad Sci U S A. 2011;108 Suppl 1:4578–85.
15. Dominguez-Bello MG, Costello EK, Contreras M, Magris M, Hidalgo G, Fierer N, et al. Delivery mode shapes the acquisition and structure of the initial microbiota across multiple body habitats in newborns. Proc Natl Acad Sci U S A. 2010;107(26):11971–5.
16. Harmsen HJ, Wildeboer-Veloo AC, Raangs GC, Wagendorp AA, Klijn N, Bindels JG, et al. Analysis of intestinal flora development in breast-fed and formula-fed infants by using molecular identification and detection methods. J Pediatr Gastroenterol Nutr. 2000;30(1):61–7.
17. Weinstock GM. Genomic approaches to studying the human microbiota. Nature. 2012;489(7415):250–6.
18. Qin J, Li R, Raes J, Arumugam M, Burgdorf KS, Manichanh C, et al. A human gut microbial gene catalogue established by metagenomic sequencing. Nature. 2010;464(7285):59–65.
19. Wu GD. Diet, the gut microbiome and the metabolome in IBD. Nestle Nutr Inst Workshop Ser. 2014;79:73–82.
20. Bellaguarda E, Chang EB. IBD and the gut microbiota—from bench to personalized medicine. Curr Gastroenterol Rep. 2015;17(4):15. doi:10.1007/s11894-015-0439-z.
21. Frank DN, St Amand AL, Feldman RA, Boedeker EC, Harpaz N, Pace NR. Molecular-phylogenetic characterization of microbial community imbalances in human inflammatory bowel diseases. Proc Natl Acad Sci U S A. 2007;104(34):13780–5.
22. Michail S, Durbin M, Turner D, Griffiths AM, Mack DR, Hyams J, et al. Alterations in the gut microbiome of children with severe ulcerative colitis. Inflamm Bowel Dis. 2012;18(10):1799–808.
23. Morgan XC, Tickle TL, Sokol H, Gevers D, Devaney KL, Ward DV, et al. Dysfunction of the intestinal microbiome in inflammatory bowel disease and treatment. Genome Biol. 2012;13(9):R79. doi:10.1186/gb-2012-13-9-r79.
24. Machiels K, Joossens M, Sabino J, De Preter V, Arijs I, Eeckhaut V, et al. A decrease of the butyrate-producing species Roseburia hominis and Faecalibacterium prausnitzii defines dysbiosis in patients with ulcerative colitis. Gut. 2014;63(8):1275–83.
25. Varela E, Manichanh C, Gallart M, Torrejon A, Borruel N, Casellas F, et al. Colonisation by Faecalibacterium prausnitzii and maintenance of clinical remission in patients with ulcerative colitis. Aliment Pharmacol Ther. 2013;38(2):151–61.

26. Rajilic-Stojanovic M, Shanahan F, Guarner F, de Vos WM. Phylogenetic analysis of dysbiosis in ulcerative colitis during remission. Inflamm Bowel Dis. 2013;19(3):481–8.
27. Lepage P, Hasler R, Spehlmann ME, Rehman A, Zvirbliene A, Begun A, et al. Twin study indicates loss of interaction between microbiota and mucosa of patients with ulcerative colitis. Gastroenterology. 2011;141(1):227–36.
28. Hedin C, van der Gast CJ, Rogers GB, Cuthbertson L, McCartney S, Stagg AJ, et al. Siblings of patients with Crohn's disease exhibit a biologically relevant dysbiosis in mucosal microbial metacommunities. [Published online Apr. 8, 2015] Gut 2015. doi: 10.1136 gutjnl-2014–308896.
29. Sokol H, Pigneur B, Watterlot L, Lakhdari O, Bermudez-Humaran LG, Gratadoux JJ, et al. Faecalibacterium prausnitzii is an anti-inflammatory commensal bacterium identified by gut microbiota analysis of Crohn disease patients. Proc Natl Acad Sci U S A. 2008;105(43):16731–6.
30. Gevers D, Kugathasan S, Denson LA, Vazquez-Baeza Y, Van Treuren W, Ren B, et al. The treatment-naive microbiome in new-onset Crohn's disease. Cell Host Microbe. 2014;15(3):382–92.
31. Lewis JD. A review of the epidemiology of inflammatory bowel disease with a focus on diet, infections and antibiotic exposure. Nestle Nutr Inst Workshop Ser. 2014;79:1–18.
32. Ng SC. Emerging leadership lecture: inflammatory bowel disease in Asia: emergence of a "western" disease. J Gastroenterol Hepatol. 2015;30(3):440–5.
33. De Filippo C, Cavalieri D, Di Paola M, Ramazzotti M, Poullet JB, Massart S, et al. Impact of diet in shaping gut microbiota revealed by a comparative study in children from Europe and rural Africa. Proc Natl Acad Sci U S A. 2010;107(33):14691–6.
34. David LA, Maurice CF, Carmody RN, Gootenberg DB, Button JE, Wolfe BE, et al. Diet rapidly and reproducibly alters the human gut microbiome. Nature. 2014;505(7484):559–63.
35. Devkota S, Wang Y, Musch MW, Leone V, Fehlner-Peach H, Nadimpalli A, et al. Dietary-fat-induced taurocholic acid promotes pathobiont expansion and colitis in Il10-/- mice. Nature. 2012;487(7405):104–8.
36. Wu GD, Chen J, Hoffmann C, Bittinger K, Chen YY, Keilbaugh SA, et al. Linking long-term dietary patterns with gut microbial enterotypes. Science. 2011;334(6052):105–8.
37. Dixon LJ, Kabi A, Nickerson KP, McDonald C. Combinatorial effects of diet and genetics on inflammatory bowel disease pathogenesis. Inflamm Bowel Dis. 2015;21(4):912–22.
38. Amre DK, D'Souza S, Morgan K, Seidman G, Lambrette P, Grimard G, et al. Imbalances in dietary consumption of fatty acids, vegetables, and fruits are associated with risk for Crohn's disease in children. Am J Gastroenterol. 2007;102(9):2016–25.
39. Ananthakrishnan AN, Khalili H, Konijeti GG, Higuchi LM, de Silva P, Korzenik JR, et al. A prospective study of long-term intake of dietary fiber and risk of Crohn's disease and ulcerative colitis. Gastroenterology. 2013;145(5):970–7.
40. Erickson AR, Cantarel BL, Lamendella R, Darzi Y, Mongodin EF, Pan C, et al. Integrated metagenomics/metaproteomics reveals human host-microbiota signatures of Crohn's disease. PLoS One. 2012;7(11):e49138.
41. Atarashi K, Tanoue T, Oshima K, Suda W, Nagano Y, Nishikawa H, et al. Treg induction by a rationally selected mixture of clostridia strains from the human microbiota. Nature. 2013;500(7461):232–6.
42. Smith PM, Howitt MR, Panikov N, Michaud M, Gallini CA, Bohlooly-Y M, et al. The microbial metabolites, short-chain fatty acids, regulate colonic treg cell homeostasis. Science. 2013;341(6145):569–73.
43. Lindsay JO, Whelan K, Stagg AJ, Gobin P, Al-Hassi HO, Rayment N, et al. Clinical, microbiological, and immunological effects of fructo-oligosaccharide in patients with Crohn's disease. Gut. 2006;55(3):348–55.
44. Benjamin JL, Hedin CR, Koutsoumpas A, Ng SC, McCarthy NE, Hart AL, et al. Randomised, double-blind, placebo-controlled trial of fructo-oligosaccharides in active Crohn's disease. Gut. 2011;60(7):923–9.
45. Casellas F, Borruel N, Torrejon A, Varela E, Antolin M, Guarner F, et al. Oral oligofructose-enriched inulin supplementation in acute ulcerative colitis is well tolerated and associated with lowered faecal calprotectin. Aliment Pharmacol Ther. 2007;25(9):1061–7.

46. Welters CF, Heineman E, Thunnissen FB, van den Bogaard AE, Soeters PB, Baeten CG. Effect of dietary inulin supplementation on inflammation of pouch mucosa in patients with an ileal pouch-anal anastomosis. Dis Colon Rectum. 2002;45(5):621–7.
47. Bamba T, Kanauchi O, Andoh A, Fujiyama Y. A new prebiotic from germinated barley for nutraceutical treatment of ulcerative colitis. J Gastroenterol Hepatol. 2002;17(8):818–24.
48. Faghfoori Z, Navai L, Shakerhosseini R, Somi MH, Nikniaz Z, Norouzi MF. Effects of an oral supplementation of germinated barley foodstuff on serum tumour necrosis factor-alpha, inter-leukin-6 and -8 in patients with ulcerative colitis. Ann Clin Biochem. 2011;48(Pt 3):233–7.
49. Kanauchi O, Suga T, Tochihara M, Hibi T, Naganuma M, Homma T, et al. Treatment of ulcer-ative colitis by feeding with germinated barley foodstuff: first report of a multicenter open control trial. J Gastroenterol. 2002;37 Suppl 14:67–72.
50. Ananthakrishnan AN, Khalili H, Konijeti GG, Higuchi LM, de Silva P, Fuchs CS, et al. Long-term intake of dietary fat and risk of ulcerative colitis and Crohn's disease. Gut. 2014;63(5):776–84.
51. Gruber L, Kisling S, Lichti P, Martin FP, May S, Klingenspor M, et al. High fat diet accelerates pathogenesis of murine Crohn's disease-like ileitis independently of obesity. PLoS One. 2013;8(8):e71661.
52. Hou JK, Abraham B, El-Serag H. Dietary intake and risk of developing inflammatory bowel disease: a systematic review of the literature. Am J Gastroenterol. 2011;106(4):563–73.
53. Reif S, Klein I, Lubin F, Farbstein M, Hallak A, Gilat T. Pre-illness dietary factors in inflam-matory bowel disease. Gut. 1997;40(6):754–60.
54. Calder PC. Fatty acids and inflammation: the cutting edge between food and pharma. Eur J Pharmacol. 2011;668 Suppl 1:S50–8.
55. Huang S, Rutkowsky JM, Snodgrass RG, Ono-Moore KD, Schneider DA, Newman JW, et al. Saturated fatty acids activate TLR-mediated proinflammatory signaling pathways. J Lipid Res. 2012;53(9):2002–13.
56. Martinez-Medina M, Denizot J, Dreux N, Robin F, Billard E, Bonnet R, et al. Western diet induces dysbiosis with increased E coli in CEABAC10 mice, alters host barrier function favouring AIEC colonisation. Gut. 2014;63(1):116–24.
57. Tilg H, Moschen AR. Food, immunity, and the microbiome. Gastroenterology. 2015;148(6):1107–19.
58. Myles IA, Fontecilla NM, Janelsins BM, Vithayathil PJ, Segre JA, Datta SK. Parental dietary fat intake alters offspring microbiome and immunity. J Immunol. 2013;191(6):3200–9.
59. Berni Canani R, Terrin G, Borrelli O, Romano MT, Manguso F, Coruzzo A, et al. Short- and long-term therapeutic efficacy of nutritional therapy and corticosteroids in paediatric Crohn's disease. Dig Liver Dis. 2006;38(6):381–7.
60. Kaakoush NO, Day AS, Leach ST, Lemberg DA, Nielsen S, Mitchell HM. Effect of exclusive enteral nutrition on the microbiota of children with newly diagnosed Crohn's disease. Clin Gastroenterol Hepatol. 2015;6:e71.
61. Soo J, Malik BA, Turner JM, Persad R, Wine E, Siminoski K, et al. Use of exclusive enteral nutrition is just as effective as corticosteroids in newly diagnosed pediatric Crohn's disease. Dig Dis Sci. 2013;58(12):3584–91.
62. Ruemmele FM, Pigneur B, Garnier-Lengline H. Enteral nutrition as treatment option for Crohn's disease: in kids only? Nestle Nutr Inst Workshop Ser. 2014;79:115–23.
63. Lionetti P, Callegari ML, Ferrari S, Cavicchi MC, Pozzi E, de Martino M, et al. Enteral nutri-tion and microflora in pediatric Crohn's disease. JPEN J Parenter Enteral Nutr. 2005;29(4 Suppl):S173–5; discussion S175–8, S184–8.
64. Nahidi L, Leach ST, Mitchell HM, Kaakoush NO, Lemberg DA, Munday JS, et al. Inflammatory bowel disease therapies and gut function in a colitis mouse model. BioMed Res Int. 2013;2013:909613.
65. Shiga H, Kajiura T, Shinozaki J, Takagi S, Kinouchi Y, Takahashi S, et al. Changes of faecal microbiota in patients with Crohn's disease treated with an elemental diet and total parenteral nutrition. Dig Liver Dis. 2012;44(9):736–42.

66. Leach ST, Mitchell HM, Eng WR, Zhang L, Day AS. Sustained modulation of intestinal bacteria by exclusive enteral nutrition used to treat children with Crohn's disease. Aliment Pharmacol Ther. 2008;28(6):724–33.
67. Gerasimidis K, Bertz M, Hanske L, Junick J, Biskou O, Aguilera M, et al. Decline in presumptively protective gut bacterial species and metabolites are paradoxically associated with disease improvement in pediatric Crohn's disease during enteral nutrition. Inflamm Bowel Dis. 2014;20(5):861–71.
68. Kiss EA, Vonarbourg C, Kopfmann S, Hobeika E, Finke D, Esser C, et al. Natural aryl hydrocarbon receptor ligands control organogenesis of intestinal lymphoid follicles. Science. 2011;334(6062):1561–5.
69. Li Y, Innocentin S, Withers DR, Roberts NA, Gallagher AR, Grigorieva EF, et al. Exogenous stimuli maintain intraepithelial lymphocytes via aryl hydrocarbon receptor activation. Cell. 2011;147(3):629–40.
70. Monteleone I, Rizzo A, Sarra M, Sica G, Sileri P, Biancone L, et al. Aryl hydrocarbon receptor-induced signals up-regulate IL-22 production and inhibit inflammation in the gastrointestinal tract. Gastroenterology. 2011;141(1):237–48; 248.e1.
71. Zelante T, Iannitti RG, Cunha C, De Luca A, Giovannini G, Pieraccini G, et al. Tryptophan catabolites from microbiota engage aryl hydrocarbon receptor and balance mucosal reactivity via interleukin-22. Immunity. 2013;39(2):372–85.
72. Fukumoto S, Toshimitsu T, Matsuoka S, Maruyama A, Oh-Oka K, Takamura T, et al. Identification of a probiotic bacteria-derived activator of the aryl hydrocarbon receptor that inhibits colitis. Immunol Cell Biol. 2014;92(5):460–5.
73. Ananthakrishnan AN, Khalili H, Higuchi LM, Bao Y, Korzenik JR, Giovannucci EL, et al. Higher predicted vitamin D status is associated with reduced risk of Crohn's disease. Gastroenterology. 2012;142(3):482–9.
74. Bernstein CN. Should patients with inflammatory bowel disease take vitamin D to prevent cancer? Clin Gastroenterol Hepatol. 2014;12(5):828–30.
75. Wang L, Wang ZT, Hu JJ, Fan R, Zhou J, Zhong J. Polymorphisms of the vitamin D receptor gene and the risk of inflammatory bowel disease: a meta-analysis. Genet Mol Res. 2014;13(2):2598–610.
76. Wu S, Zhang YG, Lu R, Xia Y, Zhou D, Petrof EO, et al. Intestinal epithelial vitamin D receptor deletion leads to defective autophagy in colitis. Gut. 2015;64(7):1082–94. doi:10.1136/gutjnl-2014-307436.
77. Assa A, Vong L, Pinnell LJ, Rautava J, Avitzur N, Johnson-Henry KC, et al. Vitamin D deficiency predisposes to adherent-invasive escherichia coli-induced barrier dysfunction and experimental colonic injury. Inflamm Bowel Dis. 2015;21(2):297–306.
78. Balamurugan R, Mary RR, Chittaranjan S, Jancy H, Shobana Devi R, Ramakrishna BS. Low levels of faecal lactobacilli in women with iron-deficiency anaemia in south India. Br J Nutr. 2010;104(7):931–4.
79. Tompkins GR, O'Dell NL, Bryson IT, Pennington CB. The effects of dietary ferric iron and iron deprivation on the bacterial composition of the mouse intestine. Curr Microbiol. 2001;43(1):38–42.
80. Werner T, Wagner SJ, Martinez I, Walter J, Chang JS, Clavel T, et al. Depletion of luminal iron alters the gut microbiota and prevents Crohn's disease-like ileitis. Gut. 2011;60(3):325–33.
81. Erichsen K, Hausken T, Ulvik RJ, Svardal A, Berstad A, Berge RK. Ferrous fumarate deteriorated plasma antioxidant status in patients with Crohn disease. Scand J Gastroenterol. 2003;38(5):543–8.
82. Gisbert JP, Bermejo F, Pajares R, Perez-Calle JL, Rodriguez M, Algaba A, et al. Oral and intravenous iron treatment in inflammatory bowel disease: hematological response and quality of life improvement. Inflamm Bowel Dis. 2009;15(10):1485–91.

83. Lindgren S, Wikman O, Befrits R, Blom H, Eriksson A, Granno C, et al. Intravenous iron sucrose is superior to oral iron sulphate for correcting anaemia and restoring iron stores in IBD patients: a randomized, controlled, evaluator-blind, multicentre study. Scand J Gastroenterol. 2009;44(7): 838–45.
84. Zimmermann MB, Chassard C, Rohner F, N'goran EK, Nindjin C, Dostal A, et al. The effects of iron fortification on the gut microbiota in African children: a randomized controlled trial in Cote d'ivoire. Am J Clin Nutr. 2010;92(6):1406–15.
85. Cassat JE, Skaar EP. Iron in infection and immunity. Cell Host Microbe. 2013;13(5):509–19.
86. Beal J, Silverman B, Bellant J, Young TE, Klontz K. Late onset necrotizing enterocolitis in infants following use of a xanthan gum-containing thickening agent. J Pediatr. 2012;161(2):354–6.
87. Moyana TN, Lalonde JM. Carrageenan-induced intestinal injury in the rat—a model for inflammatory bowel disease. Ann Clin Lab Sci. 1990;20(6):420–6.
88. Nickerson KP, Chanin R, McDonald C. Deregulation of intestinal anti-microbial defense by the dietary additive, maltodextrin. Gut Microbes. 2015;6(1):78–83.
89. Swidsinski A, Ung V, Sydora BC, Loening-Baucke V, Doerffel Y, Verstraelen H, et al. Bacterial overgrowth and inflammation of small intestine after carboxymethyl cellulose ingestion in genetically susceptible mice. Inflamm Bowel Dis. 2009;15(3):359–64.
90. Nickerson KP, McDonald C. Crohn's disease-associated adherent-invasive escherichia coli adhesion is enhanced by exposure to the ubiquitous dietary polysaccharide maltodextrin. PLoS One. 2012;7(12):e52132.
91. Thymann T, Moller HK, Stoll B, Stoy AC, Buddington RK, Bering SB, et al. Carbohydrate maldigestion induces necrotizing enterocolitis in preterm pigs. Am J Physiol Gastrointest Liver Physiol. 2009;297(6):G1115–25.
92. Sigall-Boneh R, Pfeffer-Gik T, Segal I, Zangen T, Boaz M, Levine A. Partial enteral nutrition with a Crohn's disease exclusion diet is effective for induction of remission in children and young adults with Crohn's disease. Inflamm Bowel Dis. 2014;20(8):1353–60.

Chapter 2
Dietary Risk Factors for the Onset and Relapse of Inflammatory Bowel Disease

Andrew R. Hart and Simon S.M. Chan

Introduction

The aetiology of Crohn's disease (CD) and ulcerative colitis (UC), and the factors that influence disease relapse are largely unknown. Identifying the relevant exposures is vital, so that measures may be instituted to prevent inflammatory bowel disease (IBD) in high-risk groups, and interventions recommended to help patients remain in clinical remission. Diet is an obvious exposure to investigate as there are plausible biological mechanisms for how this may be involved in both the pathogenesis and natural history. The potential biological mechanisms will be discussed in the following sections, but diet can affect: the composition of the gut microbiota, have direct toxic actions on intestinal cells and influence the local mucosal inflammatory mechanisms. A role for diet in IBD pathogenesis is supported by the results from ecological epidemiological studies. The incidence of both CD and UC is higher in Western than Eastern countries, which may reflect variations in dietary patterns [1]. In the East, the increasing adoption of westernised diets could be contributing to the rising incidence there. In Europe, where there are differences in patterns of food consumption across the continent, the incidence in northern European countries, compared to those in the south, is 80 % higher for CD and 40 % higher for UC [2]. Migrants to new countries adopt the incidence pattern of their host nation [3]. Finally, the dramatic increases in incidence in IBD, particularly during the latter part of the twentieth century [1] may hypothetically be explained by

A.R. Hart, M.B. Ch.B., M.D., F.R.C.P. • S.S.M. Chan, M.B. B.Chir., Ph.D., M.R.C.P. (✉)
University of East Anglia, Bob Champion Research and Education Building,
James Watson Road, Norwich Research Park, Norwich, Norfolk NR4 7TJ, UK

Department of Gastroenterology, Norfolk and Norwich University Hospital, NHS Foundation Trust, Colney Lane, Norwich, Norfolk NR4 7UY, UK
e-mail: a.hart@uea.ac.uk; simon.chan@doctors.org.uk

© Springer International Publishing Switzerland 2016
A.N. Ananthakrishnan (ed.), *Nutritional Management of Inflammatory Bowel Diseases*, DOI 10.1007/978-3-319-26890-3_2

Table 2.1 Summary of the evidence for foods in the aetiology of IBD

Nutrient/food group	Evidence to date	Suggestions for future work
Fatty acids	PUFAs are precursors of inflammatory and anti-inflammatory mediators affect the gut microbiota and influence obesity. Epidemiological evidence from two cohort studies suggest a beneficial effect of a low n-6/n-3 PUFA ratio in UC, but the findings are inconsistent for UC	Cohort studies to investigate the effects of particular PUFAs and to consider if there are interactions between different groups
Vitamin D	In vitro studies have demonstrated the anti-inflammatory effects of vitamin D via modulating toll-like receptor activation and antibacterial responses. Descriptive epidemiological studies report a north–south gradient in incidence which may reflect variations in sunlight exposure. Data from the US cohort study showing inverse associations between predicted total vitamin D status and CD, and dietary vitamin D and UC	Investigation of vitamin D status and dietary intake in other cohort studies
Fibre	Fibre is converted to short-chain fatty acids, such as butyrate, which is the energy source for colonocytes and have immunomodulatory properties including inhibition of *NF-KB*. The two cohort investigations report no associations between dietary fibre and UC. The US work found inverse associations between fibre from fruit and CD	Investigation of fibre intake from different sources in CD in other cohort studies
Sulphur, iron and zinc	Toxic effects on the mucosa including sulphur inhibiting butyrate metabolism and pro-oxidant effects of iron. Conversely, zinc appears to be required for maintenance of intestinal barrier integrity and down-regulation of pro-inflammatory cytokines	Observational epidemiological work to justify any clinical interventions

dietary changes. This chapter will review the current evidence on how food and its components may be involved in both the aetiology of IBD and affect the natural history of established disease in patients and suggest what further research is required for clarification (Table 2.1).

Methodology to Investigate Diet

The ideal methodology to investigate if diet influences the aetiology of incident IBD and clinical outcomes in patients is to adopt randomised controlled trials of either dietary supplementations or exclusions. However, for investigating aetiology and diet, randomised controlled trials are unethical and non-pragmatic. The practical difficulties are that hundreds of thousands of initially well people would need to be recruited and then followed up for many years for adequate numbers to develop IBD to ensure that the trial had sufficient power. Asking well people to continuously modify their diet over many years is unrealistic, and it is unethical to encourage participants to eat foods which may be deleterious. Therefore, to study IBD aetiology, non-interventional observational investigations are required, where participants' habitual diet is recorded and compared between those with and without IBD. The two types of observational study design available are retrospective case–control studies and prospective cohort investigations. The latter are more scientifically robust for nutritional epidemiological work, as they reduce both selection and recall biases for diet which are associated with case–control work. In a cohort study, many thousands of well people complete information on their habitual diet and are then followed up over many years to identify those who develop IBD. As participants are recording their current diet at recruitment, there is less recall bias for eating habits, than in case–control work, where patients have difficulties accurately recalling their diet months or years before the onset of their symptoms. Furthermore, in prospective studies as both future cases and those who remain as controls are recruited from the same baseline population then selection bias is minimised. Whilst cohort studies are more time consuming and expensive to conduct than case–control work, they are the preferred methodology for investigating diet and IBD aetiology. To date, two such studies exist: EPIC-IBD (European Prospective Investigation into Cancer and Nutrition) in a cohort of 401,326 men and women in eight European countries and secondly the US Nurses' Health Study (NHS) of 238,386 female nurses.

For studying dietary modifications and the subsequent clinical outcomes in patients with established disease, randomised controlled clinical trials are possible as sufficient numbers of patients can be recruited. An approach to deciding which foods to investigate can be based on firstly plausible mechanisms and secondly surveys of patients who report foods which they feel may exacerbate their symptoms. In a survey of 244 French patients with IBD, 40 % identified food as a risk factor for precipitating relapse, and 47.5 % reported that the disease had changed the pleasure of eating [4]. In a cohort study from the USA, diet was measured with both semi-quantitative food frequency questionnaires and open-ended questions [5]. Foods reported to frequently worsen symptoms included: vegetables, spicy foods, fruit, nuts, milk, red meat, soda, popcorn, dairy, alcohol, high-fibre foods, coffee and beans and those which improved symptoms included: yogurt, rice and bananas.

When investigating aetiology or treatments, whether the findings in individual studies are indeed casual need to be considered in the context of The Bradford Hill Criteria [6]. These state that causality is implied if: there are plausible biological mechanisms for any findings, the effect sizes are large with dose–response effects, there are consistent findings across many studies, co-variates are considered and the data on exposures are recorded before the onset of symptoms. The sections below summarise the prospective cohort studies which have investigated diet in the aetiology of IBD and also the few randomised controlled clinical trials of dietary interventions in patients with UC and CD. Whether the findings are causal will be discussed in the context of the Bradford Hill Criteria, and where appropriate we suggest what further research or clarification is required.

Hypothesis Generating Studies

One approach to studying dietary factors in IBD aetiology is to investigate if there are any associations with many nutrients, namely a hypothesis-free approach. Although this may generate several false-positive findings, any associations detected may stimulate further work to explore potential biological mechanisms for nutrients to investigate in greater detail. As discussed above, the preferred aetiological methodology for this are prospective cohort investigations. Such data were first reported from the EPIC-IBD study in 2008 where in a subcohort of EPIC, 260,686 initially well men and women were followed up for a median time of 3.8 years during which 139 participants developed incident UC [7]. A total of 18 nutrients, vitamins and minerals were studied and no associations were detected, apart from a borderline significant positive association with an increasing percentage energy intake from total polyunsaturated fatty acids (PUFAs) (trend across quartiles OR = 1.19, 95 % CI = 0.99–1.43, P = 0.07). These macronutrients may influence the inflammatory process, and this association led to further work investigating PUFAs [8–11], which is discussed in the following section. A similar exploratory analysis for many nutrients has not yet been conducted for EPIC participants who subsequently developed Crohn's disease. In the US Nurses' Health Study, such a global nutrient analysis has not yet been reported, although the effects of particular food groups including dietary fat [12], fibre [13] and vitamin D [14] have been published. The EPIC-IBD study investigated dietary carbohydrate intake and the risk of CD and UC and reported no associations with either total sugar, carbohydrate or starch intakes [15]. Conversely, several previous case–control investigations had documented positive associations between a high sugar intake and the development of CD [16–19], although the definitions of sugar varied in different investigations. However, the positive links in the latter study design may be due to recall bias, where subjects with CD reported their current rather than their pre-symptomatic diet that included soluble sugars which they could tolerate. This potential recall bias for sugar intake emphasises the importance of prospective cohort studies for investigating diet and the risk of IBD. The aetiological prospective epidemiological studies investigating specific dietary hypothesis in both cohort investigations are now discussed.

Fatty Acids

The different PUFAs chiefly omega-6 (n-6 PUFAs) and omega-3 (n-3 PUFAs) are characterised by the position of the double bond on their long aliphatic tail. The synthesis of both groups is limited in humans and dietary intakes are the main sources. Significant quantities of n-6 PUFAs are found in red meat, certain cooking oils (e.g. sunflower and corn oils) and some margarines. Similarly, foods rich in n-3 PUFAs are oily fish, rape-seed oil and soya bean oil. In Western countries, the ratio of n-6/n-3 dietary PUFA intakes is higher in comparison to those people living in developing countries, and there is emerging evidence that these macronutrients may play a role in IBD aetiology. The pathophysiological effects of PUFAs may hypothetically be via a variety of mechanisms that affect inflammatory processes in different ways. Firstly, both n-6 and n-3 PUFAs are precursors to a large range of key mediators involved in modulating the intensity and duration of inflammatory responses [20]. Lipid mediators derived from n-6 PUFAs are converted via the arachidonic acid pathway to substrates for the enzymes cyclooxygenase and lipoxygenase which leads to the production of prostaglandins and leukotrienes with pro-inflammatory effects. Conversely, the same enzymes metabolise n-3 PUFAs to lipid mediators with biologically less potent inflammatory properties than those derived from n-6 PUFAs. Competitive inhibition may exist between n-6 and n-3 metabolism as a consequence of dietary intakes which affects the relative production of the different prostaglandins and leukotrienes. More recently, n-3 PUFAs are reported to give rise to a novel class of lipid mediators that limit the inflammatory process [21]. A second possible mechanism of PUFAs is diets containing differing proportions of fatty acids may shape the composition of the gut microbiota to one that predisposes to the development or relapse of IBD. The nature of the diet affects the composition of the gut microbiota and the metabolites they produce, which may have diverse effects on host immune and inflammatory responses [22]. Thirdly, excess intakes of fat can lead to obesity which itself is associated with increased markers of bowel inflammation and intestinal permeability, both hallmarks of IBD [23]. Finally, n-3 PUFAs can act directly on inflammatory cells to inhibit key transcription factors such as PPARγ and NFκB, required for the intracellular signalling cascade that activates inflammation [24]. However, the effects of these fatty acids may be dependent on having a background of susceptible genetics as a study in children reported that those who consumed a higher ratio of n-6:n-3 and were carriers of specific single nucleotide polymorphisms in the genes *CYP4F3* and *FADS2* had an increased susceptibility to paediatric Crohn's disease [25].

There are several epidemiological studies which report that PUFAs are associated with IBD aetiology, although the evidence is more compelling for UC than CD. In the EPIC-IBD study, the highest quintile for dietary intakes of the n-6 PUFA linoleic acid, as measured by food frequency questionnaires (FFQs) were associated with an increased odds of developing UC (OR = 2.49, 95 % CI = 1.23–5.07) [10]. Conversely, the same EPIC-IBD nested case–control study reported that the highest quintile for dietary intakes of docosahexaenoic acid, an n-3 PUFA, were associated with a decreased odds of developing UC (OR = 0.32, 95 % CI = 0.06–0.97) [10]. In addition to FFQs, a subcohort of the EPIC-IBD study from Denmark has used biomarker measurements of n-6 PUFA intakes from gluteal fat biopsies, which provide a more accurate assessment of longer term dietary intake compared to FFQs [9]. In this particular study, an association with increased arachidonic acid intake, an n-6 PUFA, measured from gluteal fat biopsies and odds of developing UC was reported

(P_{trend} per 0.1 % unit increase in arachidonic acid concentration=0.0001). The US prospective Nurses' Health Study cohort has also found associations between PUFAs and the risk of developing IBD having observed that participants in the highest quintile of n3/n6 PUFA ratio intake had a decreased risk of developing UC (HR=0.69, 95 % CI=0.49–0.98, P for trend=0.03) [13]. No associations were seen for the intakes of the n-6 PUFAs, arachidonic acid and linoleic acid or the total intake of long-chain n-3 PUFAs (docosapentaenoic acid, eicosapentaenoic acid and docosahexaenoic acid). For CD only the EPIC-IBD study has reported an association between PUFAs and CD aetiology, with participants in the highest quintile of docosahexaenoic acid intake having a decreased odds for CD (OR=0.06, 95 % CI=0.01–0.72) [11]. The dissimilarities in the n-3 PUFA results with the Nurses' Health Study Cohort may be due to differences in the reporting of individual n-3 PUFAs as opposed to total n-3 PUFAs. The only consistent finding from the two cohort studies was that no associations were seen for n-6 PUFAs and the development of CD. Clarification of the inconsistencies of the role of all PUFAs in UC aetiology, and n-3 PUFAs in CD are required by providing more precise estimates of the intakes from biomarker studies.

In the clinical setting, there is currently no evidence to support the use of actual PUFA *dietary modifications* in preventing the relapse of either UC or CD in patients. Most clinical trials have assessed fish oil *supplements*, rich in n-3 PUFAs with the results having shown no benefits. These trials in UC and CD are summarised in Cochrane reviews [26, 27], although the conclusions are limited by heterogeneity in study design and in several the small sample sizes. To date, *large* randomised controlled clinical trials (EPIC-1 and EPIC-2) investigating fish oils for the maintenance of disease remission have been performed in CD only [28]. Each of these enrolled over 350 CD patients in remission who were randomised to receive either placebo or gelatin capsules containing fish oils. The Kaplan–Meier analyses showed no differences in the time to relapse between these interventions in either study (EPIC-1, $p=0.30$; EPIC-2, $p=0.48$). Similar large trials need to be conducted in patients with UC.

Vitamin D

Vitamin D is a hormone with a broad range of biological activities that are mediated via signalling of the vitamin D receptor (VDR), which belongs to the nuclear hormone receptor superfamily. Cells of the immune system including T cells and antigen-presenting cells all express VDR as do intestinal epithelial cells. Whilst the role of VDR signalling in the gut has not been fully elucidated, there are plausible biological mechanisms for how vitamin D may prevent IBD via modulating innate and adaptive immune responses between toll-like receptors (TLR) and the TLR-induced antibacterial responses. Other potential protective mechanisms include a synergistic interaction with NF-κb inducing expression of B-defensin [29] which facilitates autophagy in macrophages [30] and preventing the production of TNFα in monocytes [31]. Vitamin D has further effects on both B and T cells [32], including tolerance to self-antigens and inhibition of IL-2 production required for lymphocyte proliferation. Deficiency of vitamin D, which is derived predominantly from exposure to sunlight and in smaller amounts from diet, may therefore predispose to IBD through over activation of the immune system or lack of a response to foreign antigens. These anti-inflammatory mechanisms are supported by animal work reporting mice lacking VDR are more susceptible to dextran sodium sulphate colitis which may be due to disruption in epithelial junctions [33].

There is supportive evidence for a role for vitamin D deficiency in the aetiology of IBD from descriptive, aetiological and genetic epidemiological studies. There is a north–south gradient in IBD incidence in both the USA [34] and Europe [2], which may reflect differences in exposure to sunlight. Furthermore, there may be a link between polymorphisms in the VDR gene on chromosome 12 and the development of IBD [35, 36]. The US Nurses' Health Study has investigated a validated score predictive of plasma vitamin D status and the subsequent risk of CD and UC in their cohort of 72,719 women aged 40–73 years recruited in 1986 and followed up to 2008 [14]. The predicted vitamin D status was based on a combination of variables including: dietary intake and supplements, body mass index, racial origin, exposure to sunlight and regional ultraviolet radiation intensity [14]. During the follow-up of 1,492,811 person-years, there were 122 documented incident cases of CD and 123 of UC. For CD, there was a significant inverse association for total predicted vitamin D status (highest vs. lowest quartile HR$=0.54$, 95 % CI$=0.30$–0.99, $P_{trend}=0.02$), but none for UC. However, for vitamin D intake from dietary and supplement sources, there were statistically nonsignificant inverse associations with CD, but an inverse trend across quartiles for UC ($P_{trend}=0.04$). The reasons for the discrepancies between vitamin D sources for the two forms of IBD are unknown, but the possibilities include firstly varying biological properties of vitamin D derived from different sources and secondly residual confounding. The latter are other factors associated with vitamin D status, which themselves influence the development of IBD. In the first report from the EPIC-IBD study, no association was found for dietary vitamin D intake and UC (excluding supplement use) [7]. In the clinical setting, as far as we are aware there are no randomised controlled trials of foods rich in vitamin D in the treatment of either the relapse or maintenance of remission in patients with IBD. The results from such trials would be difficult to interpret as foods rich in vitamin D also contain n-3 PUFAs, the latter which could also have therapeutic benefits. Furthermore, the relevance of such work could be questionable as exposure to sunlight is a major source of vitamin D. There is only one controlled trial assessing dietary supplements of vitamin D, which randomised 104 patients with CD in remission to receive either 1200 IU of oral vitamin D3 plus 1200 mg of calcium daily, or 1200 mg calcium alone, as a maintenance therapy for 1 year [37]. There were fewer relapses during follow-up in the test group compared to controls (13 % vs. 29 %, $P=0.06$). We believe there is no similar work in UC, and these plus confirmatory clinical trials in CD are needed to confirm if there any therapeutic benefits of vitamin D supplementation.

In summary, there is emerging but as yet insufficient evidence to state vitamin D is involved in either preventing the development of IBD or has any therapeutic properties. Laboratory and animal studies have reported many biological mechanisms for how vitamin D may have beneficial effects on the immune system and protect against the development of intestinal inflammation. To fulfil the Bradford Hill Criteria as to whether vitamin D deficiency is important, confirmatory prospective cohort studies are required to confirm the results reported in the US Nurses' Health Study and further clinical trials in patients.

Fibre

Dietary fibre may protect against the development of IBD, through several mechanisms, through its conversion to the short-chain fatty acids (SCFAs) acetate, butyrate and propionate. Butyrate is the main energy source for colonocytes and is associated with the maintenance of the intestinal epithelium, whilst SCFAs have immunomodulatory roles including inhibition of the transcription factor NF-*KB* [38]. The fermentation of fibre is dependent on the gut microbiota, including *Bacteroidetes* species, which some studies report are deficient in patients with IBD [39]. The intake of total dietary fibre, and that from different food sources, was recorded in FFQs completed every 4 years, in the US Nurses' Health Study of 170,776 women with 3,317,425 person-years of follow-up over 26 years [13]. In this report, there were 269 incident cases of CD diagnosed and 338 cases of UC. For UC, there were no associations with either total dietary fibre intake or that from any specific food groups. However, for CD the highest quintile of energy-adjusted cumulative average dietary fibre intake, namely 24.3 g/day, was associated with a 41 % reduction in risk compared with the lowest quintile (HR=0.59, 95 % CI=0.39–0.90). This reduction was largely due to the fibre content from fruits (highest vs. lowest quintile HR=0.57, 95 % CI=0.38–0.85), with no associations detected for fibre from either: vegetables, cereals or legumes. The dose–effect relationship across quintiles (P=0.02) for fruit fibre adds support for a causal association. In the EPIC-IBD study, no associations were reported for total fibre intake (OR trend across quartiles=1.03, 95 % CI=0.84–1.25) and the odds of developing UC, although fibre intake from specific foods nor fibre in CD have yet been investigated [7]. To date, no clinical trials have investigated dietary fibre as a treatment for IBD. In summary, although there are biological mechanisms for fibre deficiency in IBD, these are not fully supported by the epidemiological evidence. To clarify if there is a causal association in CD, further prospective aetiological data are required and evidence from randomised controlled clinical trials of fibre supplements in patients.

Sulphur, Iron and Zinc

Excess dietary sulphur may be involved in the aetiology of IBD as it is converted to hydrogen sulphide which may be deleterious to the colon through inhibiting butyrate oxidation, the principal energy source for colonocytes [40]. The mineral is obtained from several sources: namely sulphated amino acids (cysteine and methionine in red meat, cheese, whole milk, eggs, fish and nuts), and inorganic sulphur present firstly in Brassica vegetables, (cauliflower, cabbage, broccoli and sprouts) and secondly in preservatives in processed foods (breads, beers, sausages and dried fruit). Excess hydrogen sulphide is present in the faeces of patients with ulcerative colitis [41] and is the principal by-product of sulphate-reducing bacteria. These obligate anaerobic flagellated organisms are present in higher numbers in the faeces of patients with ulcerative colitis than in healthy controls [42]. However, faecal flora cultures do not accurately reflect bacteria colonising both the intestinal mucous gel layer and tissues themselves. Tissue colonisation was investigated by using FISH (fluorescent in situ hybridisation) to determine the presence of sulphate-reducing bacteria microbial composition in specimens resected from patients with IBD. In a small study, whose findings need confirmation from larger work, such bacteria were not detected in control tissues, but were in 3 of 12 patients with UC and 1 of 8 patients with colonic CD, but none in ileal specimens [43]. To the best of our knowledge, there are no epidemiological studies which have assessed if dietary sulphur is involved in the aetiology of either UC or CD. However, the effect of dietary sulphur intake was investigated, as measured by food-frequency questionnaires, in 183 patients with known UC in remission and their subsequent rates of relapse [44]. During the 1-year follow-up period, 52 % of patients relapsed and for those in the top tertile of sulphur intake, compared to the lowest, the odds ratio for relapse was nearly trebled (OR = 2.76, 95 % CI = 1.19–6.40) and for sulphate intake (OR = 2.61, 95 % CI = 1.08–6.30). For red and processed meat intakes which contain sulphur, higher intakes were associated with more than a fivefold chance of relapse (OR = 5.19, 95 % CI = 2.09–12.9). To advance our knowledge of whether sulphur is important, validated dietary questionnaires need to be developed to measure dietary sulphur intake and randomised controlled clinical trials performed in patients of a diet low in sulphur.

For dietary iron, there are plausible mechanisms for a potential role in aetiology and relapse due to the mineral's pro-oxidant properties resulting in tissue damage to: proteins, DNA and lipids. Iron may induce oxidant activity in the intestinal mucosa by enhancing the conversion of hydrogen peroxide to the highly reactive hydroxyl-free radical. Of note the aminosalicylate drugs used to treat IBD possess antioxidant properties [45]. In vitro work on colonic biopsies from patients with UC and normal control subjects, reported the amounts of mucosal reactive oxygen species, as measured by luminol-amplified chemiluminescence, were significant lowered by the iron-chelating agent desferrioxamine in inactive and active disease, respectively [46]. To date, the cohort investigations have not currently assessed dietary iron in either UC or CD, although the positive associations in work on relapse in UC with red meat intake could plausibly involve haem [44]. Clarification of any possible mechanisms of iron and data from observational work are required to fully justify randomised controlled trials of iron-chelating therapies.

The micronutrient zinc also has strong biological plausibility in the development and risk of IBD relapse. At present, this is limited to in vitro work and animal models of colitis reporting that zinc is required to maintain the integrity of the intestinal mucosal barrier and down-regulation of pro-inflammatory cytokines [47–49]. Notably zinc deficiency is associated with severity of colitis in animal models [50].

To date, there are no published cohort studies investigating the association between zinc and IBD aetiology or relapse. However, unpublished work from the US prospective Nurses' Health Study cohort suggests that intakes of zinc are inversely associated with the risk of developing CD but not UC.

Conclusions

There are many plausible mechanisms for how several dietary constituents, namely PUFAs, vitamin D, fibre, sulphur, iron and zinc may influence the development of UC and CD. The effects of specific nutrients needs to be further studied in both the European and US follow-up studies, which currently does not exist for all nutrients, to see if the findings are consistent. Dietary interventions in patients cannot be recommended at present. Interventional studies would require representative patient groups, a precise dietary modification to be determined and involve a sufficiently large sample size. Work investigating diet needs to progress as it is eminently modifiable if it is found to be associated with both the development and natural history of IBD.

References

1. Molodecky N, Soon I, Rabi D, Ghali W, Ferris M, Chernoff G, et al. Increasing incidence and prevalence of the inflammatory bowel diseases with time, based on systematic review. Gastroenterology. 2012;142:46–54.
2. Shivananda S, Lennard-Jones JE, Logan R, Fear N, Price A, Carpenter L, et al. Incidence of inflammatory bowel disease across Europe: is there a difference between north and south? Results of the European collaborative study on inflammatory bowel disease (EC-IBD). Gut. 1996;39:690–7.
3. Probert C, Jayanthi V, Pinder D, Wicks A, Mayberry J. Epidemiological study of ulcerative proctocolitis in Indian migrants and the indigenous population of Leicestershire. Gut. 1992;33:687–93.
4. Zallot C, Quilliot D, Chevaux J, Peyrin-Biroulet C, Gueant-Rodriquez R, Freling E, et al. Dietary beliefs and behaviour among inflammatory bowel disease patients. Inflamm Bowel Dis. 2013;19:66–72.
5. Cohen A, Lee D, Long M, Kappelman M, Martin C, Sandler R, et al. Dietary patterns and self-reported associations of diet with symptoms of inflammatory bowel disease. Dig Dis Sci. 2013;58:1322–8.
6. Hill AB. The environment and disease: association or causation. Proc R Soc Med. 1965;58:295–300.
7. Hart A, Luben R, Olsen A, Tjonneland A, Linseisen J, Nagel G, et al. Diet in the aetiology of ulcerative colitis—a European prospective cohort study. Digestion. 2008;77:57–64.
8. John S, Luben R, Shrestha S, Welch A, Khaw K-T, Hart A. Dietary n-3 polyunsaturated fatty acids and the aetiology of ulcerative colitis: a UK prospective cohort study. Eur J Gastroenterol Hepatol. 2010;22:602–6.
9. De Silva PSA, Olsen A, Christensen J, Berg Schmidt E, Overvad K, Tjonneland A, et al. An association between dietary arachidonic acid, measured in adipose tissue, and ulcerative colitis. Gastroenterology. 2010;139:1912–7.

10. Hart AR. The IBD in EPIC study investigators. Linoleic acid, a dietary n-6 polyunsaturated fatty acid, and the aetiology of ulcerative colitis: a nested case-control study within a European prospective cohort study. Gut. 2009;58:1606–11.
11. Chan SS, Luben R, Olsen A, Tjonneland A, Kaaks R, Lindgren S, et al. Association between high dietary intake of the n-3 polyunsaturated fatty acid docosahexaenoic acid and reduced risk of Crohn's disease. Aliment Pharmacol Ther. 2014;39:834–42.
12. Ananthakrishnan A, Khalili H, Konijeti G, Higuchi L, de Silva P, Fuchs C, et al. Long-term intake of dietary fat and risk of ulcerative colitis and Crohn's disease. Gut. 2014;63:776–84.
13. Ananthakrishnan A, Khalili H, Konijeti G, Higuchi L, de Silva P, Korzenik J, et al. A prospective study of long-term intake of dietary fibre and risk of Crohn's disease and ulcerative colitis. Gastroenterology. 2013;145:970–7.
14. Ananthakrishnan A, Khalili H, Higuchi L, Bao Y, Korzenik J, Giovannucci E, et al. Higher predicted vitamin D status is associated with reduced risk of Crohn's disease. Gastroenterology. 2012;142:482–9.
15. Chan SS, Luben R, van Schaik F, Oldenburg B, Bueno-de-Mesquita B, Hallmans G, et al. Carbohydrate intake in the etiology of Crohn's disease and ulcerative colitis. Inflamm Bowel Dis. 2014;20:2013–21.
16. Tragnone A, Valpiani D, Miglio F, Elmi G, Bazzocchi G, Pipitone E, et al. Dietary habits as risk factors for inflammatory bowel disease. Eur J Gastroenterol Hepatol. 1995;7:47–51.
17. Jarnerot G, Jarnmark I, Nilsson K. Consumption of refined sugar by patients with Crohn's disease, ulcerative colitis and irritable bowel syndrome. Scand J Gastroenterol. 1983;18:999–1002.
18. Kasper H, Sommer H. Dietary fibre and nutrient intake in Crohn's disease. Am J Clin Nutr. 1979;32:1898–901.
19. Silkoff K, Hallak A, Yegena L, Rozen P, Mayberry JF, Rhodes J. Consumption of refined carbohydrate by patients with Crohn's disease in Tel-Aviv-Yafo. Postgrad Med J. 1980;56:842–6.
20. Fritsche K. Fatty acids as modulators of the immune response. Annu Rev Nutr. 2006;26:45–73.
21. Serhan C, Chiang N, van Dyke T. Resolving inflammation: dual anti-inflammatory and pro-resolution lipid mediators. Nat Rev Immunol. 2008;8:349–61.
22. De Filippo C, Cavalieri D, Di Paola M, Ramazzotti M, Poullet J, Massart S. Impact of diet in shaping gut microbiota revealed by a comparative study in children from Europe and rural africa. Proc Natl Acad Sci U S A. 2010;107:14691–6.
23. Moreno-Navarrete J, Sabater M, Ortega F, Ricart W, Fernandez-Real J. Circulating zonulin, a marker of intestinal permeability, is increased in association with obesity-associated insulin resistance. PLoS One. 2012;7, e37160.
24. Novak T, Babcock T, Jho D, Helton W, Espat N. NF-kappa B inhibition by omega-3 fatty acids modulates LPS-stimulated macrophage TNF-alpha transcription. Am J Physiol. 2003;284:L84–9.
25. Costea I, Mack D, Lemaitre R, Israel D, Marcil V, Ahmad A, et al. Interactions between the dietary polyunsaturated fatty acid ratio and genetic factors determine susceptibility to pediatric Crohn's disease. Gastroenterology. 2014;146:929–31.
26. Turner D, Steinhart A, Griffiths A. Omega 3 fatty acids (fish oil) for maintenance of remission in ulcerative colitis. Cochrane Database Syst Rev. 2007;(3):CD006443.
27. Lev-Tzion R, Griffiths A, Leder O, Turner D. Omega 3 fatty acids (fish oil) for maintenance of remission in Crohn's disease. Cochrane Database Syst Rev. 2014;(28):CD006320.
28. Feagan BG, Sandborn WJ, Mittmann U, Bar-Meir S, D'Haens G, Bradette M, et al. Omega-3 free fatty acids for the maintenance of remission in Crohn's disease: the EPIC randomized controlled trials. JAMA. 2008;299:1690–7.
29. Liu P, Schenk M, Walker V, Dempsey P, Kanchanapoomi M, Heelwright M, et al. Convergence of IL-1beta and VDR activation pathways in human TLR2/1-induced antimicrobial responses. PLoS One. 2009;4, e5810.
30. Yuk J, Shin DM, Lee HM, Yang CS, Jin H, Kim KK, et al. Vitamin D3 induces autophagy in human monocytes/macrophages via cathelicidin. Cell Host Microbe. 2009;6:231–43.

31. Zhang Y, Leung D, Richers B, Liu Y, Remigio LK, Riches DW, et al. Vitamin D inhibits mono-cyte/macrophage proinflammatory cytokine production by targeting MAPK phosphatase-1. J Immunol. 2012;188:2127–35.
32. Lemire J, Adams J, Kermani-Arab V, Bakke A, Sakai R, Jordan S. 1,25-dihydroxyvitamin D3 suppresses human T helper/inducer lymphocyte activity in vitro. J Immunol. 1985;134: 3032–5.
33. Kong J, Zhang Z, Mea M. Novel role of the vitamin D receptor in maintaining the integrity of the intestinal mucosal barrier. Am J Physiol Gastrointest Liver Physiol. 2008;294:G208–16.
34. Khalili H, Huang E, Ananthakrishnan A, Higuchi L, Richter J, Fuchs C, et al. Geographical variation and incidence of inflammatory bowel disease among US women. Gut. 2012;61:1686–92.
35. Simmons D, Mullighan C, Welsh K, Jewell D. Vitamin D receptor gene polymorphism: asso-ciation with Crohn's disease susceptibility. Gut. 2000;47:211–4.
36. Dresner-Pollak R, Ackerman Z, Eliakim R, Karban A, Chowers YFH. The BsmI vitamin D receptor gene polymorphism is associated with ulcerative colitis in Jewish Ashkenazi patients. Genet Test. 2004;8:417–20.
37. Jorgensen S, Agnholt J, Glerup H, Lyhne S, Villadsen GE, Hvas C, et al. Clinical trial: vitamin D3 treatment in Crohn's disease—a randomised double-blind placebo-controlled study. Aliment Pharmacol Ther. 2010;32:377–83.
38. Maslowski K, Mackay C. Diet, gut microbiota and immune responses. Nat Immunol. 2011;12:5–9.
39. Nagalingam N, Lynch S. Role of the microbiota in inflammatory bowel diseases. Inflamm Bowel Dis. 2012;18:968–84.
40. Roediger WE, Duncan S, Kapaniris O, Millard S. Reducing sulfur compounds of the colon impair colonocyte nutrition: implications for ulcerative colitis. Gastroenterology. 1993;104: 802–9.
41. Pitcher M, Beatty E, Cummings J. The contribution of sulphate reducing bacteria and 5-aminosalicyclic acid to faecal sulphide in patients with ulcerative colitis. Gut. 2000;46: 64–72.
42. Gibson G, Cummings J, MacFarlane G. Growth and activities of sulphate-reducing bacteria in gut contents of healthy subjects and patients with ulcerative colitis. FEMS Microbiol Lett. 1991;86:103–12.
43. Kleessen B, Kroesen A, Buhr H, Blaut M. Mucosal and invading bacteria in patients with inflammatory bowel disease compared with controls. Scand J Gastroenterol. 2002;37(9): 1034–41.
44. Jowett S, Seal C, Pearce M, Phillips E, Gregory W, Barton J, et al. Influence of dietary factors on the clinical course of ulcerative colitis: a prospective cohort study. Gut. 2004;53:1479–84.
45. Grisham MB. Oxidants and free radicals in inflammatory bowel disease. Lancet. 1994;344: 859–61.
46. Millar A, Rampton D, Blake D. Effects of iron and iron chelation in vitro on mucosal oxidant activity in ulcerative colitis. Aliment Pharmacol Ther. 2000;14:1163–8.
47. Bao B, Prasad AS, Beck FW, et al. Zinc decreases C-reactive protein, lipid peroxidation, and inflammatory cytokines in elderly subjects: a potential implication of zinc as an atheroprotec-tive agent. Am J Clin Nutr. 2010;91:1634–41.
48. Bao B, Prasad AS, Beck FW, et al. Zinc supplementation decreases oxidative stress, incidence of infection, and generation of inflammatory cytokines in sickle cell disease patients. Transl Res. 2008;152:67–80.
49. Barollo M, Medici V, D'Inca R, et al. Antioxidative potential of a combined therapy of anti TNFalpha and Zn acetate in experimental colitis. World J Gastroenterol. 2011;17:4099–103.
50. Chen BW, Wang HH, Liu JX, et al. Zinc sulphate solution enema decreases inflammation in experimental colitis in rats. J Gastroenterol Hepatol. 1999;14:1088–92.

Part II
Nutritional Deficiencies in Inflammatory Bowel Diseases

Chapter 3
Vitamin D and Inflammatory Bowel Disease

Athanasios P. Desalermos, Francis A. Farraye, and Hannah L. Miller

Introduction

Vitamin D Synthesis and Metabolism

Vitamin D is an essential vitamin for humans. It plays a crucial role in calcium homeostasis and bone metabolism. Furthermore, vitamin D has key effects on the immune system, muscle function, and brain development [1]. It consists of a group of fat-soluble molecules with a four-ringed cholesterol backbone. The main circulating molecule is the 25-hydroxyvitamin D [25(OH)D] (calcidiol). The active form of vitamin D is 1,25-dihydroxyvitamin D [1,25(OH)2D] (calcitriol). 1,25(OH)2D acts intracellularly, through the vitamin D receptor (VDR), and regulates gene transcription. VDR is a nuclear hormone receptor, can be found in all nucleated cells, and belongs to class II steroid hormone receptor [2].

Vitamin D can be found in a limited number of foods. Its main natural source is the dermal synthesis. Vitamin D in the skin is formed as vitamin D3 (cholecalciferol). 7-dehydrocholesterol in skin cells under exposure to solar ultraviolet B radiation converted to pre-vitamin D_3, which is transformed to vitamin D3 after a thermal induction. Skin production is very efficient and minimal exposure of arms and face can produce vitamin D equivalent of 200 international units (IU) from food

A.P. Desalermos, M.D.
Division of Gastroenterology, University of California, San Diego, USA
e-mail: adesalermos@ucsd.edu

F.A. Farraye, M.D., M.Sc. (✉)
Section of Gastroenterology, Boston University Medical Center, Boston, MA, USA
e-mail: francis.farraye@bmc.org

H.L. Miller, M.D.
Connecticut Gastroenterology Consultants, 40 Temple St, New Haven, CT 06510, USA

© Springer International Publishing Switzerland 2016
A.N. Ananthakrishnan (ed.), *Nutritional Management of Inflammatory Bowel Diseases*, DOI 10.1007/978-3-319-26890-3_3

consumption [3]. Nevertheless, the specific amount of vitamin D produced by sun exposure cannot be estimated with accuracy as it is dependent on the season, latitude, time of the day, the presence of sunscreen and skin type [4]. Of note, melanin lessens the dermal production of vitamin D3. People with limited exposure to sunlight such as disabled persons and older people with less effective cutaneous production are prone to vitamin D deficiency. Vitamin D_2 (ergocalciferol) and vitamin D3 (cholecalciferol) can be found in very few foods, including salmon, tuna, and mushrooms. Human-made ergocalciferol and cholecalciferol supplements have been developed, and fortified food with ergocalciferol and cholecalciferol is common in many countries including the United States [1]. Vitamin D3 and D2 are of similar potency. The absorption of the vitamin D contained in food is performed by enterocytes. Micelles are formed in the gut, absorbed by the enterocytes, and incorporated into chylomicrons. Various diseases affecting the fat absorption distress the vitamin D absorption, examples include Crohn's disease (CD), pancreatic insufficiency, celiac disease, cholestatic liver disease, and cystic fibrosis [1, 5]. Dermal produced and diet delivered inactive vitamin D is metabolized to the liver and kidneys to its active forms, by two enzymatic hydroxylation reactions, which form 25(OH)D and 1,25(OH)2D, respectively (Fig. 3.1). Synthesis of the active form of vitamin D, calcitriol, is performed by the kidneys, and is regulated by two hormones, the parathyroid hormone (PTH) which increases the production, and fibroblast-like growth factor-23 (FGF23), which decreases it [1]. The half-life of 25(OH)D is 2–3 weeks, while for 1,25(OH)2D it is between 4 and 6 h.

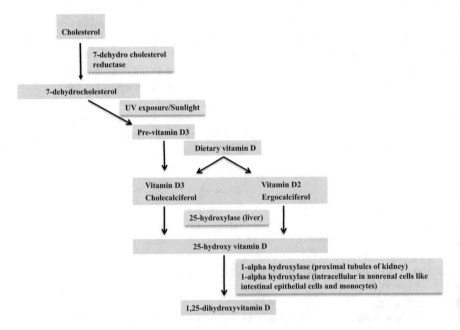

Fig. 3.1 Vitamin D metabolism

IBD and Vitamin D Deficiency

Vitamin D Requirements and Deficiency

The ideal level of vitamin D is an area of controversy and under research. Levels of 25(OH)D are used as an estimation of vitamin D adequacy, as this is the best indicator of vitamin D status. Levels lower than 20 ng/mL (50 nmol/L) are generally considered deficient, levels between 21 and 29 ng/mL (52.5 and 72.5 nmol/L) are insufficient and levels between 30 and 100 ng/mL (75 and 250 nmol/L) are considered normal [1, 5–7]. Interestingly, these numbers are based on observations that do not take into account extra-skeletal health. Those observations include sufficient production by the kidneys of 1,25(OH)2D for optimal calcium absorption from the gut, maximum level of suppression of PTH, and a protective level against a clinical end point, such as a fracture. Racial differences in vitamin D levels have been observed. African Americans have lower total serum 25(OH)D concentrations than other races without the consequences of vitamin D deficiency as the bioavailable 25(OH)D is similar between the different ethnic groups. The phenomenon is explained by lower levels of vitamin D-binding protein in this ethnic group as well [8].

Deficiency to vitamin D among people of all ages is very common and has multiple pathogenetic mechanisms [1, 5, 6, 9–11]. Impaired cutaneous production, insufficient dietary intake, and fat malabsorption decrease the availability of the vitamin. Residents of northern latitudes, dark skinned, hospitalized, or institutionalized individuals, and older adults have suboptimal dermal production of vitamin D. Furthermore, older adults minimize the vitamin D containing food intake. Disorders in the metabolism of the vitamin D, like hydroxylation by the liver or kidney, affect the active forms of the vitamin. Finally, in hereditary diseases, such as hereditary vitamin D-resistant rickets, where the VDR is defective and resistant to vitamin D, patients develop rickets within the first 2 years of life. Moreover, obese people, and patients taking medications that increase the metabolism of vitamin D, like phenytoin, are prone to low levels of the vitamin [1, 5, 6, 9–11]. Research data underline the correlation between obesity and vitamin D deficiency, and causative mechanisms include preferred deposition of vitamin D in fatty tissue, making it unavailable, or volumetric dilution, as higher body mass can cause a dilution effect [12–15].

Prevalence of Vitamin D Deficiency in IBD

A particularly at risk population for vitamin D deficiency are patients with inflammatory bowel disease (IBD). In addition to environmental and genetic factors mentioned above, IBD-specific factors include an inflamed bowel causing losses through the gastrointestinal tract, resected bowel causing reduced absorption, medication use that affects vitamin D absorption from the intestine, and anorexia from severely active disease. A recent study in pediatric patients with IBD showed an abnormal metabolism of vitamin D, where the PTH is not rationally elevated in the setting of a low vitamin D, compared with healthy controls. Furthermore, conversion of 25(OH)D to 1,25(OH)2D appeared impaired. In the study elevated tumor necrosis factor α (TNF-α) levels were statistically associated with lower 1,25(OH)2D levels. PTH and renal 1-α-hydroxylase suppression from inflammatory cytokines, like TNF-α, may be the cause for abnormal metabolism of vitamin D in IBD patients [16]. Multiple studies have assessed the prevalence of vitamin D deficiency among individuals with IBD, ranging from 22 to 70 % for CD, and as high as 45 % for ulcerative colitis (UC) [17]. In a study of 242 patients with CD from Canada, 8 % of the patients were found to be vitamin D deficient and 22 % of the patients were vitamin D insufficient, defined as 25(OH)D less than 25 nmol/L, and less than 40 nmol/L, respectively. In this patient cohort, predictors of vitamin D deficiency were smoking status, nutrition, and sunlight exposure of the patient [18]. A Norwegian study of 120 IBD adult patients found vitamin D deficiency in 27 % of subjects with CD, and 15 % with UC. The difference was statistically significant between the two groups, $P < 0.05$. Of note, 37 % of the individuals with CD, who had small bowel resection, were found to have secondary hyperparathyroidism [19].

Metabolic Bone Disease in IBD Patients

Vitamin D and Metabolic Bone Disease

Among the main reasons for the clinically significant metabolic bone disease in IBD patients, vitamin D deficiency plays a crucial role. As a critical risk factor for bone disease, a severe and prolonged vitamin D deficiency can cause hypocalcemia by a decreased intestinal absorption of calcium. Low levels of calcium cause upregulation of the production of PTH, and secondary hyperparathyroidism. This can lead to demineralization of bones and eventually, osteomalacia in adults and rickets and osteomalacia in children. Osteomalacia can be asymptomatic or produce various symptoms like bone pain and muscle weakness, difficulty walking, and fracture [1, 5]. Typical levels of vitamin D (25-hydroxyvitamin D) in the setting of osteomalacia are less than 10 ng/mL.

The prevalence of osteopenia and osteoporosis among patients with IBD appears high. In a study of 63 patients with CD and 41 with UC, 42 % of the patients had osteopenia of the femoral neck [−2.5 Standard Deviation (SD) < bone mineral density (BMD) *T* score < −1 SD] and 41 % had osteoporosis (BMD *T* score < −2.5) [20]. In another study of 44 patients with CD and 35 with UC, a high prevalence of osteopenia and osteoporosis were also found, *T* scores < −1.0 from 51 to 77 %; *T* scores < −2.5 from 17 to 28 % [21]. A recent study of 143 patients, determined that

48.07 %, and 18.26 % of UC patients had osteopenia and osteoporosis, respectively. For CD patients, 56.41 % had osteopenia, and 15.38 % had osteoporosis [22]. These observations underline the crucial role of adequate vitamin D intake for optimal bone that in turn can improve the overall quality of life for individuals with IBD.

Clinical Consequences of Metabolic Bone Disease in IBD Patients

The clinical significance of osteopenia and osteoporosis of patients with IBD, and the associated risk of fracture have been studied extensively over the past 10 years. The results are conflicting, however, overall an increased risk for fracture among people of IBD has been observed. Several studies highlight the risk of fracture. A large study from the University of Manitoba using an extensive IBD database with 6027 patients, found an increased incidence of fractures, 40 % higher compared with the general population, especially among people older than 60 years of age. More specifically, fractures of the spine, hip, wrist, forearm, and rib were all increased, with incidence ratios 1.74, 1.59, 1.33, 1.25, respectively. Notably, there was no difference between CD and UC, and similar fracture rates were calculated in each age stratum [23]. An analysis of 434 patients with UC, 383 with CD, and 635 controls showed an increased risk of fracture among females with CD, with a relative risk of 2.5. The difference was not statistically significant for male patients with CD or patients with UC [24]. Furthermore, a cohort of CD patients, showed an elevated prevalence of vertebral fractures. Notably, the incidence was similar among patients with normal BMD, and patients with osteopenia and osteoporosis. In the study, the inflammatory process expressed by the C-reactive protein (CRP) positively correlated with height reductions of vertebrae [25]. Subsequent studies have not been able to validate the increased risk of fracture. For example, in a population based study in Olmsted County Minnesota of 238 CD patients were compared with controls matched by sex and age, and the risk of fracture was not increased, compared with the matched controls [26].

The importance of screening for osteoporosis in IBD patients was underlined by the American Gastroenterological Association (AGA). Based on their recommendations, patients with IBD should be screened with dual energy X-ray absorptiometry (DXA) if they have one or more risk factors for osteoporosis, which include postmenopausal women, male older than 50, history of vertebral fractures, hypogonadism, or chronic corticosteroid therapy. Furthermore, they recommend repeat of the test after 2–3 years if the initial test was normal. For patients found with osteoporosis or low trauma fracture, workup for secondary causes of osteoporosis should be initiated, including complete blood count, serum calcium, 25(OH)D, creatinine, alkaline phosphatase, testosterone in males, and serum protein electrophoresis [27]. In the setting of an increased risk of fracture, the impact of osteoporosis and osteopenia on the general health and quality of life of IBD individuals is significant, especially for older adults.

Vitamin D and Immune Response

Vitamin D plays an important role in innate and adaptive immunity [28–30]. VDR is expressed in the majority of immune system cells like macrophages, monocytes, dendritic cells, T and B cells. Immune cells have the necessary enzymes to convert 25(OH)D to its active form of 1,25(OH)2D. Locally produced active vitamin D has autocrine and paracrine effects, direct and indirect effect on B and T activated cells, modulating effect on the adaptive immune response and on antigen-presenting cells, like dendritic and macrophages, all of which regulate the innate immunity [31]. Largely, this effect facilitates mucosa integrity, supports a balanced microbiome, and promotes an immunosuppressive state by switching from a helper T cell (Th) 1 and 17 profile to Th 2 cell and T regulator (Treg) cell profile.

Antibacterial Activity of Vitamin D

Vitamin D upregulates the innate immune system and coordinates the immune response to bacterial infections. Therefore, vitamin D antibacterial properties regulate a balanced microbiome. Intracellular bacteria, like *Mycobacterium tuberculosis* activate Toll-like receptors (TLRs), which institute a direct antimicrobial action against those pathogens. Activation of TLRs of macrophages, by *M. tuberculosis* derived lipopeptide, upregulates VDR gene and vitamin D-1α-hydroxylase (CYP27b1 in humans) gene, which converts the 25(OH)D to the active 1,25(OH)2D. A cascade of reactions occurs which produce an immune response of the host towards the pathogen, including cathelicidin, an antimicrobial peptide [32]. Vitamin D directly influences cathelicidin production [33]. Moreover, vitamin D stimulates the upregulation of pattern recognition receptor NOD2. Muramyl dipeptide is a product of Gram-negative and Gram-positive bacteria and activates the NOD2 receptor. As a consequence, the nuclear transcription factor kappa-light-chain-enhancer of activated B cells (NF-κB) is stimulated, which causes expression of the gene *DEFB2*, encoding antimicrobial peptide defensin β2. Importantly, the pathogenesis of CD has been linked with the impaired function of NOD2 and DEFB2 [34].

Autophagy and Vitamin D

Autophagy is an important part of immune innate system. Vitamin D plays a crucial role as it induces and regulates this catabolic process [35]. By affecting different pathways which induce autophagy, vitamin D regulates immune and inflammatory responses. More specifically, 1,25(OH)2D via cathelicidin helps the co-localization of mycobacterial phagosomes with autophagosomes in human macrophages [36].

Vitamin D and Dendritic Cells

Vitamin D has significant effects on adaptive immunity, as it acts as an immune modulator. VDR can be found in activated B and T cells, and dendritic cells [37]. Dendritic cells, as antigen-presenting cells, act as a messenger between innate and adaptive immune system and play a significant role in the regulation of adaptive immunity. Vitamin D decreases the proliferation, differentiation, and maturation of dendritic cells. Dendritic cells are stimulated by lipopolysaccharide, part of the Gram-negative bacteria cell wall, and are able to produce more 1,25(OH)2D after an increased expression of vitamin D 1α-hydroxylase [38]. Monocytic differentiation to dendritic cells is suppressed by vitamin D action, and in this way the ability of dendritic cells to stimulate T-cell proliferation is reduced. Vitamin D decreases the production of interleukin (IL) 12, and the upregulation of the co-stimulatory molecules cluster of differentiation 40 (CD40), CD80, CD86, and class II major histocompatibility complex (MHC) molecules. Vitamin D also increases the production of IL-10 by the dendritic cells. Overall, the effect is immunosuppressive, as IL-12 induces Th 1 cells, and upregulation of CD40, CD80, and CD86 in antigen-presenting cells activates Th 1 cells. Moreover, vitamin D increases the production of Treg, by an upregulation of Fox2 and IL-10 [39]. In this way, vitamin D supports a nonspecific antigen response and drives a possible over response of the immune system that could lead to pathologic conditions [40, 41].

Vitamin D and Macrophages

Vitamin D upregulates the differentiation of monocytes to macrophages, increases the production of prostaglandin E2, which has immunosuppressant properties, and decreases the granulocyte macrophage colony stimulating factor (GM-CSF). Furthermore, it reduces proinflammatory cytokines like interferon (IFN) γ, lysosomal acid phosphatase, hydrogen peroxide, and macrophage-specific membrane antigens production from macrophages. Of note, decreased production of INF-γ causes impaired activation of macrophages [42]. Also, vitamin D can reduce the antigen-presenting ability of macrophages by blocking the expression of MHC-2 antigens. In addition, 1,25(OH)2D impairs the expression of TLR2, TLR4, and TLR9, and as an effect less IL-6 is produced after a TLR9 challenge [43]. In antigen-presenting cells like macrophages, vitamin D impairs the IL-6 and IL-23 production, thus blocking the Th 17 cells response [39].

Vitamin D and T Cells Differentiation

Vitamin D key targets are the Th 1, 2, and 17 cells, follicular helper T cells (T_{FH}) and Treg cells, and their differentiation. Type 1 Th cells act on cell-mediated immune responses and produce pro-inflammatory cytokines like IFN-γ and lymphotoxin. In

IBD, Th1 cells are directed against self-proteins. Type 2 Th cells play a role on antibody-mediated immunity and produce anti-inflammatory cytokines, IL-4, IL-5, and IL-13. Examples of diseases influenced by type 2 Th cells are asthma and food allergies [28]. 1,25(OH)2D suppresses Th1 cells activity, and in this way decreases their production of pro-inflammatory cytokines like IFN-γ, IL-2, and TNF-α. Also, it inhibits the Th 17 and T_{FH} cells pro-inflammatory cytokine production, IL-17 and IL-21, respectively [44]. Vitamin D controls the overproduction of these cytokines, and appears to have a potential role in controlling IBD [30]. Vitamin D acts on the differential of T cells in favor of Th 2, and Treg cells over Th 1 and Th 17 cells. Thus, a balance is achieved between an inflammatory and immunosuppressive response of the immune system. In parallel, vitamin D acts directly on B cells, inhibiting the proliferation and increasing the apoptosis of activated B cells. Also, cytotoxic activity of CD+ T cells is reduced by the action of vitamin D [44–46]. Moreover, 1,25(OH)2D limits the production of plasma cells, immunoglobulin production, and post-switch memory B cells [47].

Vitamin D and IBD Pathogenesis

Vitamin D deficiency has been proposed as a pathogenetic mechanism of IBD (Table 3.1). Multiple studies and observations underline the significance of vitamin D deficiency in the development of IBD, and possible mechanisms have been suggested. However, only one clinical study has examined the vitamin D level in relation to risk of IBD. A large prospective cohort study of more than 70,000 women found that sufficient levels of vitamin D were linked with statistically significant lower incidence of CD, $P<0.02$ [48].

North–South Gradient of IBD

Studies in Europe and United States have observed a geographical distribution and variation of UC and CD. The incidence of IBD is higher in northern latitudes [49–52]. The putative explanation for this north–south gradient is the exposure to UVB radiation, which is lower in northern latitudes. Dermal vitamin D production depends on the sunlight exposure, and populations of southern latitudes have lower risk of developing IBD, and low sun exposure has been proven as risk factor for IBD [53, 54].

Distorted Immunity in Vitamin D Deficiency

Experimental models have been developed to assess the relation of vitamin D status with the pathogenesis of IBD. An experimental IBD animal model was developed using IL-10 knockout mice, who displayed diarrhea, enterocolitis, and weight loss.

Table 3.1 Vitamin D and IBD pathogenesis

1. Epidemiological studies	A north–south gradient and a geographical distribution and variation of UC[a] and CD[b] have been observed. The incidence of IBD[c] is higher in northern latitudes, likely due to less sunlight exposure and impaired production of vitamin D	[49–54]
2. Distorted immunity in vitamin D deficiency		
(a) Control of the inflammation	VDR[d], IL[e]-10 double KO[f] mice colitis model found with high expression of inflammatory cytokines (INF[g]-γ, IL-1β, IL-2, IL-12, TNF[h]-α). VDR was essential in the model to control the inflammation in the KO mice	[57, 65–67]
	Serum 25(OH)D[i] is inversely correlated with calprotectin, in IBD patients	
	VDR downregulates the NF-κB[j] by increasing the production of the inhibitor of κBα, an endogenous inhibitor of NF-κB, thus reduces the inflammation in the intestine	
	Epithelial VDR has an anticolitic potential, reduces apoptosis by downregulating pre-apoptotic modulator, PUMA	
(b) Maintenance of epithelial barrier	Vitamin D supports epithelial junctions of mucosa, and upregulates junction proteins, like claudins, ZO-1, and occludins. Disruption of the mucosal barrier has been noted in IBD	[58–60]
(c) Dysbiosis	In a VDR, IL-10 double KO colitis model, a 50-fold bacteria increase in the colon, a change in the gut microbiome, and a reduced angiogenin-4, was found in vitamin D deficient mice	[63]
(d) Innate immune response	Autophagy gene *ATG16L1*, which affects Paneth cells antimicrobial action and autophagy, is regulated by vitamin D. Bacterial products upregulate VDR and *ATG16L1* and decrease inflammation. Vitamin D deficiency impairs autophagy, and influences chronic mucosal inflammation, and potentially IBD	[64]
(e) Adaptive immune response	A trinitrobenzene sulfonic acid Th 1 cell-mediated colitis in mice found that vitamin D inhibits the Th 1 cell production, promotes the Th[k] 2 cell action, and enhances regulatory T cell functions	[39]
3. Genetic associations, polymorphism	IBD susceptibility has a strong genetic component. Examples: VDR and DBP[l] gene polymorphism	[68–72]
4. Animal studies	Animal IBD model with IL-10 KO mice develop more severe symptoms if were vitamin D deficient	[39, 55, 56, 61, 62]
	Mice model of dextran sodium sulfate-induced colitis sufficient vitamin D levels improved the colitis. Moreover, the secretion of TNF-α was reduced	
	A trinitrobenzene sulfonic acid Th 1 cell-mediated colitis in mice found that 1,25(OH)2D[m] improves the severity of the colitis	

(continued)

Table 3.1 (continued)

5. Clinical studies	A prospective cohort study of more than 70,000 women found an inverse relationship between vitamin D levels and risk of CD	[48 73, 74, 83, 84]
	13 % of patients with IBD treated with 1200 IU[n] of 1,25(OH)2D and 1200 mg of calcium had a relapse after a year, compared with 29 % of IBD patients treated with calcium alone ($P=0.06$)	
	Individuals with IBD receiving 1,25(OH)2D for 6 weeks had significantly decreased Crohn's disease activity index, C-reactive protein, and markers of bone turnover ($P<0.05$), but no significant differences after 12 months	
	Low pretreatment levels of vitamin D are associated with earlier discontinuation of anti-TNF-α therapy ($P<0.05$)	
	Low vitamin D appears as a risk factor for IBD-related surgery in IBD, improvement of the 25(OH)D serum level reduces the risk in CD	

[a]Ulcerative colitis
[b]Crohn's disease
[c]Inflammatory bowel disease
[d]Vitamin D receptor
[e]Interleukin
[f]Knockout
[g]Interferon
[h]Tumor necrosis factor
[i]25-Hydroxyvitamin D
[j]Nuclear transcription factor kappa-light-chain-enhancer of activated B cells
[k]T helper cell
[l]Vitamin D-binding protein
[m]1,25-Dihydroxyvitamin D
[n]International units

The researchers showed that vitamin D deficient mice had more severe symptoms than vitamin D sufficient mice, and the difference was statistically significant [55, 56]. Interestingly, in a similar experimental model with VDR and IL-10 double knockout mice, high expression of inflammatory cytokines, such as IFN-γ, IL-1β, IL-2, IL-12, and TNF-α, was observed in the experimental colitis, and VDR was essential in the model to control the inflammation in the knockout mice [57]. Furthermore, vitamin D appears vital for the preservation of an intact intestinal barrier in the intestine, as it supports the integrity of junction complexes of the mucosa. This was shown in a colitis model using dextran sulfate sodium as stressor for the mucosa of the intestine. Mice deficient of VDR developed severe colitis, characterized by diarrhea, rectal bleeding, and death. These mice were shown to have severe disruption in epithelial junctions and reduction in the junction proteins like claudins, ZO-1, and occludins [58–60]. Interestingly, a disrupted and malfunctioning intestinal epithelial barrier, with distorted tight junctions, has been found in CD, in parallel with impaired expression and distribution of claudin 2, 5, and 8 [60]. Further research with the model of dextran sodium sulfate-induced colitis in mice showed that 1,25(OH)2D produced locally in the colon, and distally in the kidneys affect the severity of the colitis, and mice with normal vitamin D levels demonstrate less histological evidence of colitis, symptom of weight loss, and expression of inflammatory cytokines [61]. In the same animal model, vitamin D has been shown to ameliorate the symptoms of colitis and reduce secretion of TNF-α. The reduction of TNF-α was performed by downregulating a number of genes, which are associated with TNF-α production, a crucial factor of inflammation in IBD [62].

Vitamin D, Dysbiosis, and IBD

Low vitamin D levels can alter the enteric flora and distort the microbiome. Recent studies have proposed an interesting link between vitamin D status, dysbiosis, and IBD. Using the VDR and IL-10 double knockout model, vitamin D deficient mice showed 50-fold bacteria increase in the colon and in parallel, angiogenin-4, an antibacterial protein associated with enteric bacteria control, was reduced. It was hypothesized that vitamin D deficiency influenced a colitis, which was driven by a distorted antibacterial activity and a change in the gut microbiota [63]. In addition, autophagy, as we mentioned earlier, is regulated by vitamin D, and insufficient vitamin D can affect autophagy. This can change the microbiome, the intestinal homeostasis, and contribute to the pathophysiology of IBD. A correlation between vitamin D, dysbiosis, autophagy, and genetic susceptibility for IBD has been observed. Another study demonstrated that vitamin D regulates autophagy gene *ATG16L1*. This is a susceptibility gene for IBD, which affects the antimicrobial action of Paneth cells and autophagy by decreased lysozyme activity. At the same time, the bacterial product butyrate positively influences VDR and expression of *ATG16L1* and reduces inflammation in an experimental colitis model. Vitamin D deficiency could affect intestinal homeostasis by decreased autophagy and lead to development of states of chronic mucosal inflammation, and potentially IBD [64].

Intestinal Inflammation and Vitamin D

The research findings highlight the vital role of VDR for the homeostasis of the mucosal barrier of the intestine and inflammation of the epithelium. A correlation between intestinal inflammation markers, like calprotectin, and vitamin D status has been noted, and underlines the link between vitamin D and gut inflammation. In a study of patients with UC and CD, the serum 25(OH)D was inversely correlated with fecal calprotectin, but not with other systemic inflammation markers like CRP. This correlation was statistical significant [65]. In addition, NF-κB has a critical role in inflammation. VDR negatively regulates the NF-κB by positively modulating the inhibitor of κBα, an endogenous inhibitor of NF-κB, and in this way regulates the inflammation level in the intestine [66]. Moreover, a study showed the anticolitic potential of epithelial VDR, which reduces apoptosis by acting on a crucial pre-apoptotic modulator PUMA, which downregulates and hence decreases the colonic inflammation and protects the intestinal mucosa [67].

Vitamin D Receptor Gene Polymorphism

IBD susceptibility appears to have a strong genetic component. Examples of genetic components are VDR and vitamin D-binding protein (DBP) gene polymorphism. VDR gene is located in a region on chromosome 12, and genome screening techniques have found a linkage between the polymorphism of VDR gene with the pathogenesis of IBD [68–70]. A recent meta-analysis evaluated the relation between IBD and four genetic polymorphisms in VDR gene, ApaI, BsmI, FokI, and TaqI. Based on their subgroup analysis, a significant link found between VDR ApaI polymorphism and an increased risk for CD, as well as the TaqI polymorphism and a decreased risk for UC. Furthermore, the study highlights the varying genetic fingerprinting of different ethnic groups [71]. Moreover, DBP gene polymorphism has been associated with IBD. A statistical analysis of 884 individuals, including 636 IBD individuals showed that DBP 420 variant Lys found more frequently in non-IBD controls than in IBD patients [72].

Vitamin D Status and IBD Severity

Multiple clinical studies have been conducted to assess a possible correlation between vitamin D level and severity of IBD. The results of the studies are conflicting, but overall highlight the significance of sufficient vitamin D level for optimal control of IBD. A recent multi-institution IBD cohort with 3217 patients demonstrated that vitamin D deficiency is an independent risk factor for IBD-related surgery. A dose–response correlation was found in the CD cohort, and restoration of normal levels of vitamin D was associated with reduced risk for subsequent surgery [73]. A retrospective cohort study of 101 IBD patients from a single academic tertiary referral center examining the vitamin D status in patients with IBD on anti-TNF-α therapy found vitamin D insufficiency in the cohort of both primary nonresponders and those with a loss of response [74]. Severity of disease activity was found to negatively correlate with 25(OH)D levels in a cohort study of 34 patients with CD [75]. A cross-sectional study of 182 patients with CD found disease activity, assessed by the CD activity index and CRP levels, correlated with lower vitamin D levels [76]. Moreover, in a cohort of 220 IBD patients, 141 with CD and 79 with UC, serum concentration of vitamin D correlates with health-related quality of life in UC and CD during the winter and spring period [77].

Fewer studies explored the significance of optimum vitamin D level for the severity of UC. Vitamin D status and clinical disease activity using the six-point partial Mayo index were assessed in a cross-sectional study with 34 patients with UC, and individuals with low levels of 25(OH)D were statistically more likely to have elevated severity of UC [78]. Recently, preliminary results of a 5-year prospective study of over 1000 patients with IBD found that lower vitamin D levels correlated with poor quality of life, increased utilization of health care system by 44 %, and increased use of medications like steroids, biologics, and narcotics [79]. Although these studies show positive correlations, many studies have found no association between vitamin D status and disease severity, even though a large portion of patients were vitamin D deficient [80, 81].

Vitamin D as Therapeutic Modality for IBD

Published data from experimental models of colitis, and observational studies, have shown that vitamin D could be used as a potential therapeutic agent for IBD [39, 58, 82]. Two main treatment studies have examined the effect of vitamin D supplementation on CD and UC, and the potential of its use as a therapeutic modality. A multicenter, randomized, double-blind, placebo-controlled study in Denmark was performed in 180 patients with CD in remission. In the two treatment groups, 1200 IU of 1,25(OH)2D with 1200 mg of calcium or 1200 mg of calcium (placebo group) were administered daily for 1 year. Twenty nine percent of the individuals on calcium alone had a relapse, compared with 13 % for the group of vitamin D, which was not statistically significant ($P=0.06$) [83]. A second prospective study in patients with CD compared the efficacy of 1,25(OH)2D and 25(OH)D as a therapeutic intervention for disease activity and bone health [84]. In the short term, after 6 weeks CD activity index, CRP protein, and markers of bone turnover were significantly decreased ($P<0.05$) in the 1,25(OH)2D treatment arm. Of note, no significant differences were noted for the 25(OH)D treatment group at 6 weeks, and for either group at 12 months [84].

Vitamin D and Risk of *Clostridium difficile* Infection in IBD Patients

Patients with IBD are at increased risk for *Clostridium difficile* infection (CDI) [85, 86]. Vitamin D influences the antibacterial properties of the intestine, and production of antimicrobial compounds like cathelicidins. It acts prophylactically against infections and as modulator of the microbiome [32, 33, 87]. A recent multi-institutional IBD cohort study found that sufficient plasma 25(OH)D level was associated with lower risk of CDI in IBD patients [88]. Vitamin D could potentially be used to aid in the prevention of CDI.

Vitamin D and Risk of Colon Cancer in IBD Patients

Individuals with IBD are in increased risk for colorectal cancer (CRC). CRC is one of the main causes for mortality among patients with IBD [89]. Inflammation is a risk factor for the development of CRC and frequent relapses of IBD add significantly to that risk [90, 91]. Vitamin D through its anti-inflammatory properties may act as potential protective agent against CRC in IBD. In vitro studies have shown 1,25(OH)2D reduces the growth and promotes differentiation of colon cancer cell lines [92–94]. A study using the human colon cancer line, HT-29, found an impaired growth of HT-29 cells treated with vitamin D. The study proposes a putative target of vitamin D, via the TLR4 pathway, against CRC in populations with IBD [95]. UC patients have lower expression of VDR, and have been shown to have a higher risk of CRC, and thus, a low VDR expression has been proposed as marker of dysplasia and cancer in individuals with UC [96]. A meta-analysis of case–control studies found that daily vitamin D supplementation could decrease the CRC incidence, as patients with sufficient vitamin D serum levels had a 50 % lower risk of CRC compared with patients with low vitamin D levels [97]. Furthermore, daily intake of 1000 IU of vitamin D could reduce the risk for CRC by 50 % [98]. Conversely, a randomized, double-blind, placebo-controlled clinical study of 36,282 postmenopausal women didn't demonstrate a significance reduction of the risk of CRC among postmenopausal women receiving 400 IU/day of vitamin D for 7 years [99]. Notably, the study has significant limitations as the dose of vitamin D, 400 IU/day, appears lower than the current recommendations, and the serum level of vitamin D was not assessed during the study.

Clinical Recommendations

The significance of optimal vitamin D status for intestinal health and homeostasis is well known and accepted among clinical experts. Even though more research is needed to prove the link between vitamin D deficiency and gut inflammation, it is appropriate to ensure that every patient with IBD has an optimal serum 25(OH)D level (Table 3.2). At this point, no gastroenterology guidelines have been proposed for the assessment of vitamin D status in subjects with IBD. The Clinical Guidelines Subcommittee of The Endocrine Society recommends testing serum 25(OH)D level for every patient with IBD on steroid therapy [6]. We believe that a reasonable approach consists of screening for vitamin D deficiency yearly. More frequent testing is needed in deficient patients with or without metabolic bone disease, and in those with active IBD on steroids. The ideal timing to screen patients is the late winter or early spring when the level of vitamin D is the lowest, especially in patients living in northern latitudes [100]. The U.S. Preventive Services Task Force recently released its recommendations where screening for vitamin D deficiency for asymptomatic adults is not recommended as the current evidence is insufficient to assess the balance of benefit and harm.

Table 3.2 Clinical recommendations for IBD patients

Whom to test for vitamin D deficiency?	Every patient with IBD[a]	[6]
When should we test?	Yearly, or more often based on the level of vitamin D and risk for deficiency. Better time to test in late winter or early spring, when level in nadir	[100]
Serum 25(OH)D level		[1, 5–7]
Deficiency	<25 nmol/L (10 ng/mL) (IOM[b])	
	<50 nmol/L (20 ng/mL) (Endocrine society)	
Insufficiency	25 to <50 nmol/L (10–20 ng/mL) (IOM)	[1, 5–7]
	50 to <75 nmol/L (20–30 ng/mL) (Endocrine society)	
Sufficiency	≥50 nmol/L (20 ng/mL) (IOM)	[1, 5–7]
	≥75 nmol/L (30 ng/mL) (Endocrine society)	
Vitamin D intake recommendations		
Age <1 year of age with sufficient levels	400 IU[c]/day	[6, 101]
Age 1–70 years of age with sufficient levels	600 IU/day	
Age >70 years of age with sufficient levels	800 IU/day	
Adults in risk for vitamin D deficiency	1000 IU/day	
Adults with vitamin D deficiency	6000 IU/day for 6 weeks, or 50,000 IU once a week for 8 weeks	

[a]Inflammatory bowel disease
[b]Institute of Medicine
[c]International units

The ideal daily vitamin D intake for patients with IBD depends on age and level of serum 25(OH)D. For patients with normal vitamin D levels, infants should receive 400 IU of vitamin D per day, children 1 year and older and adults should receive 600 IU, and the elderly over 70 years 800 IU, based on the recommendations from the Institute of Medicine and the Endocrine Practice Guidelines [101]. For patients at risk for vitamin D deficiency, the recommendation is for at least 1000 IU/day. For adults with documented low levels of 25(OH)D 6000 IU/day for 6 weeks, or 50,000 IU/week for 8 weeks is recommended [6]. The most appropriate vitamin D regimen for patients with IBD was tested in a randomized, controlled, non-blinded, clinical trial. Three different oral regimens were used for 6 weeks, including 2000 IU of vitamin D2 daily, 2000 IU of vitamin D3 daily, and 50,000 IU of vitamin D2 weekly. All 3 regimens were well tolerated, but two oral regimens of 2000 IU of vitamin D3 daily and 50,000 IU of vitamin D2 weekly were superior in raising the 25(OH)D serum levels [102].

Table 3.3 Future areas of research

1. Vitamin D deficiency and IBD[a] pathogenesis: confirmation of the causative association
2. Vitamin D supplementation as therapeutic modality for IBD prevention, control, and treatment
3. Verification of the optimal serum vitamin D level for the control of intestinal inflammation
4. Link of dysbiosis with vitamin D deficiency and IBD pathogenesis
5. Vitamin D status and risk of colon cancer
6. Association between severity and relapse of IBD and vitamin D serum level
7. *Clostridium difficile* colitis in IBD and vitamin D as possible protective factor

[a]Inflammatory bowel disease

Future Areas of Research

Future research is needed to expand our understanding on various aspects of the interaction between vitamin D status and IBD pathogenesis and its effect on the natural course of IBD (Table 3.3). It is still unclear if low vitamin D is a risk factor for the development of CD and UC. Experimental models have shown a possible relationship but very few clinical studies have been performed and demonstrate a causative association [48]. Most of those studies are cross-sectional and underpowered. More prospective, well-designed studies are needed to clarify the consequences of vitamin D deficiency and answer if vitamin D can prevent the development of the disease. Additional studies are needed to investigate if vitamin D deficiency promotes IBD relapses, or if low vitamin D level is just the result of an inflamed gut with impaired absorption. Data from published research works suggest this association but larger, high quality studies are required to prove the theoretical risk of a more severe disease in the setting of vitamin D deficiency [73–76, 78, 103]. Moreover, the optimal dosing of vitamin D and appropriate vitamin D serum level for ideal intestinal health are additional research areas. The use of vitamin D as a potential therapeutic modality for the treatment of IBD comes with advantages, as it is cheap, easily tolerated and has a safe pharmaceutical profile. Fortunately, research efforts are underway to improve our knowledge of vitamin D deficiency and its effects, and new progress will be made in the prevention and treatment of IBD.

References

1. Holick MF. Vitamin D deficiency. N Engl J Med. 2007;357(3):266–81.
2. Lowe KE, Maiyar AC, Norman AW. Vitamin D-mediated gene expression. Crit Rev Eukaryot Gene Expr. 1992;2(1):65–109.
3. Haddad JG. Vitamin D—solar rays, the Milky Way, or both? N Engl J Med. 1992;326(18):1213–5.
4. Binkley N, Novotny R, Krueger D, et al. Low vitamin D status despite abundant sun exposure. J Clin Endocrinol Metab. 2007;92(6):2130–5.

5. Rosen CJ. Clinical practice. Vitamin D insufficiency. N Engl J Med. 2011;364(3):248–54.
6. Holick MF, Binkley NC, Bischoff-Ferrari HA, et al. Evaluation, treatment, and prevention of vitamin D deficiency: an Endocrine Society clinical practice guideline. J Clin Endocrinol Metab. 2011;96(7):1911–30.
7. Institute Of Medicine, Taylor CL, Ross AC, Yaktine AL, Del Valle HB, editors. Dietary reference intakes calcium vitamin D. Washington, DC: National Academies Press; 2011.
8. Powe CE, Evans MK, Wenger J, et al. Vitamin D-binding protein and vitamin D status of black Americans and white Americans. N Engl J Med. 2013;369(21):1991–2000.
9. Holick MF, Siris ES, Binkley N, et al. Prevalence of Vitamin D inadequacy among postmenopausal North American women receiving osteoporosis therapy. J Clin Endocrinol Metab. 2005;90(6):3215–24.
10. Lips P, Hosking D, Lippuner K, et al. The prevalence of vitamin D inadequacy amongst women with osteoporosis: an international epidemiological investigation. J Intern Med. 2006;260(3):245–54.
11. Holick MF. High prevalence of vitamin D inadequacy and implications for health. Mayo Clin Proc. 2006;81(3):353–73.
12. Peterson CA, Tosh AK, Belenchia AM. Vitamin D insufficiency and insulin resistance in obese adolescents. Ther Adv Endocrinol Metab. 2014;5(6):166–89.
13. Drincic AT, Armas LA, Van Diest EE, et al. Volumetric dilution, rather than sequestration best explains the low vitamin D status of obesity. Obesity (Silver Spring). 2012;20(7):1444–8.
14. Mawer EB, Backhouse J, Holman CA, et al. The distribution and storage of vitamin D and its metabolites in human tissues. Clin Sci. 1972;43(3):413–31.
15. Blum M, Dolnikowski G, Seyoum E, et al. Vitamin D(3) in fat tissue. Endocrine. 2008;33(1):90–4.
16. Prosnitz AR, Leonard MB, Shults J, et al. Changes in vitamin D and parathyroid hormone metabolism in incident pediatric Crohn's disease. Inflamm Bowel Dis. 2012;19(1):45–53.
17. Pappa HM, Grand RJ, Gordon CM. Report on the vitamin D status of adult and pediatric patients with inflammatory bowel disease and its significance for bone health and disease. Inflamm Bowel Dis. 2006;12(12):1162–74.
18. Siffledeen JS, Siminoski K, Steinhart H, et al. The frequency of vitamin D deficiency in adults with Crohn's disease. Can J Gastroenterol. 2003;17(8):473–8.
19. Jahnsen J, Falch JA, Mowinckel P, et al. Vitamin D status, parathyroid hormone and bone mineral density in patients with inflammatory bowel disease. Scand J Gastroenterol. 2002;37(2):192–9.
20. Pollak RD, Karmeli F, Eliakim R, et al. Femoral neck osteopenia in patients with inflammatory bowel disease. Am J Gastroenterol. 1998;93(9):1483–90.
21. Bjarnason I, Macpherson A, Mackintosh C, et al. Reduced bone density in patients with inflammatory bowel disease. Gut. 1997;40(2):228–33.
22. Dumitrescu G, Mihai C, Dranga M, et al. Bone mineral density in patients with inflammatory bowel disease from north-eastern Romania. Rev Med Chir Soc Med Nat Iasi. 2014;117(1):23–8.
23. Bernstein CN, Blanchard JF, Leslie W, et al. The incidence of fracture among patients with inflammatory bowel disease. A population-based cohort study. Ann Intern Med. 2000;133(10):795–9.
24. Vestergaard P, Krogh K, Rejnmark L, et al. Fracture risk is increased in Crohn's disease, but not in ulcerative colitis. Gut. 2000;46(2):176–81.
25. Siffledeen JS, Siminoski K, Jen H, et al. Vertebral fractures and role of low bone mineral density in Crohn's disease. Clin Gastroenterol Hepatol. 2007;5(6):721–8.
26. Loftus Jr EV, Crowson CS, Sandborn WJ, et al. Long-term fracture risk in patients with Crohn's disease: a population-based study in Olmsted County, Minnesota. Gastroenterology. 2002;123(2):468–75.
27. Bernstein CN, Leslie WD, Leboff MS. AGA technical review on osteoporosis in gastrointestinal diseases. Gastroenterology. 2003;124(3):795–841.

28. Cantorna MT, Zhu Y, Froicu M, et al. Vitamin D status, 1,25-dihydroxyvitamin D3, and the immune system. Am J Clin Nutr. 2004;80(6 Suppl):1717S–20.
29. Cantorna MT, Mahon BD. D-hormone and the immune system. J Rheumatol Suppl. 2005;76:11–20.
30. Reich KM, Fedorak RN, Madsen K, et al. Vitamin D improves inflammatory bowel disease outcomes: basic science and clinical review. World J Gastroenterol. 2014;20(17):4934–47.
31. Guillot X, Semerano L, Saidenberg-Kermanac'h N, et al. Vitamin D and inflammation. Joint Bone Spine. 2010;77(6):552–7.
32. Liu PT, Stenger S, Li H, et al. Toll-like receptor triggering of a vitamin D-mediated human antimicrobial response. Science. 2006;311(5768):1770–3.
33. Adams JS, Ren S, Liu PT, et al. Vitamin d-directed rheostatic regulation of monocyte antibacterial responses. J Immunol. 2009;182(7):4289–95.
34. Wang TT, Dabbas B, Laperriere D, et al. Direct and indirect induction by 1,25-dihydroxyvitamin D3 of the NOD2/CARD15-defensin beta2 innate immune pathway defective in Crohn disease. J Biol Chem. 2010;285(4):2227–31.
35. Wu S, Sun J. Vitamin D, vitamin D receptor, and macroautophagy in inflammation and infection. Discov Med. 2011;11(59):325–35.
36. Yuk JM, Shin DM, Lee HM, et al. Vitamin D3 induces autophagy in human monocytes/macrophages via cathelicidin. Cell Host Microbe. 2009;6(3):231–43.
37. Provvedini DM, Tsoukas CD, Deftos LJ, et al. 1,25-dihydroxyvitamin D3 receptors in human leukocytes. Science. 1983;221(4616):1181–3.
38. Fritsche J, Mondal K, Ehrnsperger A, et al. Regulation of 25-hydroxyvitamin D3-1 alpha-hydroxylase and production of 1 alpha,25-dihydroxyvitamin D3 by human dendritic cells. Blood. 2003;102(9):3314–6.
39. Daniel C, Sartory NA, Zahn N, et al. Immune modulatory treatment of trinitrobenzene sulfonic acid colitis with calcitriol is associated with a change of a T helper (Th) 1/Th17 to a Th2 and regulatory T cell profile. J Pharmacol Exp Ther. 2008;324(1):23–33.
40. Canning MO, Grotenhuis K, de Wit H, et al. 1-alpha,25-Dihydroxyvitamin D3 (1,25(OH)(2)D(3)) hampers the maturation of fully active immature dendritic cells from monocytes. Eur J Endocrinol. 2001;145(3):351–7.
41. Penna G, Adorini L. 1 Alpha,25-dihydroxyvitamin D3 inhibits differentiation, maturation, activation, and survival of dendritic cells leading to impaired alloreactive T cell activation. J Immunol. 2000;164(5):2405–11.
42. Helming L, Bose J, Ehrchen J, et al. 1alpha,25-Dihydroxyvitamin D3 is a potent suppressor of interferon gamma-mediated macrophage activation. Blood. 2005;106(13):4351–8.
43. Dickie LJ, Church LD, Coulthard LR, et al. Vitamin D3 down-regulates intracellular Toll-like receptor 9 expression and Toll-like receptor 9-induced IL-6 production in human monocytes. Rheumatology (Oxford). 2010;49(8):1466–71.
44. Jeffery LE, Burke F, Mura M, et al. 1,25-Dihydroxyvitamin D3 and IL-2 combine to inhibit T cell production of inflammatory cytokines and promote development of regulatory T cells expressing CTLA-4 and FoxP3. J Immunol. 2009;183(9):5458–67.
45. Meehan MA, Kerman RH, Lemire JM. 1,25-Dihydroxyvitamin D3 enhances the generation of nonspecific suppressor cells while inhibiting the induction of cytotoxic cells in a human MLR. Cell Immunol. 1992;140(2):400–9.
46. Barrat FJ, Cua DJ, Boonstra A, et al. In vitro generation of interleukin 10-producing regulatory CD4(+) T cells is induced by immunosuppressive drugs and inhibited by T helper type 1 (Th1)- and Th2-inducing cytokines. J Exp Med. 2002;195(5):603–16.
47. Chen S, Sims GP, Chen XX, et al. Modulatory effects of 1,25-dihydroxyvitamin D3 on human B cell differentiation. J Immunol. 2007;179(3):1634–47.
48. Ananthakrishnan AN, Khalili H, Higuchi LM, et al. Higher predicted vitamin D status is associated with reduced risk of Crohn's disease. Gastroenterology. 2012;142(3):482–9.
49. Shivananda S, Lennard-Jones J, Logan R, et al. Incidence of inflammatory bowel disease across Europe: is there a difference between north and south? Results of the European collaborative study on inflammatory bowel disease (EC-IBD). Gut. 1996;39(5):690–7.

50. Armitage EL, Aldhous MC, Anderson N, et al. Incidence of juvenile-onset Crohn's disease in Scotland: association with northern latitude and affluence. Gastroenterology. 2004;127(4):1051–7.
51. Khalili H, Huang ES, Ananthakrishnan AN, et al. Geographical variation and incidence of inflammatory bowel disease among US women. Gut. 2012;61(12):1686–92.
52. Nerich V, Monnet E, Etienne A, et al. Geographical variations of inflammatory bowel disease in France: a study based on national health insurance data. Inflamm Bowel Dis. 2006;12(3):218–26.
53. Jantchou P, Clavel-Chapelon F, Racine A, et al. High residential sun exposure is associated with a low risk of incident Crohn's disease in the prospective E3N cohort. Inflamm Bowel Dis. 2014;20(1):75–81.
54. Nerich V, Jantchou P, Boutron-Ruault MC, et al. Low exposure to sunlight is a risk factor for Crohn's disease. Aliment Pharmacol Ther. 2011;33(8):940–5.
55. Kuhn R, Lohler J, Rennick D, et al. Interleukin-10-deficient mice develop chronic enterocolitis. Cell. 1993;75(2):263–74.
56. Cantorna MT, Munsick C, Bemiss C, et al. 1,25-Dihydroxycholecalciferol prevents and ameliorates symptoms of experimental murine inflammatory bowel disease. J Nutr. 2000;130(11):2648–52.
57. Froicu M, Zhu Y, Cantorna MT. Vitamin D receptor is required to control gastrointestinal immunity in IL-10 knockout mice. Immunology. 2006;117(3):310–8.
58. Kong J, Zhang Z, Musch MW, et al. Novel role of the vitamin D receptor in maintaining the integrity of the intestinal mucosal barrier. Am J Physiol Gastrointest Liver Physiol. 2008;294(1):G208–16.
59. Henderson P, van Limbergen JE, Schwarze J, et al. Function of the intestinal epithelium and its dysregulation in inflammatory bowel disease. Inflamm Bowel Dis. 2011;17(1):382–95.
60. Zeissig S, Burgel N, Gunzel D, et al. Changes in expression and distribution of claudin 2, 5 and 8 lead to discontinuous tight junctions and barrier dysfunction in active Crohn's disease. Gut. 2007;56(1):61–72.
61. Liu N, Nguyen L, Chun RF, et al. Altered endocrine and autocrine metabolism of vitamin D in a mouse model of gastrointestinal inflammation. Endocrinology. 2008;149(10):4799–808.
62. Zhu Y, Mahon BD, Froicu M, et al. Calcium and 1 alpha,25-dihydroxyvitamin D3 target the TNF-alpha pathway to suppress experimental inflammatory bowel disease. Eur J Immunol. 2005;35(1):217–24.
63. Lagishetty V, Misharin AV, Liu NQ, et al. Vitamin D deficiency in mice impairs colonic antibacterial activity and predisposes to colitis. Endocrinology. 2010;151(6):2423–32.
64. Wu S, Zhang YG, Lu R, et al. Intestinal epithelial vitamin D receptor deletion leads to defective autophagy in colitis. Gut. 2015;64(7):1082–94.
65. Garg M, Rosella O, Lubel JS, et al. Association of circulating vitamin D concentrations with intestinal but not systemic inflammation in inflammatory bowel disease. Inflamm Bowel Dis. 2013;19(12):2634–43.
66. Wu S, Xia Y, Liu X, et al. Vitamin D receptor deletion leads to reduced level of IkappaBalpha protein through protein translation, protein-protein interaction, and post-translational modification. Int J Biochem Cell Biol. 2010;42(2):329–36.
67. Liu W, Chen Y, Golan MA, et al. Intestinal epithelial vitamin D receptor signaling inhibits experimental colitis. J Clin Invest. 2013;123(9):3983–96.
68. Simmons JD, Mullighan C, Welsh KI, et al. Vitamin D receptor gene polymorphism: association with Crohn's disease susceptibility. Gut. 2000;47(2):211–4.
69. Dresner-Pollak R, Ackerman Z, Eliakim R, et al. The BsmI vitamin D receptor gene polymorphism is associated with ulcerative colitis in Jewish Ashkenazi patients. Genet Test. 2004;8(4):417–20.
70. Naderi N, Farnood A, Habibi M, et al. Association of vitamin D receptor gene polymorphisms in Iranian patients with inflammatory bowel disease. J Gastroenterol Hepatol. 2008;23(12):1816–22.

71. Wang L, Wang ZT, Hu JJ, et al. Polymorphisms of the vitamin D receptor gene and the risk of inflammatory bowel disease: a meta-analysis. Genet Mol Res. 2014;13(2):2598–610.
72. Eloranta JJ, Wenger C, Mwinyi J, et al. Association of a common vitamin D-binding protein polymorphism with inflammatory bowel disease. Pharmacogenet Genomics. 2011;21(9):559–64.
73. Ananthakrishnan AN, Cagan A, Gainer VS, et al. Normalization of plasma 25-hydroxy vitamin D is associated with reduced risk of surgery in Crohn's disease. Inflamm Bowel Dis. 2013;19(9):1921–7.
74. Zator ZA, Cantu SM, Konijeti GG, et al. Pretreatment 25-hydroxyvitamin D levels and durability of anti-tumor necrosis factor-alpha therapy in inflammatory bowel diseases. JPEN J Parenter Enteral Nutr. 2014;38(3):385–91.
75. Joseph AJ, George B, Pulimood AB, et al. 25 (OH) vitamin D level in Crohn's disease: association with sun exposure & disease activity. Indian J Med Res. 2009;130(2):133–7.
76. Jorgensen SP, Hvas CL, Agnholt J, et al. Active Crohn's disease is associated with low vitamin D levels. J Crohns Colitis. 2013;7(10):e407–13.
77. Hlavaty T, Krajcovicova A, Koller T, et al. Higher vitamin D serum concentration increases health related quality of life in patients with inflammatory bowel diseases. World J Gastroenterol. 2014;20(42):15787–96.
78. Blanck S, Aberra F. Vitamin D deficiency is associated with ulcerative colitis disease activity. Dig Dis Sci. 2013;58(6):1698–702.
79. Kabbani TA, Rivers C, Swoger J, et al. Association of mean vitamin D level with clinical status in inflammatory bowel disease: a 5-year prospective study. In: 79th Annual scientific meeting of the American College of Gastroenterology; 2014.
80. El-Matary W, Sikora S, Spady D. Bone mineral density, vitamin D, and disease activity in children newly diagnosed with inflammatory bowel disease. Dig Dis Sci. 2011;56(3):825–9.
81. Levin AD, Wadhera V, Leach ST, et al. Vitamin D deficiency in children with inflammatory bowel disease. Dig Dis Sci. 2011;56(3):830–6.
82. Narula N, Marshall JK. Management of inflammatory bowel disease with vitamin D: beyond bone health. J Crohns Colitis. 2012;6(4):397–404.
83. Jorgensen SP, Agnholt J, Glerup H, et al. Clinical trial: vitamin D3 treatment in Crohn's disease—a randomized double-blind placebo-controlled study. Aliment Pharmacol Ther. 2010;32(3):377–83.
84. Miheller P, Muzes G, Hritz I, et al. Comparison of the effects of 1,25 dihydroxyvitamin D and 25 hydroxyvitamin D on bone pathology and disease activity in Crohn's disease patients. Inflamm Bowel Dis. 2009;15(11):1656–62.
85. Trifan A, Stanciu C, Stoica O, et al. Impact of *Clostridium difficile* infection on inflammatory bowel disease outcome: a review. World J Gastroenterol. 2014;20(33):11736–42.
86. Regnault H, Bourrier A, Lalande V, et al. Prevalence and risk factors of Clostridium difficile infection in patients hospitalized for flare of inflammatory bowel disease: a retrospective assessment. Dig Liver Dis. 2014;46(12):1086–92.
87. Guo C, Gombart AF. The antibiotic effects of vitamin D. Endocr Metab Immune Disord Drug Targets. 2014;14(4):255–66.
88. Ananthakrishnan AN, Cagan A, Gainer VS, et al. Higher plasma vitamin D is associated with reduced risk of *Clostridium difficile* infection in patients with inflammatory bowel diseases. Aliment Pharmacol Ther. 2014;39(10):1136–42.
89. Triantafillidis JK, Nasioulas G, Kosmidis PA. Colorectal cancer and inflammatory bowel disease: epidemiology, risk factors, mechanisms of carcinogenesis and prevention strategies. Anticancer Res. 2009;29(7):2727–37.
90. Federico A, Morgillo F, Tuccillo C, et al. Chronic inflammation and oxidative stress in human carcinogenesis. Int J Cancer. 2007;121(11):2381–6.
91. Ahmadi A, Polyak S, Draganov PV. Colorectal cancer surveillance in inflammatory bowel disease: the search continues. World J Gastroenterol. 2009;15(1):61–6.
92. Cross HS, Pavelka M, Slavik J, et al. Growth control of human colon cancer cells by vitamin D and calcium in vitro. J Natl Cancer Inst. 1992;84(17):1355–7.

93. Hofer H, Ho G, Peterlik M, et al. Biological effects of 1alpha-hydroxy- and 1beta-(hydroxymethyl)-vitamin D compounds relevant for potential colorectal cancer therapy. J Pharmacol Exp Ther. 1999;291(2):450–5.
94. Bischof MG, Redlich K, Schiller C, et al. Growth inhibitory effects on human colon adenocarcinoma-derived Caco-2 cells and calcemic potential of 1 alpha,25-dihydroxyvitamin D3 analogs: structure-function relationships. J Pharmacol Exp Ther. 1995;275(3):1254–60.
95. Murillo G, Nagpal V, Tiwari N, et al. Actions of vitamin D are mediated by the TLR4 pathway in inflammation-induced colon cancer. J Steroid Biochem Mol Biol. 2010;121(1–2):403–7.
96. Wada K, Tanaka H, Maeda K, et al. Vitamin D receptor expression is associated with colon cancer in ulcerative colitis. Oncol Rep. 2009;22(5):1021–5.
97. Gorham ED, Garland CF, Garland FC, et al. Optimal vitamin D status for colorectal cancer prevention: a quantitative meta analysis. Am J Prev Med. 2007;32(3):210–6.
98. Gorham ED, Garland CF, Garland FC, et al. Vitamin D and prevention of colorectal cancer. J Steroid Biochem Mol Biol. 2005;97(1–2):179–94.
99. Wactawski-Wende J, Kotchen JM, Anderson GL, et al. Calcium plus vitamin D supplementation and the risk of colorectal cancer. N Engl J Med. 2006;354(7):684–96.
100. Pappa H. Vitamin D deficiency and supplementation in patients with IBD. Gastroenterol Hepatol (N Y). 2014;10(2):127–9.
101. Ross AC, Manson JE, Abrams SA, et al. The 2011 report on dietary reference intakes for calcium and vitamin D from the Institute of Medicine: what clinicians need to know. J Clin Endocrinol Metab. 2011;96(1):53–8.
102. Pappa HM, Mitchell PD, Jiang H, et al. Treatment of vitamin D insufficiency in children and adolescents with inflammatory bowel disease: a randomized clinical trial comparing three regimens. J Clin Endocrinol Metab. 2012;97(6):2134–42.
103. Ulitsky A, Ananthakrishnan AN, Naik A, et al. Vitamin D deficiency in patients with inflammatory bowel disease: association with disease activity and quality of life. JPEN J Parenter Enteral Nutr. 2011;35(3):308–16.

Chapter 4
Diagnosis and Management of Iron Deficiency in Inflammatory Bowel Disease

Thomas Greuter and Stephan R. Vavricka

Introduction

Iron is a critical element and essential for fundamental metabolic processes in cells with a major role in oxygen (O_2) carry (hemoglobin), muscle function (myoglobin), and mitochondrial processes [1]. Despite this fundamental role in human metabolism, there is a narrow balance between iron supply and absorption on one side, and iron demand on the other. Iron deficiency is the most common nutritional deficiency [2] and the leading cause of anemia worldwide [3–5]. In the United States, prevalence of iron deficiency ranges from 4.5 to 18.0 % [6–8], while 50 % of anemia worldwide is thought to be caused by iron deficiency [9]. A number which seems huge given 2.2 billion people globally affected by anemia [4].

While iron deficiency is a common medical condition, clinical presentation is rather nonspecific with most of cases remaining undiagnosed therefore. Among the most frequently reported symptoms are paleness, fatigue, headache, and dyspnea [2, 10–12]. In contrast, more typical findings such as tachycardia, vertigo, or even syncope are less often reported and suggest severe states of anemia [13, 14]. Due to its mostly chronic and asymptomatic disease course, a majority of cases are identified

T. Greuter, M.D.
Division of Gastroenterology and Hepatology, University Hospital Zurich,
Rämistrasse 100, Zurich 8091, Switzerland
e-mail: th_greuter@bluewin.ch

S.R. Vavricka, M.D. (✉)
Division of Gastroenterology and Hepatology, University Hospital Zurich,
Rämistrasse 100, Zurich 8091, Switzerland

Division of Gastroenterology and Hepatology, Triemli Hospital Zurich,
Birmensdorferstrasse 497, Zurich 8063, Switzerland
e-mail: stephan.vavricka@usz.ch

© Springer International Publishing Switzerland 2016
A.N. Ananthakrishnan (ed.), *Nutritional Management of Inflammatory Bowel Diseases*, DOI 10.1007/978-3-319-26890-3_4

based on routine laboratory work-up including hemoglobin and ferritin. Thus, regular laboratory testing including screening for iron deficiency and anemia is indicated particularly in those patients with a high risk of decreased iron supply such as vegetarians or children, those with impaired intestinal absorption (celiac disease or inflammatory bowel disease), increased blood (intestinal tumors or intestinal parasites), or the presence of chronic inflammation with a combination of anemia of chronic disease and iron deficiency anemia. However, most of the cases with iron deficiency anemia are seen in otherwise healthy patients showing an increased iron demand such as pregnant women, adolescents, or athletes [2]. Awareness of a mostly chronic and asymptomatic disease course is especially important regarding the possible consequences of iron deficiency, among which are impaired quality of life and the ability to work, increased hospitalizations and health care costs [15–17].

In inflammatory bowel disease patients, anemia is the most common systemic complication and extraintestinal manifestation [18–21]. Prevalence ranges from 9 to 74 % [22]. Iron deficiency anemia accounts for the majority of anemic patients followed by anemia of chronic disease [23, 24]. While the former develops as the consequence of iron deficiency (decreased intake or intestinal absorption, continuous or recurrent blood loss), the latter is caused by inflammatory processes. However, the two types are frequently overlapping [23]. Other causes are vitamin B12 deficiency, folic acid deficiency or toxic effects of medications. Given the above-mentioned consequences of untreated iron deficiency and anemia, these two IBD complications are more than just laboratory markers [20]. Prevention and treatment of those conditions is key in the management of IBD patients and awareness of those is especially important given the frequent recurrence despite adequate and successful anti-inflammatory therapy [25].

In this chapter, we focus mainly on iron deficiency anemia and discuss the most important physiological mechanisms in human iron cycle, diagnostic steps in clinical practice, and therapeutic approaches in IBD patients with iron deficiency. Recommendations regarding screening, treatment, and prevention of iron deficiency and anemia are mainly based on the current European Crohn's and Colitis Organisation (ECCO) Guidelines [25].

The Iron Cycle

The only physiological way of iron uptake is via intestinal absorption, which additionally represents the critically controlled process in iron metabolism [1]. In contrast, excretion of iron is not regulated and loss of iron happens in a non-controlled way via desquamation of skin, intestinal epithelial cells, or blood loss (e.g., menstruation). Normally, 1–2 mg iron is lost through these mechanisms [26]. While human body contains 3–5 g total iron, 20–25 mg is needed for production of red blood cells and cellular metabolism daily [26]. Most of the needed iron can be recycled from senescent blood cells by the reticuloendothelial system (RES) [1]. However, uncontrolled loss of iron has to be compensated by intestinal absorption only.

Thus, margins between intestinal uptake und iron requirements are narrow. Dietary iron is available in two forms as heme and non-heme iron; the former consists of Fe^{2+} (ferrous iron) and can be found in animal food sources such as meat or poultry, the latter consists of the ferric ion (Fe^{3+}), which is present in vegetarian foods [2, 27]. Iron is transported through the intestinal brush border via a divalent metal transporter (DMT1) only in its ferrous form; [28] Iron from vegetarian food has to be reduced by a membrane-associated ferrireductase DcytB first [29]. Thus, absorption rates of iron from animal sources are generally higher [2]. At the basolateral membrane, Ferroportin transports iron into systemic circulation [30, 31] where it is transformed to its ferrous form again by a multicopper oxidase homologous to ceruloplasmin [1]. In its ferrous form, iron is finally able to bind to Transferrin, an iron-transporting protein. The iron-Transferrin complex consequently binds cells expressing a Tf-binding protein on its surface, among which erythroblasts in the bone marrow are the most important and most frequent [1].

Iron absorption needs a close control in order to up- or down-regulate intestinal uptake in accordance with body requirements. This narrow homeostasis is basically controlled by hepcidin, a peptide hormone synthesized in the liver, which allows immediate adjustments of iron fluctuation by binding to and inducing degradation of ferroportin [32]. Hepcidin itself is increased in the presence of iron overload, systemic inflammation, and/or infection [1, 33], which partly explains the overlap of anemia of chronic disease in inflammatory disorders and iron deficiency. In contrast, Hepcidin decreases in the presence of iron deficiency, tissue hypoxia, or increased erythropoiesis [1, 3].

Iron Deficiency and Anemia in IBD Patients

Extraintestinal manifestations (EIM) of IBD are frequently observed with a prevalence ranging from 6 to 47 % [34–41]. They considerably affect morbidity and mortality in IBD patients [42, 43]. Besides typical EIM such as arthritis, uveitis, or skin changes, which are seen as reactive to underlying IBD, systemic manifestations may also include IBD-related complications due to metabolic abnormalities such as nephrolithiasis, amyloidosis, osteopathy, or anemia [41]. Nonetheless, compared to classical EIM, anemia in IBD has received only little attention [23], as it may be too common to be specifically recognized as a complication [44]. In addition, treating anemia has often low priority [44]. However, prevalence of anemia in IBD seems to be high, although studies show differences ranging from 9 to 74 % [22]. A recent review showed a mean prevalence of 17 %, increasing up to 68 % in those patients hospitalized for IBD [21]. Thus, anemia can be considered as one of the most common systemic complications of acute IBD [23]. Iron deficiency, which is the most frequent cause of anemia in IBD, is seen in 36–90 % of all IBD patients [19]. Although chronic blood loss and decreased iron absorption leads to iron deficiency with a consecutively developing anemia, anemia in IBD patients is often multifactorial with the two main causes of iron deficiency [45] and anemia of chronic disease [46]. Further possible causes are drug toxicity (sulfasalazine, thiopurines), IBD-associated autoimmune hemolysis, myelodysplastic syndrome, or impaired absorption of vitamin B12 or folate [23].

Independent of the underlying mechanism, anemia has been recognized as a key symptom in IBD [44]. Furthermore, the impact of anemia on quality of life of IBD patients is substantial [25]. Several studies have shown impaired quality of life for anemia in general patients [47, 48] and in those affected with IBD [17, 18, 22, 44]. Even in the absence of specific symptoms, anemia seems to impair quality of life [15, 17, 23]. Of note, quality of life may be as low as in anemic patients with advanced cancer and anemia in IBD patients seems to raise comparable concerns as abdominal pain or diarrhea does [44, 49]. In addition to an impaired quality of life, anemia negatively affects the ability to work, hospitalization, and health care costs [16, 25]. Thus, anemia is more than just a common feature of IBD; it is of great clinical relevance for the patient [23]. Doctors caring for IBD patients should be more aware of this frequent medical condition.

Diagnosis of Iron Deficiency and Anemia

Anemia in IBD is defined indifferent to other conditions. The cut-off limits according to the WHO definition can be applied in all IBD patients [25]. However, interindividual differences and modulating factors such as age, gender, pregnancy, high altitude, smoking, and ethnicity should be taken into account [50, 51]. According to the World Health Organization WHO, minimum hemoglobin levels used to define anemia in white people living at sea level are: 12.0 g/L for non-pregnant women, 13.0 g/L for men. Iron deficiency is usually diagnosed by serum ferritin. Lower limits are defined according to the level of systemic inflammation. In the absence of biochemical (assessed by CRP, ESR, and leukocyte count) and clinical evidence (assessed by CDAI, CDEIS, Mayo Score) of inflammation, serum ferritin cut-off level for the presence of iron deficiency is <30 µg/L [25]. Definition of iron deficiency in the presence of systemic inflammation is rather challenging. A serum ferritin up to 100 µg/L may still be consistent with iron deficiency. In such cases, concentration of soluble transferrin receptor (sTfR) in the serum and sTfR/log ferritin index have been shown to be an indicator of iron supply available for erythropoiesis and therefore to help distinguish between iron deficiency anemia and anemia of chronic disease [52–55]. A serum ferritin of more than 100 µg/L likely excludes true iron deficiency [44, 56]. In addition an sTfR/log serum ferritin ratio of less than 1 is useful to exclude true iron deficiency in anemia of chronic disease [52, 56]. However, anemia of chronic disease often goes along with functional iron deficiency, which is indicated by a transferrin saturation (TfS) <20 % [25].

Screening for anemia and iron deficiency is recommended in all IBD patients and consists of complete blood count, serum ferritin, and CRP. Screening should be repeated every 6–12 months for all patients in clinical remission, while anemia and iron deficiency screening should be at least performed every 3 months in those IBD patients with active disease [25]. In addition, vitamin B12 and folic acid should be measured regularly, at least every year, but more often in high-risk patients with ileal resection or those showing macrocytosis. Anemia work-up is indicated in all patients showing hemoglobin below normal limits and should include the following parameters: red blood cell indices (RDW, MCV), reticulocyte count, differential blood count, transferrin saturation, CRP, and serum ferritin. Based on a hematologic algorithm, most of the anemia forms can be easily classified without additional measurements. More extensive work-up includes serum concentrations of vitamin B12, folic acid, haptoglobin, the percentage of hypochromic red cells, reticulocyte hemoglobin, lactate dehydrogenase, soluble transferrin receptor, creatinine, and urea [25]. If the cause of anemia remains unclear after extensive work-up, referral to a hematologist is recommended.

Treatment of Iron Deficiency and Anemia in IBD Patients

Every IBD patients with iron deficiency anemia should be treated given significant improvements regarding quality of life [17, 57]. Intravenous iron supplementation is favored over oral supplementation in IBD patients for different reasons. The intravenous formulas are more effective, lead to a faster response, and are generally better tolerated [58–61]. They have been shown to be safe, effective, and well tolerated for the correction of iron deficiency anemia in IBD patients in several trials [57, 60, 62, 63]. In the presence of intestinal inflammation, iron absorption is limited and non-absorbed iron can be exposed to the ulcerated intestinal surface, which may lead to mucosal harm and even disease exacerbation [64–67]. Thus, oral supplementation is actually only recommended for those patients with mild anemia, absence of intestinal inflammatory activity, and no prior intolerance to oral regimens [25]. No more than 100 mg elemental iron per day is recommended; higher doses may lead to more side effects and therefore lower compliance. However, in most cases low dose oral iron is effective [68–70]. Oral iron-containing preparations differ regarding dosage, salt, chemical state of iron (ferrous or ferric), and galenic form (quick vs. prolonged release.) [71] In non-IBD iron deficiency anemia, bivalent iron preparations are of high efficacy, acceptable tolerability (especially as prolonged-release formulation), and low cost, while trivalent preparations have a poorer absorption and are more expensive [71]. The four commonly available ferrous iron supplementations are: ferrous sulfate, which is the standard treatment, ferrous sulfate exsiccated, ferrous gluconate, and ferrous fumarate [2]. In contrast to non-IBD conditions, where oral supplementation is considered first-line in most cases, intravenous iron should be considered as first-line treatment in the majority of IBD patients with iron deficiency anemia. The primary goal in IBD patients with iron deficiency anemia is normalization of hemoglobin levels and iron stores. Importantly, serum ferritin levels should not be measured within the first 8 weeks after intravenous supplementation given possible interference and false-high values [72]. Six different intravenous regimens are available for treatment of iron deficiency anemia: iron sucrose, ferric gluconate, ferric carboxymaltose, iron isomaltoside-1000, ferumoxytol, and iron dextran (low-molecular-weight forms) [2]. High-molecular-weight iron dextran has been withdrawn from the market due to higher frequency of serious adverse events including anaphylactic reactions [73], while low-molecular-weight forms show a safety profile comparable to other intravenous iron formulations [74]. Practical guidelines recommend slow infusion rates, patient observation, and administration in an adequate setting with access to resuscitation facilities to further minimize risk of serious adverse events [3, 73, 74]. Different compositions of these formula lead to different iron release rates, which determine the amount of iron given as a single dose. Table 4.1 summarizes the currently available intravenous iron formulations according to reviews by Larson [75] and Auerbach [76]. The dose needed for intravenous supplementation can be calculated with the Ganzoni's formula: body weight in kg × 2.3 × hemoglobin deficiency (target hemoglobin level—patient hemoglobin level) + 500–1000 mg iron [77]. However, a simplified scheme has been established and seems to be of better efficacy and compliance than the Ganzoni's formula [57]. The estimation of total iron need can be based on baseline hemoglobin and body weight only. Although this scheme has only been tested for ferric carboxymaltose in the FERGIcor trial [57], it can also be applied for dosing of other intravenous iron formulations.

In contrast to iron deficiency anemia, treatment recommendations for IBD patients with iron deficiency, but without anemia are rather controversial [25]. There is some evidence for a benefit of treating iron deficiency before development of anemia with studies showing improvement of fatigue or physical performance in women of reproductive age and in other conditions such as heart failure [78–80].

Table 4.1 Intravenous iron preparations (according to Larson [75] and Auerbach [76])

	Molecular weight (kDa)	Test dose	Preservatives	Maximal single dose	Higher doses (off label use)
LMW Dextran (CosmoFer®, INFeD®)	165	Yes (25 mg 15–30 min)	None	100 mg (>30 s)	Total dose infusion over 4 h
Iron sucrose (Venofer®)	34–60	No	None	200 mg (2–5 min)	300 mg over 1 h
Ferric gluconate (Ferrelcit®, Nulecit®)	289–444	No	Benzyl alcohol	125 mg (10 min)	250 mg (15 min)
Ferumoxytol (Feraheme®)	750	No	None	510 mg (<1 min)	no
Ferric carboxymaltose (Injectafer®, Ferinject®)	150	No	Intravenous iron preparationsNone	750 mg (slow push or over 15 min)	no
Iron isomaltoside (Monofer®)	150	No	None	20 mg/kg (30–60 min)	no

However, data about treating iron deficiency in IBD patients is lacking hitherto. Current guidelines recommend iron supplementation depending on patients' history, symptoms, and individual preferences [25].

How to Prevent Iron Deficiency and Anemia in IBD Patients

Given a strong correlation between intestinal disease extent and activity on one side and blood loss and severity of anemia on the other, treatment of underlying disease activity is key in both treatment and prevention of iron deficiency and anemia [19, 81, 82]. Recurrence of anemia is often an indicator for persistence of intestinal disease activity and warrants further investigation of possible subclinical disease activity [25]. After successful treatment of iron deficiency anemia, patients should be followed up closely given a high rate of recurrence in the first year thereafter [62, 83]. Guidelines recommend monitoring with full blood count and ferritin levels every 3 months for the first year and every 6–12 months thereafter [25]. Interestingly, a study could show a relation between the size of post-treatment iron stores and the speed of recurrence of iron deficiency anemia in IBD patients [83]. A cut-off level of more than 400 µg/L prevented recurrence significantly better than levels below [83]. Of note, the FERGImain trial showed significantly lower recurrence rates in those patients, where iron supplementation was reinitiated if ferritin levels fell below 100 µg/L, which was assessed at 2-months intervals [62]. In addition, those patients receiving preventive iron supplementation reported less gastrointestinal symptoms and IBD flares than those without [62]. Thus, a proactive approach is recommended rather than just a watch-and-wait strategy and such an approach seems to be cost-effective given the possible savings compared to anemic IBD patients [84].

Other anemia treatment options such as erythropoiesis-stimulating agents or even blood transfusion should be considered only in those patients with anemia of chronic disease who have shown insufficient response to intravenous iron supplementation and who continue to have low hemoglobin levels despite adequate anti-inflammatory treatment including biologic agents. Blood transfusion should be restricted to those patients with a hemoglobin concentration of less than 7 g/dL or above if anemia is symptomatic or if comorbidities such as coronary artery disease are present [85–87]. In most patients, even hemoglobin levels of less than 7 g/dL can be tolerated in the meantime. Iron supplementation remains key in those patients receiving erythropoiesis-stimulating factors or blood transfusions.

What to Tell Patients?

Screening for iron deficiency and anemia is key in management of IBD patients and should not depend on clinical symptoms given a mostly chronic and asymptomatic disease course. Dietary iron from animal food sources are better absorbed than iron present in the vegetarian diet [88]. Anemia should be seen as a systemic manifestation of IBD comparable to other EIM such as arthritis or skin problems [20]. Possible impact of anemia on quality of life and the ability to work should be discussed with IBD patients and treatment for anemia should be started in every patient fulfilling WHO criteria of iron deficiency anemia [16, 25]. Intravenous iron supplementation should be first-line therapy and oral supplementation only seems to be an option in those patients with mild anemia, absence of intestinal disease activity, and no history of prior intolerance. Oral iron supplementation may even exacerbate disease activity in IBD patients with intestinal inflammation [64–67]. Controversy about evidence of iron supplementation in patients with iron deficiency without anemia should be discussed with the patient in detail and decision about supplementation or not should be based on clinical presentation, patient's history, and individual preferences. Information about frequent and fast recurrence of anemia despite adequate treatment should be provided with a close follow-up during the first year [62, 83]. Patients with a drop-down in their serum ferritin below 100 µg/L should be motivated to reinstall intravenous iron supplementation [62]. Data about possible prevention of disease flares by this proactive approach should be provided. Last but not least, proactive prevention of recurrence of iron deficiency should be seen as cost-effective given the possibility of preventing anemic IBD patients and their consequences [84].

References

1. Hentze MW, Muckenthaler MU, Galy B, Camaschella C. Two to tango: regulation of mammalian iron metabolism. Cell. 2010;142(1):24–38.
2. Lopez A, Cacoub P, Macdougall IC, Peyrin-Biroulet L. Iron deficiency anaemia. Lancet. 2015;pii: S0140-6736(15)60865-0. doi: 10.1016/S0140-6736(15)60865-0.
3. Camaschella C. Iron-deficiency anemia. N Engl J Med. 2015;372(19):1832–43.
4. Kassebaum NJ, Jasrasaria R, Naghavi M, et al. A systematic analysis of global anemia burden from 1990 to 2010. Blood. 2014;123(5):615–24.
5. Stevens GA, Finucane MM, De-Regil LM, et al. Global, regional, and national trends in haemoglobin concentration and prevalence of total and severe anaemia in children and pregnant and non-pregnant women for 1995–2011: a systematic analysis of population-representative data. Lancet Glob Health. 2013;1(1):e16–25.
6. Looker AC, Dallman PR, Carroll MD, Gunter EW, Johnson CL. Prevalence of iron deficiency in the United States. JAMA. 1997;277(12):973–6.
7. Cogswell ME, Looker AC, Pfeiffer CM, et al. Assessment of iron deficiency in US preschool children and nonpregnant females of childbearing age: National Health and Nutrition Examination Survey 2003–2006. Am J Clin Nutr. 2009;89(5):1334–42.
8. Mei Z, Cogswell ME, Looker AC, et al. Assessment of iron status in US pregnant women from the National Health and Nutrition Examination Survey (NHANES), 1999–2006. Am J Clin Nutr. 2011;93(6):1312–20.
9. WHO, UNICEF, UNU. Iron deficiency anemia: assessment, prevention and control. Report of a joint WHO/UNICEF/UNU consultation. Geneva: World Health Organization; 1998.
10. Fourn L, Salami L. Diagnostic value of tegument pallor in anemia in pregnant women in Benin. Sante Publique. 2004;16(1):123–32.
11. Bager P. Fatigue and acute/chronic anaemia. Dan Med J. 2014;61(4):B4824.

12. Bergsjø P, Evjen-Olsen B, Hinderaker SG, Oleking'ori N, Klepp KI. Validity of non-invasive assessment of anaemia in pregnancy. Trop Med Int Health. 2008;13(2):272–7.
13. Matteson KA, Raker CA, Pinto SB, Scott DM, Frishman GN. Women presenting to an emergency facility with abnormal uterine bleeding: patient characteristics and prevalence of anemia. J Reprod Med. 2012;57(1–2):17–25.
14. Quinn JV, Stiell IG, McDermott DA, Sellers KL, Kohn MA, Wells GA. Derivation of the San Francisco Syncope Rule to predict patients with short-term serious outcomes. Ann Emerg Med. 2004;43(2):224–32.
15. Pizzi LT, Weston CM, Goldfarb NI, et al. Impact of chronic conditions on quality of life in patients with inflammatory bowel disease. Inflamm Bowel Dis. 2006;12(1):47–52.
16. Ershler WB, Chen K, Reyes EB, Dubois R. Economic burden of patients with anemia in selected diseases. Value Health. 2005;8(6):629–38.
17. Wells CW, Lewis S, Barton JR, Corbett S. Effects of changes in hemoglobin level on quality of life and cognitive function in inflammatory bowel disease patients. Inflamm Bowel Dis. 2006;12(2):123–30.
18. Gasche C. Anemia in IBD: the overlooked villain. Inflamm Bowel Dis. 2000;6(2):142–50; discussion 51.
19. Kulnigg S, Gasche C. Systematic review: managing anaemia in Crohn's disease. Aliment Pharmacol Ther. 2006;24(11–12):1507–23.
20. Gisbert JP, Gomollón F. Common misconceptions in the diagnosis and management of anemia in inflammatory bowel disease. Am J Gastroenterol. 2008;103(5):1299–307.
21. de la Morena F, Gisbert J. Anemia and inflammatory bowel disease. Rev Esp Enferm Dig. 2008;100(5):285–93.
22. Wilson A, Reyes E, Ofman J. Prevalence and outcomes of anemia in inflammatory bowel disease: a systematic review of the literature. Am J Med. 2004;116(Suppl 7A):44S–9.
23. Gomollón F, Gisbert JP. Anemia and inflammatory bowel diseases. World J Gastroenterol. 2009;15(37):4659–65.
24. Stein J, Hartmann F, Dignass AU. Diagnosis and management of iron deficiency anemia in patients with IBD. Nat Rev Gastroenterol Hepatol. 2010;7(11):599–610.
25. Dignass AU, Gasche C, Bettenworth D, et al. European consensus on the diagnosis and management of iron deficiency and anaemia in inflammatory bowel diseases. J Crohns Colitis. 2015;9(3):211–22.
26. Steinbicker AU, Muckenthaler MU. Out of balance—systemic iron homeostasis in iron-related disorders. Nutrients. 2013;5(8):3034–61.
27. McDermid JM, Lönnerdal B. Iron. Adv Nutr. 2012;3(4):532–3.
28. Gunshin H, Mackenzie B, Berger UV, et al. Cloning and characterization of a mammalian proton-coupled metal-ion transporter. Nature. 1997;388(6641):482–8.
29. McKie AT. The role of Dcytb in iron metabolism: an update. Biochem Soc Trans. 2008;36(Pt 6):1239–41.
30. McKie AT, Marciani P, Rolfs A, et al. A novel duodenal iron-regulated transporter, IREG1, implicated in the basolateral transfer of iron to the circulation. Mol Cell. 2000;5(2):299–309.
31. Donovan A, Brownlie A, Zhou Y, et al. Positional cloning of zebrafish ferroportin1 identifies a conserved vertebrate iron exporter. Nature. 2000;403(6771):776–81.
32. Nemeth E, Tuttle MS, Powelson J, et al. Hepcidin regulates cellular iron efflux by binding to ferroportin and inducing its internalization. Science. 2004;306(5704):2090–3.
33. Camaschella C. Iron and hepcidin: a story of recycling and balance. Hematology Am Soc Hematol Educ Program. 2013;2013:1–8.
34. Bernstein CN, Blanchard JF, Rawsthorne P, Yu N. The prevalence of extraintestinal diseases in inflammatory bowel disease: a population-based study. Am J Gastroenterol. 2001;96(4):1116–22.
35. Bernstein CN, Wajda A, Blanchard JF. The clustering of other chronic inflammatory diseases in inflammatory bowel disease: a population-based study. Gastroenterology. 2005;129(3):827–36.

36. Mendoza JL, Lana R, Taxonera C, Alba C, Izquierdo S, Díaz-Rubio M. Extraintestinal manifestations in inflammatory bowel disease: differences between Crohn's disease and ulcerative colitis. Med Clin (Barc). 2005;125(8):297–300.
37. Ricart E, Panaccione R, Loftus EV, et al. Autoimmune disorders and extraintestinal manifestations in first-degree familial and sporadic inflammatory bowel disease: a case-control study. Inflamm Bowel Dis. 2004;10(3):207–14.
38. Rankin GB, Watts HD, Melnyk CS, Kelley ML. National Cooperative Crohn's Disease Study: extraintestinal manifestations and perianal complications. Gastroenterology. 1979;77(4 Pt 2):914–20.
39. Su CG, Judge TA, Lichtenstein GR. Extraintestinal manifestations of inflammatory bowel disease. Gastroenterol Clin North Am. 2002;31(1):307–27.
40. Veloso FT, Carvalho J, Magro F. Immune-related systemic manifestations of inflammatory bowel disease. A prospective study of 792 patients. J Clin Gastroenterol. 1996;23(1):29–34.
41. Vavricka SR, Brun L, Ballabeni P, et al. Frequency and risk factors for extraintestinal manifestations in the Swiss inflammatory bowel disease cohort. Am J Gastroenterol. 2011;106(1):110–9.
42. Das KM. Relationship of extraintestinal involvements in inflammatory bowel disease: new insights into autoimmune pathogenesis. Dig Dis Sci. 1999;44(1):1–13.
43. Monsén U, Sorstad J, Hellers G, Johansson C. Extracolonic diagnoses in ulcerative colitis: an epidemiological study. Am J Gastroenterol. 1990;85(6):711–6.
44. Gasche C, Lomer MC, Cavill I, Weiss G. Iron, anaemia, and inflammatory bowel diseases. Gut. 2004;53(8):1190–7.
45. Semrin G, Fishman DS, Bousvaros A, et al. Impaired intestinal iron absorption in Crohn's disease correlates with disease activity and markers of inflammation. Inflamm Bowel Dis. 2006;12(12):1101–6.
46. de Silva AD, Mylonaki M, Rampton DS. Oral iron therapy in inflammatory bowel disease: usage, tolerance, and efficacy. Inflamm Bowel Dis. 2003;9(5):316–20.
47. Haas JD, Brownlie T. Iron deficiency and reduced work capacity: a critical review of the research to determine a causal relationship. J Nutr. 2001;131(2S-2):676S–88; discussion 88S–90S.
48. Goodnough LT, Nissenson AR. Anemia and its clinical consequences in patients with chronic diseases. Am J Med. 2004;116(Suppl 7A):1S–2.
49. Leitgeb C, Pecherstorfer M, Fritz E, Ludwig H. Quality of life in chronic anemia of cancer during treatment with recombinant human erythropoietin. Cancer. 1994;73(10):2535–42.
50. Beutler E, Waalen J. The definition of anemia: what is the lower limit of normal of the blood hemoglobin concentration? Blood. 2006;107(5):1747–50.
51. Perry GS, Byers T, Yip R, Margen S. Iron nutrition does not account for the hemoglobin differences between blacks and whites. J Nutr. 1992;122(7):1417–24.
52. Skikne BS, Punnonen K, Caldron PH, et al. Improved differential diagnosis of anemia of chronic disease and iron deficiency anemia: a prospective multicenter evaluation of soluble transferrin receptor and the sTfR/log ferritin index. Am J Hematol. 2011;86(11):923–7.
53. Infusino I, Braga F, Dolci A, Panteghini M. Soluble transferrin receptor (sTfR) and sTfR/log ferritin index for the diagnosis of iron-deficiency anemia. A meta-analysis. Am J Clin Pathol. 2012;138(5):642–9.
54. Oustamanolakis P, Koutroubakis IE. Soluble transferrin receptor-ferritin index is the most efficient marker for the diagnosis of iron deficiency anemia in patients with IBD. Inflamm Bowel Dis. 2011;17(12):E158–9.
55. Beguin Y. Soluble transferrin receptor for the evaluation of erythropoiesis and iron status. Clin Chim Acta. 2003;329(1–2):9–22.
56. Weiss G, Goodnough LT. Anemia of chronic disease. N Engl J Med. 2005;352(10):1011–23.
57. Evstatiev R, Marteau P, Iqbal T, et al. FERGIcor, a randomized controlled trial on ferric carboxymaltose for iron deficiency anemia in inflammatory bowel disease. Gastroenterology. 2011;141(3):846–53. e1–2.

58. Lee TW, Kolber MR, Fedorak RN, van Zanten SV. Iron replacement therapy in inflammatory bowel disease patients with iron deficiency anemia: a systematic review and meta-analysis. J Crohns Colitis. 2012;6(3):267–75.
59. Macdougall IC, Bock AH, Carrera F, et al. FIND-CKD: a randomized trial of intravenous ferric carboxymaltose versus oral iron in patients with chronic kidney disease and iron deficiency anaemia. Nephrol Dial Transplant. 2014;29(11):2075–84.
60. Onken JE, Bregman DB, Harrington RA, et al. A multicenter, randomized, active-controlled study to investigate the efficacy and safety of intravenous ferric carboxymaltose in patients with iron deficiency anemia. Transfusion. 2014;54(2):306–15.
61. Vadhan-Raj S, Strauss W, Ford D, et al. Efficacy and safety of IV ferumoxytol for adults with iron deficiency anemia previously unresponsive to or unable to tolerate oral iron. Am J Hematol. 2014;89(1):7–12.
62. Evstatiev R, Alexeeva O, Bokemeyer B, et al. Ferric carboxymaltose prevents recurrence of anemia in patients with inflammatory bowel disease. Clin Gastroenterol Hepatol. 2013;11(3):269–77.
63. Kulnigg S, Stoinov S, Simanenkov V, et al. A novel intravenous iron formulation for treatment of anemia in inflammatory bowel disease: the ferric carboxymaltose (FERINJECT) randomized controlled trial. Am J Gastroenterol. 2008;103(5):1182–92.
64. de Silva AD, Tsironi E, Feakins RM, Rampton DS. Efficacy and tolerability of oral iron therapy in inflammatory bowel disease: a prospective, comparative trial. Aliment Pharmacol Ther. 2005;22(11–12):1097–105.
65. Seril DN, Liao J, Ho KL, Warsi A, Yang CS, Yang GY. Dietary iron supplementation enhances DSS-induced colitis and associated colorectal carcinoma development in mice. Dig Dis Sci. 2002;47(6):1266–78.
66. Seril DN, Liao J, West AB, Yang GY. High-iron diet: foe or feat in ulcerative colitis and ulcerative colitis-associated carcinogenesis. J Clin Gastroenterol. 2006;40(5):391–7.
67. Oldenburg B, van Berge Henegouwen GP, Rennick D, Van Asbeck BS, Koningsberger JC. Iron supplementation affects the production of pro-inflammatory cytokines in IL-10 deficient mice. Eur J Clin Invest. 2000;30(6):505–10.
68. Rimon E, Kagansky N, Kagansky M, et al. Are we giving too much iron? Low-dose iron therapy is effective in octogenarians. Am J Med. 2005;118(10):1142–7.
69. Makrides M, Crowther CA, Gibson RA, Gibson RS, Skeaff CM. Efficacy and tolerability of low-dose iron supplements during pregnancy: a randomized controlled trial. Am J Clin Nutr. 2003;78(1):145–53.
70. Gasche C, Ahmad T, Tulassay Z, et al. Ferric maltol is effective in correcting iron deficiency anemia in patients with inflammatory bowel disease: results from a phase-3 clinical trial program. Inflamm Bowel Dis. 2015;21(3):579–88.
71. Santiago P. Ferrous versus ferric oral iron formulations for the treatment of iron deficiency: a clinical overview. ScientificWorldJournal. 2012;2012:846824.
72. Ali M, Rigolosi R, Fayemi AO, Braun EV, Frascino J, Singer R. Failure of serum ferritin levels to predict bone-marrow iron content after intravenous iron-dextran therapy. Lancet. 1982;1(8273):652–5.
73. Faich G, Strobos J. Sodium ferric gluconate complex in sucrose: safer intravenous iron therapy than iron dextrans. Am J Kidney Dis. 1999;33(3):464–70.
74. Okam MM, Mandell E, Hevelone N, Wentz R, Ross A, Abel GA. Comparative rates of adverse events with different formulations of intravenous iron. Am J Hematol. 2012;87(11):E123–4.
75. Larson DS, Coyne DW. Update on intravenous iron choices. Curr Opin Nephrol Hypertens. 2014;23(2):186–91.
76. Auerbach M, Ballard H, Glaspy J. Clinical update: intravenous iron for anaemia. Lancet. 2007;369(9572):1502–4.
77. Ganzoni AM. Intravenous iron-dextran: therapeutic and experimental possibilities. Schweiz Med Wochenschr. 1970;100(7):301–3.

78. Krayenbuehl PA, Battegay E, Breymann C, Furrer J, Schulthess G. Intravenous iron for the treatment of fatigue in nonanemic, premenopausal women with low serum ferritin concentration. Blood. 2011;118(12):3222–7.
79. Anker SD, Comin Colet J, Filippatos G, et al. Ferric carboxymaltose in patients with heart failure and iron deficiency. N Engl J Med. 2009;361(25):2436–48.
80. Favrat B, Balck K, Breymann C, et al. Evaluation of a single dose of ferric carboxymaltose in fatigued, iron-deficient women—PREFER a randomized, placebo-controlled study. PLoS One. 2014;9(4):e94217.
81. Cronin CC, Shanahan F. Anemia in patients with chronic inflammatory bowel disease. Am J Gastroenterol. 2001;96(8):2296–8.
82. Oldenburg B, Koningsberger JC, Van Berge Henegouwen GP, Van Asbeck BS, Marx JJ. Iron and inflammatory bowel disease. Aliment Pharmacol Ther. 2001;15(4):429–38.
83. Kulnigg S, Teischinger L, Dejaco C, Waldhör T, Gasche C. Rapid recurrence of IBD-associated anemia and iron deficiency after intravenous iron sucrose and erythropoietin treatment. Am J Gastroenterol. 2009;104(6):1460–7.
84. Nissenson AR, Wade S, Goodnough T, Knight K, Dubois RW. Economic burden of anemia in an insured population. J Manag Care Pharm. 2005;11(7):565–74.
85. Villanueva C, Colomo A, Bosch A, et al. Transfusion strategies for acute upper gastrointestinal bleeding. N Engl J Med. 2013;368(1):11–21.
86. Hébert PC, Wells G, Blajchman MA, et al. A multicenter, randomized, controlled clinical trial of transfusion requirements in critical care. Transfusion requirements in critical care investigators, Canadian Critical Care Trials Group. N Engl J Med. 1999;340(6):409–17.
87. Bager P, Dahlerup JF. The health care cost of intravenous iron treatment in IBD patients depends on the economic evaluation perspective. J Crohns Colitis. 2010;4(4):427–30.
88. Hurrell R, Egli I. Iron bioavailability and dietary reference values. Am J Clin Nutr. 2010;91(5):1461S–7.

Chapter 5
Other Micronutrient Deficiencies in Inflammatory Bowel Disease: From A to Zinc

Caroline Hwang and Kurt Hong

Introduction

The inflammatory bowel diseases (IBD), which include ulcerative colitis and Crohn's disease, are chronic inflammatory conditions of the gastrointestinal tract which increase patients' risk of malnutrition. Previous retrospective studies demonstrated that as many as 70–80 % of IBD patients exhibited weight loss during their disease course [1–4]. However, most of these studies were performed from the 1960–1980s and primarily included hospitalized patients with severe active disease, often on chronic steroid therapy.

In the last three decades, there have been several important advances in the treatment of IBD—namely, the development of multiple biologic drugs and increased use of "top-down" strategies with early combination therapy—that may be leading to a greater proportion of IBD patients attaining sustained clinical remission. Nutritional studies performed in the post-biologic era seem to suggest that IBD patients who are in remission generally have similar macronutrient intake [5, 6] and similar body mass indices [7, 8] as healthy controls. In fact, several recent studies have reported that there is a growing proportion of obese IBD patients [7, 9, 10].

C. Hwang, M.D. (✉)
Department of Medicine, Keck School of Medicine at University of Southern California (USC), 1510 San Pablo Street, Suite 322U, Los Angeles, CA 90033, USA
e-mail: caroline.hwang@med.usc.edu

K. Hong, M.D., Ph.D.
Department of Medicine, Keck School of Medicine at University of Southern California (USC), 1510 San Pablo Street, Suite 322U, Los Angeles, CA 90033, USA

Department of Medicine, Center for Clinical Nutrition and Applied Health Research, Keck School of Medicine at University of Southern California (USC), Los Angeles, CA, USA
e-mail: kurthong@med.usc.edu

© Springer International Publishing Switzerland 2016   65
A.N. Ananthakrishnan (ed.), *Nutritional Management of Inflammatory Bowel Diseases*, DOI 10.1007/978-3-319-26890-3_5

In general, malnutrition can be divided into forms that involve deficiencies in macronutrients (energy and protein intake) and those of micronutrients (vitamins, minerals, trace elements). Protein-energy malnutrition can result in weight loss and loss of muscle mass, and most often occurs with active, severe IBD. However, micronutrient deficiencies can occur even with disease that is relatively mild or in remission. Multiple simultaneous deficiencies in micronutrients are more common in patients with Crohn's disease (CD), especially those with fistulas, strictures, or prior surgical resections of the small bowel [2].

Numerous vitamin and mineral deficiencies have been reported in IBD patients [1–4]. Notably, the research in this area is lacking, as many of the studies are limited by small sample sizes, retrospective design, and frequent use of non-validated nutritional assessment methods and statistical analysis. In addition, laboratory testing that is clinically available (often measurements of plasma or serum levels of micronutrients) can be inaccurate in reflecting micronutrient status, and optimal levels of many micronutrients have yet to be established.

The most common micronutrient deficiencies in IBD patients are those of iron and vitamin D, which are discussed in detail in separate chapters. In this section, we will review the available data on the other micronutrient deficiencies that can occur with IBD and their clinical significance in this population.

Normal Micronutrient Absorption and Dietary Requirements

Vitamins and minerals are required for diverse biochemical functions in the body, including regulation of cell and tissue growth, energy metabolism, and direct antioxidant actions [11, 12]. Since all vitamins and many minerals (the so-called essential elements) are not sufficiently synthesized by humans, they need to be obtained from the diet.

Vitamins are organic compounds that can be classified as either water- or fat-soluble. Water-soluble vitamins (B vitamins, vitamin C) are readily absorbed in the intestinal lumen across enterocyte membranes by either diffusion (for non-charged, low-molecular vitamins such as vitamins B3, B6, and C) or by carrier-dependent active transport. The fat-soluble vitamins (A, D, E, and K) are hydrophobic substances that are dissolved first within fat droplets, then broken down by lipases and combined with bile salts in the duodenum to form mixed micelles which can diffuse across the enterocyte membrane [11].

Dietary minerals are inorganic elements that are important in the makeup of cellular structure and as cofactors and catalysts in enzymatic processes. The so-called "macro" minerals are those present in larger quantities in the body (i.e., kilo- or milligrams) and include calcium, phosphate, potassium, magnesium, and iron. Trace elements are present in very small amounts in the body (i.e., nanograms or parts per million), and include zinc, copper, and selenium. Macrominerals and trace elements are absorbed by passive or active transport through the intestinal mucosa, often using specialized transport proteins such as the calcium-specific TRPV6

(Transient Receptor Protein) or the more diverse DMT1 (divalent metal transporter 1) which transports several divalent metals including ferrous (Fe^{2+}), zinc (Zn^{2+}), and copper (Cu^{2+}) [11, 12].

Normally, over 95 % of vitamins and minerals within food are absorbed in the proximal small bowel, usually prior to reaching the mid-jejunum [11]. The exception to this is vitamin B12, which, when bound to intrinsic factor, is absorbed in the terminal ileum. In addition, the distal ileum also absorbs bile acids, which are critical for the absorption of fat and fat-soluble vitamins.

Dietary Requirements

Recommendations for the dietary intake of individual vitamins and minerals vary tremendously, ranging on the order of nanograms to milligrams per day. In the United States, the most widely accepted dietary guidelines were developed by the Institute of Medicine's Food and Nutrition Board, mainly for public health purposes such as food labeling and school meal planning. These guidelines (often termed "Dietary Reference Intakes") were expanded recently to account for new data that certain nutrients may help promote health and prevent disease [11, 12]. In addition, because of the recognition that a growing number of persons (39 % of American adults surveyed in the National Health and Nutrition Examination Survey [NHANES] [13]), take multivitamins and other dietary supplements, DRIs also now include information about levels associated with toxicity.

The DRI's are actually a set of four reference values (Table 5.2):

- *Recommended Dietary Allowance (RDA)*: Average daily dietary intake of a nutrient that is sufficient to meet the requirement of nearly all (97–98 %) healthy persons. This is the most commonly referenced DRI value.
- *Adequate Intake (AI)*: For nutrients for which an RDA cannot be determined based on a lack of available data. The AI is established based on observed intakes of that individual nutrient by a group of healthy persons.
- *Tolerable Upper Intake Level (UL)*: Highest daily intake of a nutrient that is likely to pose no risks of toxicity for almost all individuals.
- *Estimated Average Requirement (EAR)* is the amount of a nutrient that is estimated to meet the requirement of half of all healthy individuals in the population.

These values are listed in Table 5.2, and are also available online on the USDA or IOM websites:

http://fnic.nal.usda.gov/dietary-guidance/dietary-reference-intakes/dri-tables,
http://www.iom.edu/Activities/Nutrition/SummaryDRIs/DRI-Tables.aspx.

It is important to recognize that the DRI values were established based on healthy populations and thus may not reflect the needs of IBD patients. Notably, for patients with active disease and significant diarrhea, daily requirements for iron, potassium, calcium, magnesium, and zinc may increase significantly [2, 5]. In addition, many of the foods that are rich in these micronutrients may be difficult for some IBD patients to tolerate (refer to Table 5.2 for a list of foods). Therefore, oral supplementation may be required in certain situations, though caution must be taken with regard to counseling about supplementation, especially with certain micronutrients such as zinc and vitamin A, in which there is a narrow margin between the recommended dietary allowance (RDA) and the upper limit (UL) exists. In general, careful monitoring of supplementation should be practiced with any micronutrient that has an UL.

Pathophysiology of Micronutrient Deficiencies in IBD

Micronutrient deficiencies in IBD patients can occur by multiple mechanisms. As summarized in Table 5.1, there are a multitude of risk factors in IBD, which can be related to disease symptoms (i.e., diarrhea, anorexia), disease-related complications (i.e., bowel resection), and from drug treatments (i.e., sulfasalazine and folate antagonism).

One of the most important and probably underrecognized mechanisms for malnutrition in IBD is reduced food intake. Globally reduced intake and specific avoidance of foods is common among IBD patients. This may be particularly significant

Table 5.1 Pathogenesis of micronutrient deficiency in IBD

Decreased food intake	• Anorexia (TNF-mediated)
	• Avoidance of high-residue food (can worsen abdominal pain and diarrhea)
	• Avoidance of lactose-containing foods (high rates of concomitant lactose intolerance)
Increased intestinal loss	• Diarrhea (increased loss of Zn^{2+}, K^+, Mg^{2+})
	• Occult/overt blood loss (iron deficiency)
	• Exudative enteropathy (protein loss, and decrease in albumin-binding proteins (e.g., vitamin D-binding protein))
	• Steatorrhea (fat and fat-soluble vitamins)
Malabsorption	• Loss of intestinal surface area from active inflammation, resection, bypass, or fistula
	• Terminal ileal disease associated with deficiencies in B12 and fat-soluble vitamins
Hypermetabolic state	• Alterations of resting energy expenditure
Drug interactions	• Sulfasalazine and methotrexate inhibits folate absorption
	• Glucocorticoids impair Ca^{2+}, Zn^{2+}, and phosphorus absorption, vitamin C losses and vitamin D resistance
	• PPIs impair iron absorption, cholestyramine impairs absorption of fat-soluble vitamins, vitamin B12, and iron
Long-term total parenteral nutrition	• Can occur with any micronutrient not added to TPN
	Reported deficiencies include thiamine, vitamin A, and trace elements Zn^{2+}, Cu^{2+}, selenium, chromium

with active disease, due to anorexia (secondary to inflammatory cytokines, including interleukin IL-6, and tumor necrosis factor-alpha [TNF-α]) [14]. Many patients also self-restrict their diet to minimize symptoms of abdominal pain and diarrhea, commonly thought to be exacerbated by large fatty meals and high-residue diets.

A recent study showed that even in patients with disease in remission, persistent avoidance of major food groups remains common, with approximately one-third avoiding grains, another one-third avoiding dairy, and 18 % avoiding vegetables entirely [9]. In addition, multiple studies have reported that the majority of IBD patients, regardless of disease activity, intake levels of calcium and vitamin C that are significantly lower than Recommended Daily Allowance (RDA, Table 5.2). In addition, suboptimal intake of folate, thiamine (B1) and pyridoxine (vitamin B6), vitamin K, vitamin E and beta-carotene have also been reported to be prevalent amongst IBD patients [5, 15].

Two other important potential causes of malnutrition are enteric loss of nutrients (i.e., from diarrhea or fistula output) and malabsorption. Chronic diarrhea and fistula output can lead to wasting of zinc, calcium, and potassium [3] while iron deficiency is the most common nutritional deficiency in colitis, due largely to chronic gastrointestinal bleeding [16]. Malabsorption more frequently occurs in CD, due to small bowel inflammation or resection. Specifically, significant terminal ileal disease and/ or resections >40–60 cm can lead to vitamin B12 deficiency as well as bile-salt wasting and resultant impaired fat-soluble vitamin absorption [17]. In addition, patients with advanced primary sclerosing cholangitis are also at risk for malabsorption, as biliary strictures especially within the main branches of the biliary tract can lead to bile-salt insufficiency and steatorrhea [17].

Finally, several medications used commonly in IBD can interfere with normal micronutrient absorption. Glucocorticoids potently inhibit calcium, phosphorus, and zinc absorption and may also lead to impaired metabolism of vitamins C and D [4]. Methotrexate is a potent folate antagonist and sulfasalazine interferes with folate absorption [18]. Proton pump inhibitors, antacids, and calcium supplements can inhibit iron absorption, if taken simultaneously as dietary or supplemental iron [16]. Cholestyramine, which may be used as an antidiarrheal adjunct, can interfere with absorption of fat-soluble vitamins [4, 11]. Finally, the use of long-term parenteral nutrition can lead to deficiencies in any micronutrient not added in sufficient quantities, most commonly vitamins A, D, E, zinc, copper, and selenium [19].

Specific Micronutrient Deficiencies in IBD

A wide array of vitamin and mineral deficiencies may occur in IBD patients, particularly those with moderate-to-severe disease activity, small bowel Crohn's involvement, and history of bowel resection [1–4]. The most well-recognized nutritional deficiencies are those of iron, vitamin D, folate, cobalamin, and zinc [4–6]. Besides being relatively common in IBD cohorts, deficiencies in these micronutrients are associated with well-known clinical manifestations (i.e., anemia with iron or folate deficiency, and osteoporosis with vitamin D).

Table 5.2 Micronutrients: normal absorption and dietary reference intakes

	Micronutrient	Primary site of absorption	Dietary sources	Dietary reference intakes (**RDA** or *AF*[b]), <u>UL</u> listed if relevant
Vitamins: water-soluble	B1 (thiamine)	Jejunum/ileum	Pork, beef, ham, sunflower seeds	**1.1 mg** (women) **1.2 mg** (men)
	B2 (riboflavin)	Jejunum	Liver, milk, yogurt, pork	**1.1 mg** (women) **1.3 mg** (men)
	B3 (niacin)	Jejunum	Tuna, turkey, chicken, beef, peanuts, milk, cottage cheese	**14 mg** (women) **16 mg** (men) **18 mg** (pregnancy)
	B5 (pantothenic acid)	Jejunum	Mushrooms, corn, liver, broccoli	*4 mg*[b]
	B6 (pyridoxine)	Jejunum	Salmon, chicken, legumes, bananas, turnip greens	**1.3–1.5 mg** (women) **1.3–1.7 mg** (men)
	B7 (biotin)	Jejunum	Swiss chard, eggs, peanuts	*30 μg*[b]
	B9 (folate)	Jejunum/ileum	Asparagus, brussel sprouts, cereals, spinach, cantaloupe	**400 μg** (men, women) **600 μg** (pregnancy)
	B12 (cobalamin)	Terminal ileum	Trout, beef, shellfish, tuna, milk	**2.4 μg** (men, women)
	C (ascorbic acid)	Jejunum/ileum	Kiwi, orange, green peppers, cauliflower, broccoli	**75 mg** (women) **90 mg** (men)

Vitamins: fat-soluble	A	Ileum	Carrots, sweet potatoes, spinach, cantaloupe, liver	RAE[e]: **700 µg** (women) **900 µg** (men) (UL[d] 3000 µg)
	D	Ileum	Salmon, tuna, milk	**15 µg/600 IU** (<70 years old) **20 µg/800 IU** (>70 years old) (UL[d] 100 µg)
	E	Ileum	Sunflower seeds, almonds, sweet potato, shellfish	**15 mg** (men, women) (UL[d] 1000 mg)
	K	Ileum	Kale, spinach, broccoli	90 µg[b] (women) 120 µg[b] (men)
Minerals: macro elements	Calcium	Duodenum/ Jejunum	Yogurt, milk, cheese, collard greens, tofu	**1000 mg** (men aged 19–70, women aged 19–50) **1200 mg** (men>70 years, women >51 years old)
	Magnesium	Duodenum/ jejunum	Peanuts, bran, legumes, bean sprouts, tofu	**420 mg** (men) **320 mg** (women)
Minerals: trace elements	Iron	Duodenum	Fortified cereal, liver, beef, baked beans, pork, prune juice, apricots	**8 mg** (men, women >50 years) **18 mg** (women <50 years)
	Zinc	Unclear	Beef, crab, ham, pork, wheat germ, pecans	**8 mg** (women), **10 mg** (men) (UL[d] 40 mg)
	Chromium	Proximal small bowel	Beef, chicken, eggs, spinach, bananas, apples, wheat germ	20–35 µg[b]
	Copper	Duodenum	Oysters, beans, cashews	**900 µg** (UL[d] 10,000 µg)
	Manganese	Unclear	Pineapple, brown rice, beans	1.8–2.3 mg[b]
	Selenium	Ileum	Lobster, tuna, shrimp, ham	**55 µg** (UL[d] 400 µg)

[a]Dietary Reference Intake values, as recommended by Food and Nutrition Board and Institute of Medicine [11, 12]. Specified as Recommended Dietary Allowances (RDA, the nutrient needs of 98 % of the population), unless otherwise specified

[b]AI adequate intake (insufficient evidence to establish RDA)

[c]RAE retinol activity equivalent (1 µg RAE = 1 µg retinol = 12 µg β-carotene = 24 µg α-carotene = 5 IU)

[d]UL upper limit (highest daily intake above which side effects/toxicity may occur)

For many of the other micronutrients, the literature is sparse and the results of existing studies are often difficult to interpret, as there is significant variation with regard to the definitions of deficiency (i.e., inadequate dietary intake vs. serum levels vs. suspected clinical syndrome) and the type of IBD cohort studied (pediatric vs. adult, active disease vs. remission).

In this section, we will review the data available on the major essential micronutrients and the risk of deficiency for each in IBD. Specifically, we will focus on the prevalence, risk factors, clinical manifestations, diagnostic testing, and treatment with both diet and supplementation (summarized also in Tables 5.2, 5.3, and 5.4).

Major B Vitamins

Folate (Vitamin B9)

Folic acid plays an important role in erythrocyte metabolism, serving as a cofactor in DNA synthesis and erythrocyte division [11, 18]. Consequently, folate deficiency is classically associated with a macrocytic megaloblastic anemia. In addition, because folate is an important cofactor in the conversion of homocysteine to methionine, folate deficiency can lead to accumulation of homocysteine levels in the blood. Hyperhomocysteinemia is a known risk factor for arterial and potentially venous thromboembolism [28, 29]. In patients with IBD there is an increased prevalence of hyperhomocysteinemia (defined as fasting plasma level >15 ng/mL), with reported frequency between 11 and 52 %, compared with 3.3–5 % in the control population [30–33], which may at least partially account for the increased risk of thromboembolic disease in IBD patients.

A controversial association between folate deficiency and increased colorectal cancer risk in IBD has also been reported. Folate may play an important role in colonic inflammation and carcinogenesis, since it participates in biological methylation and nucleotide synthesis. In animal models, deficiencies have been associated with reduced levels of p53 mRNA, increased DNA strand breaks, and DNA hypomethylation in the colon [33, 34]. In human epidemiologic studies, low dietary folate intake has been associated with sporadic colorectal cancer [35–38]. Within the IBD population, there have been two case-control studies and a retrospective analysis that have shown decreased serum folate levels in patients with premalignant lesions or cancer in the colon, compared with colitis patients without neoplasms [39–41].

Folate deficiency can occur rather rapidly without regular daily intake, since total body stores only averages ~500–20,000 μg in healthy individuals and may be much lower in patients with acute illness or with malabsorptive disease [18]. Recommended Daily Allowance (RDA) for folic acid is 400 μg for healthy adults and 500–600 μg during pregnancy and lactation [11]. Daily intake up to 1000 μg might be required for individuals at higher risk for deficiency, including those on folate antagonist drugs such as methotrexate or sulfasalazine and those who consume

Table 5.3 Micronutrients with reported deficiency in IBD

		Pathophysiology	Symptoms of deficiency	Diagnosis	Prevalence
B Vitamins: water-soluble	B1 (thiamine)	Unclear mechanism	Peripheral neuropathy, cardiomyopathy (beri beri)	Mainly clinical; Consider serum B1 if symptoms severe	32 % of CD patients, unknown prevalence in UC patients
	B9 (folate)	Malabsorption (associated with ileitis/small bowel resection)	Megaloblastic anemia	Serum folate <2.5 ng/mL (can be falsely low, homocysteine >16 mmol/L confirms) RBC folate <140	40–78 % of IBD patients with inadequate folate intake; 0–26 % of Crohn's disease patients with deficiency
		Drugs (MTX, sulfasalazine)	Hyperhomocysteinemia		
		All pregnant IBD patients	Glossitis, angular stomatitis, depression		
	B12	Active ileitis	Megaloblastic anemia, pancytopenia	Serum B12 <200 pg/mL (may lack sensitivity)	11–22 % of Crohn's patients
		History of ileal/ileocolonic resection? ileoanal pouch	Peripheral neuropathy, dementia	If B12 <400, consider methylmalonic acid, homocysteine levels	100 % of patients with ileal resections >60 cm
					48 % of resections 20–40 cm
	C	Inadequate dietary intake	Poor wound healing	Mainly clinical	>50 % of Crohn's patients
			Gingivitis, scaly skin, arthralgias	Serum ascorbate <11.4 µmol/L	

(continued)

Table 5.3 (continued)

		Pathophysiology	Symptoms of deficiency	Diagnosis	Prevalence
Vitamins: Fat-soluble	A	Inadequate dietary intake	Poor wound healing	Serum tests can be unreliable	35–90 % of IBD patients with inadequate daily intake; 0–44 % with low serum levels
		Steatorrhea/fat malabsorption	Night blindness, xerophthalmia	Serum retinol, retinol-binding protein, β-carotene	
		Bile salt deficiency (wasting, use of cholestyramine)			
	D	Same as above AND	Abnormal bone metabolism (likely contributes to osteopenia/osteoporosis)	Serum 25OHD	22–70 % of CD patients and up to 45 % of UC patients deficient [20–23]
		Decreased sunlight exposure/ inadequate dietary intake	May increase IBD inflammation	<15 Deficiency	
				<20 Insufficiency	
				(>30 Optimal)	
	E	Steatorrhea/bile salt deficiency	Neuropathies, retinopathy, anemia	Serum α -tocopherol <5 μg/mL	Unclear prevalence, but one study found to serum levels lower in CD (vs. controls)
	K	Inadequate dietary intake	Likely contributes to abnormal bone metabolism (lesser degree than vit D)	Bone levels:	Unclear prevalence, but uncarboxylated osteocalcin levels lower in CD (vs. UC patients and controls)
		Steatorrhea/fat malabsorption	Bleeding, cartilage/arterial	Uncarboxylated osteocalcin (% or total)	
		Bile salt deficiency (wasting, use of cholestyramine)		Serum phylloquinone PT/ INR	

Category	Nutrient	Etiology	Clinical manifestation	Measurement	Prevalence
Minerals: Macro	Calcium	Inadequate dietary intake	Decreased bone density	Bone density scan	80–86 % of IBD patients with inadequate daily intake [5, 24]
		Vitamin D deficiency (decreased intestinal/renal absorption)	Hypoparathyroidism, hypertension, muscle spasm/twitching	Serum calcium not reflective	22–55 % of CD and 32–67 % of UC patients with osteopenia
		Hypomagnesemia (from diarrhea)	May increase sporadic polyp/CRC risk		
	Magnesium	Inadequate dietary intake	Minor contributor to bone health	24 urine magnesium most accurate	Unclear (likely very common)
		Losses from diarrhea	Hypocalcemia/hypoparathyroidism		
	Iron	Chronic blood loss	Microcytic anemia	Transferrin sat <16 %	36–90 % of IBD patients with iron-deficiency anemia
		Impaired iron metabolism (IL6, TNFα, hepcidin upregulation, inadequate intake)	Fatigue, glossitis, angular cheilitis, restless leg syndrome	Serum ferritin <30 (inactive disease, normal CRP)	
				<100 (active, ↑ CRP)	
Minerals: Trace elements	Zinc	Chronic diarrhea	Poor wound healing	Mainly clinical	Unclear (likely very common)
		Malabsorption (small bowel)	Acrodermatitis, poor taste	No accurate measurement	
		Increased need in hypermetabolic states (sepsis, critical illness)			
	Selenium	Long-term TPN	Cardiomyopathy, cartilage degeneration, hypothyroidism	Serum Se < 130 ng/mL	Unclear prevalence, but mean levels lower in both CD/UC [25–27]
		Unknown in non-TPN patients			

Table 5.4 Screening and treatment strategies for micronutrient deficiencies

		Consider empiric[a] supplementation	Consider screening for deficiency	Treatment strategies for deficiency
B Vitamins: Water-Soluble	B1 (thiamine)	Consider in patients with active ileitis or multiple jejunal/ileal resections (B-complex vitamin usually sufficient)	Usually no need to check levels Supplement if clinically suspicious	Thiamine 100 mg/day (or vitamin B complex supplement often sufficient)
	B3 (niacin)	Not sufficient evidence	Not sufficient evidence	–
	B6 (pyridoxine)	Patients on isoniazid or corticosteroids (50–100 mg pyridoxine/day) Consider in patients with elevated homocysteine or history of thromboembolic disease (B-complex vitamin usually sufficient)	Usually no need to check levels, but can consider if clinically suspicious	Pyridoxine 50–100 mg/day (or vitamin B complex supplement often sufficient)
	B9 (folate)	Patients on methotrexate or sulfasalazine (folate 1 mg/day usually sufficient) Can consider for CRC prevention, though not been validated in RCT	Definite: Patients with new anemia	Folate 1 mg/day; 2 weeks sufficient if normal jejunal absorption Consider rechecking folate in 4–6 weeks if concerned about absorption (active ileitis, multiple resections)
	B12	All patients with ileal resections >60 cm will need lifelong IM B12	Definite: Patients with new anemia Probable: Regular screening in all patients with active ileitis or small bowel resection Probable: Periodic screening in all Crohn's patients	Intramuscular B12 1000 μg monthly preferred in patients with ileal disease/resections; monitor annually in high-risk patients Oral and intranasal B12 has been studied in non-IBD patients and likely equally efficacious in patients without ileal disease

(B9 folate screening additional rows: Probable: Regular screening in patients with active ileitis or small bowel resections; Possible: Periodic screening in all Crohn's patients)

Vitamins: Fat-Soluble	C	Patients with fistulas or recent surgery (500 mg/day × 10 days)	Usually no need to check levels / Supplement if clinically suspicious	Vitamin C 100 mg/day, can be indefinite as low risk of toxicity
	A	Patients with fistulas or recent surgery (10,000 IU/day oral/IM×10 days; 15,000 IU/day for patients on steroids)	Significant steatorrhea/malabsorption, and/or multiple ileal resections	Vitamin A 10,000 IU/day orally/IM×10 days
	D	Most IBD patients (600 IU–2000 IU/day indefinitely; 2–3× higher for patients on glucocorticoids or who are obese)	All IBD patients should be screened periodically	Vitamin D2 50,000 IU 1–2 times/week for 8 weeks until serum 25OH levels >30 achieved
			Closer monitoring for patients with osteopenia/osteoporosis or risk factors (steroids, obesity, malabsorption)	Alternatively, 6000 IU daily (cholecalciferol), 2–3× higher in patients with obesity, malabsorption or steroid use
				Consider checking vitamin D q8 weeks in patients being treated and then q6mo–annually
	E	No sufficient evidence	Significant steatorrhea/malabsorption, and/or multiple ileal resections	α-tocopherol 15–25 mg/kg po once/day; parental forms may need to be given in server deficiency (rare)
	K	Not sufficient evidence currently	Significant steatorrhea/malabsorption, and/or multiple ileal resections	If bleeding complications, phytonadione 5–20 mg orally × 3 days; monitor PT/INR
		May consider in patients with osteoporosis (small studies show increased bone density with menaquinone-4 (soybeans)) monitor closely for toxicity		
Minerals: Macro	Calcium	Most IBD patients	Serum calcium not reflective	1000–1500 mg calcium (with vitamin D)
		1000 mg in women aged 18–25, men <65	Regular bone DEXA in patients with osteoporosis/osteoporosis with h/o significant steroid exposure, postmenopausal women, family history	
		1300 mg in women 25-menopause		
		1500 mg in postmenopausal women, men>65		
	Magnesium	Patients with active diarrhea (>300 g/day) or draining fistulae (elemental 5–20 mmol/day)	Active diarrhea, fistulas	5–20 mmol/day; consider checking serum/urinary magnesium in cases of severe/persistent diarrhea or fistulas

(continued)

Table 5.4 (continued)

		Consider empiric[a] supplementation	Consider screening for deficiency	Treatment strategies for deficiency
Minerals: Trace elements	Iron	Not recommended	Definite: All patients with anemia	IV iron formulations preferred
			Probable: Regular screening in patients with active inflammation, bleeding symptoms	Ferric sucrose traditional IV form (200 mg/infusion, given until anemia resoled)
			Possible: Periodic screening in all IBD patients	Ferric carboxymaltose recently developed and superior in 1 RCT (1000 mg/infusion)
				Oral iron often poorly tolerated and may increase inflammation
				Monitor iron/CBC every 4 weeks after treatment initiation asymptomatic patients (earlier in severe cases)
				Treatment goal is to restore Hgb >12 in women, >13 men
	Zinc	Patients with fistulas or recent surgery, to improve wound healing (220 mg twice daily × 10 days)	No accurate screening test available	Can consider 220 mg 1–2 times daily for patients with active, severe diarrhea, unclear length of supplementation acceptable
		Patients with severe diarrhea		
	Selenium	All TPN formulations	Possible: Consider periodic screening in all patients with IBD	Selenium 100 µg/day × 2–3 weeks; unclear monitoring intervals
	Chromium	Consider adding to TPN, though contaminants often present	Probable: Monitor in patients on TPN	
	Manganese	Consider adding to TPN, though contaminants often present; monitor for toxicity	Probable: Monitor in patients on TPN	

[a]Empiric = without clinical or laboratory evidence of deficiency; nutritional supplementation for health promotion or prevention of complications

significant and regular alcohol. Foods naturally rich in folic acid include dark leafy greens (spinach, collard, and turnip greens), asparagus, broccoli, citrus fruits, avocado, beets, and lentils (refer to Table 5.2). In the United States and Canada, nearly all cereals and enriched grain products are enriched with folate, due to national mandated programs launched in the 1980s to decrease rates of neural tube birth defects [42].

In spite of these folate fortification programs, IBD patients may be at increased risk of folic acid deficiency compared with the general population. While more recent studies demonstrate that folate deficiency is less prevalent than was previously reported in historical IBD cohort studies (51–80 %) [3, 4, 18], folate deficiency still appears to be relatively common, particularly in CD. In a recent retrospective case-control study performed in 2010, abnormal serum folate levels (<3 ng/mL) were found in 28.8 % of the CD patients, 8.8 % of ulcerative colitis (UC) patients, and 3 % of controls [43]. Three studies performed in CD—one of which only included patients with disease in remission—reported similar rates (20–26 %) of subnormal folate levels [24, 43, 44]. It should be noted that all of the above studies used serum folate level, although red blood cell (RBC) folate levels is a superior test as it averages folate levels over the preceding 3 months. There have been two studies utilizing RBC folate levels in IBD patients, showing much lower rates of deficiency seen (0–7 %) [45].

Potential mechanisms of folate deficiency in IBD include inadequate dietary intake, malabsorption, and medication interactions. Inadequate intake is likely a major contributor, as supported by two studies in which prospective food records of outpatient IBD showed inadequate folate intake in 40–78 % [5, 45]. Active Crohn's ileitis and history of small bowel resection have been demonstrated to be risk factors for folate deficiency, supporting malabsorptive mechanisms [24, 43]. Finally, sulfasalazine and methotrexate both can cause folate deficiency, as both are inhibitors of dihydrofolate reductase and cellular uptake of folate [46].

Currently, there are no clear guidelines on screening for folate deficiency in IBD patients, especially in patients with disease in remission and who report no major restrictions in their diet. However, measuring folate levels (RBC levels preferred over serum) is definitely indicated in all anemic IBD patients, particularly those with CD. In addition, if patients display other clinical symptoms of folate deficiency, such as glossitis, angular stomatitis, or depression, checking folate status is warranted [11]. If RBC folate level is normal, but suspicion for folate deficiency is high, homocysteine levels can also be assessed. Elevated serum homocysteine is potentially more sensitive, although less specific for folate deficiency, since hyperhomocysteinemia can also occurs with deficiencies of vitamin B6 and B12 [18].

Once folate deficiency is diagnosed, folate supplementation of 1 mg/day is usually sufficient to replenish deficient folate stores within 2–3 weeks [47]. Following repletion of folate stores, folate intake at the DRI levels of 400–600 μg should be sufficient in the long term. The exception to this is patients who are on folate antagonist drugs (methotrexate or sulfasalazine), pregnant IBD patients, and those on long-term TPN [48]. These higher-risk patients should receive at least 1 mg/day of folate indefinitely or for as long as their risk factor is present (i.e., until they are taken off folate antagonist/TPN or give birth).

Another potential indication for folate supplementation in IBD patients is the prevention of colitis-associated colorectal cancer (CRC), although this is more controversial. There have been several small studies that have suggested folate may potentially have chemopreventative effects, at least on the molecular level. In one small prospective, placebo-controlled study of patients with sporadic adenomas, it was found that daily supplementation with 5 mg of folate was associated with an increase in genomic DNA methylation and a decrease in the extent of p53 strand breaks, after 6 and 12 months [33]. In UC patients, supplementation with folate at doses of 15 mg/day resulted in reduced cell proliferation/kinetics in the rectal mucosa [49]. Despite these preclinical studies, the findings of several meta-analyses cannot convincingly demonstrate a clear chemopreventative effect for folate [50, 51]. However, given the safety and low cost of folate, additional folate supplementation of at least 1 mg/day (or at least counseling about adequate dietary intake) should be considered in patients with multiple years of pancolitis or other risk factors for CRC.

Cyanocobalamin (Vitamin B12)

Vitamin B12, also known as cyanocobalamin, is an essential nutrient which serves as an important cofactor in normal energy metabolism as well as amino acid and fatty acid metabolism. Additionally, B12 is vital in a myriad of other vital physiological processes such as neuron function, blood formation, bone marrow health, and DNA synthesis/regulation.

Although probably less common than folate deficiency in the general population, vitamin B12 deficiency is an especially important consideration in patients with Crohn's disease and in all elderly IBD patients. Similar to folate, deficiency in vitamin B12 is associated with a megaloblastic anemia and hyperhomocysteinemia [17, 30]. In addition to these hematological abnormalities, other clinical manifestations of B12 deficiency include neurologic and skeletal changes. Vitamin B12 deficiency appears to be associated with an increased risk of osteoporosis [52] and hip and spine fractures [53], possibly due to suppression of osteoblast activity [54]. In patients with neuropsychiatric manifestations, deficiency in vitamin B12 likely impacts neuronal myelin formation, leading to a syndrome marked by dementia, paresthesias, ataxia, weakness, and spasticity [11, 55].

Dietary sources of B12 principally come from animal products, particularly red meats, and marine sources such as mackerel, salmon, and sardine. Other sources of vitamin B12 are listed in Table 5.2. Gastrointestinal absorption of vitamin B12 occurs by a fairly complex process. Dietary cobalamin is cleaved from R factor by pancreatic proteases and binds to intrinsic factor, which is produced in the stomach. The IF-cobalamin compound then travels to the ileum where it binds to a specific receptor, cobalamin, and then is absorbed through the distal ileal mucosa. Since CD frequently affects the ileum, with 25–35 % of patients with isolated ileal inflammation and another 30–40 % with ileocolonic involvement [1], long-term inflammation can lead to impaired absorption of vitamin B12. Therefore, patients with CD are thought to be at significant risk for developing vitamin B12 deficiency [43].

In IBD cohorts, there have been few recent studies evaluating vitamin B12 status. In patients with CD, deficiency was reported in 11–22 % [17, 43, 56]. In the largest of these studies, Headstrom et al. [56] found in a retrospective multivariate analysis of 200 CD patients that the greatest risk factors for B12 deficiency were prior ileal resection (odds ratio [OR] 7.22; 95 % confidence interval [CI], 1.97–26.5) or ileocolonic resection (OR 5.81; 95 % CI, 2.09–10.12). Neither disease location nor duration was independently associated with risk of B12 deficiency. In contrast, UC is always confined to inflammation within the colon, and thus rates of B12 deficiency have generally been found to be comparable to that of the general population [43, 44]. However, there have been several reports of B12 deficiency in UC patients who have undergone proctocolectomy with ileoanal pouch anastomosis, although it is unclear if this may be related to the small amount of ileum resected during this anastomotic reconstruction ($\approx$20–40 cm) or small bowel overgrowth of the pouch [57].

Diagnosis of vitamin B12 deficiency has traditionally been based on serum vitamin B12 levels, usually defined as less than 200 pg/mL (150 pmol/L), along with clinical evidence of disease. However, in many individuals, particularly elderly patients, irreversible neuropsychiatric manifestations can begin to occur, even in the absence of hematological manifestations of B12 deficiency [55]. Therefore, it is advocated that if serum B12 levels are normal in at-risk populations (Crohn's disease patients with ileal disease, elderly IBD patients), that methylmalonic acid and homocysteine levels—metabolites of vitamin B12—be assessed next, as these appear to be more sensitive [55, 56].

Assessing for vitamin B12 status is definitively indicated in all IBD patients with anemia. In addition, any patient with new onset of depression, memory difficulties, motor dysfunction, severe fatigue, or personality changes should also be tested for B12 deficiency. In addition, periodic screening should be considered in all CD patients, especially those with active ileal CD or history of ileal resection, although the recommended intervals for screening have not been established. Previous studies have demonstrated that patients with terminal ileal resections of >60 cm will need lifelong B12 replacement, while up to 48 % of patients with shorter resection lengths of 20–40 cm are at risk of eventually developing B12 deficiency [58, 59].

In CD patients with intact ileum and whose disease is in remission, either oral or sublingual vitamin B12 supplementation can be considered. In patients with ileal resection or those with severe ileal inflammation, the optimal method for supplementation is less clear. Traditionally, the preferred approach has been monthly parenteral injections, as this route is inexpensive and is effective in quickly correcting B12 deficiency [47]. A recent Cochrane meta-analysis suggested that high-dose oral cobalamin of 1000–2000 μg (initially daily, then weekly, then monthly) was as effective as intramuscular injections in patients with B12 deficiency, although the studies did not include patients with CD [60]. However, it seems reasonable to assume that patients with IBD, especially active small bowel disease, may have impaired absorption of oral cobalamin. Therefore, at the current time further studies need to be performed before oral supplements can be widely recommended to IBD patients with B12 deficiency.

Pyridoxine (Vitamin B6)

Vitamin B6 (pyridoxine) is a water-soluble B vitamin that comes in several forms, including pyridoxine, pyridoxal, and pyridoxamine, as well as 5′ phosphates. Pyridoxal-5-phosphate (PLP), the biologically active form of vitamin B6, is a cofactor for over 140 biochemical reactions, including those involved in carbohydrate and protein metabolism, neuronal function, and RBC production. In addition, vitamin B6 may also play a role in inflammation, as Plasma PLP concentrations are inversely related to markers of inflammation such as C-reactive protein [61].

Since vitamin B6 is absorbed by passive diffusion in both jejunum and ileum, deficiency is less common than other B vitamins and rarely occurs in isolation. Although severe vitamin B6 deficiency is rare in the general population, mild inadequacy [plasma pyridoxal 5′-phosphate (PLP) <20 nmol/L] is observed in 19–27 % of the US population [62]. In IBD patients, only two studies to date have looked at vitamin B6 status. From these small studies, it appears that rates of vitamin B6 deficiency were 10–13 %, with one study demonstrating a greater risk in patients (27 % vs. 2.9 %, $p<0.01$) with active disease compared with those with quiescent disease [63, 64]. Similar to earlier observations in rheumatoid arthritis, it has been suggested that inflammation can deplete plasma vitamin B6. Lastly, certain drugs, including corticosteroids and isoniazid, may interfere with B6 metabolism [46].

The RDA for vitamin B6 is 1.3–1.7 mg/day (Table 5.2) and sources can be found in both plant and animal sources, including grains, nuts, vegetable such as spinach and cabbage, and meats such as tuna, turkey, and beef. Food preparation and processing—particularly overcooking—can significantly reduce vitamin B6 availability up to 50 % [62].

Classic manifestations of vitamin B6 deficiency include a seborrheic dermatitis-like rash, atrophic glossitis, and neurological symptoms including neuropathy. Vitamin B6 status can be assessed by measuring PLP level (deficiency defined as <10 ng/mL). In certain IBD patients with suggestive symptoms, erythrocyte transaminase activity, with and without PLP added, can also used as a functional test of pyridoxine status, and may be a more accurate reflection of vitamin B6 status in critically ill patients [61, 62]. Vitamin B6 deficiency can be treated with 50–100 mg/day of pyridoxine daily [11].

Other B Vitamins

Thiamine (Vitamin B1)

Thiamine is a water-soluble vitamin that is important in the catabolism of sugars and amino acids, and in which severe deficiencies are associated with peripheral neuropathy and cardiomyopathy (beri-beri) [11]. Thiamine is found in multiple dietary sources (eggs, meats, bread, nuts), and high temperature cooking and baking as well as pasteurization can destroy thiamine. Similar to vitamin B6, thiamine absorption mainly occurs in the jejunum by varying degrees of active and passive transport, depending on body stores and luminal concentrations of thiamine.

There have been two small studies demonstrating that thiamine deficiency may be more common in CD patients compared with controls [5, 63]. The more recent of these studies was performed within the last decade on 54 CD patients whose disease was in remission. Even in this group, dietary thiamine intake was significantly lower than controls and low serum vitamin B1 was found in 32 % of patients [5]. The rate of thiamine deficiency in either active CD or in patients with UC is not known. In another study, IBD patients with fatigue attribute to mild intracellular thiamine deficiency were treated with oral or parenteral thiamine with reported improved in symptom [65]. The RDA for thiamine is 1.2–1.4 mg/day for the general population [11] and at least this amount should be recommended for patients with IBD. If patients are unable to meet these requirements through dietary sources, most B-complex multivitamins will provide sufficient amounts of thiamine.

Riboflavin (Vitamin B2)

Vitamin B2 (riboflavin) is a water-soluble vitamin that acts as an oxidant in several important reactions, including fatty acid oxidation, reduction of glutathione, and pyruvate decarboxylation. Dietary sources of vitamin B2 include meats, fish, eggs and milk, green vegetables, yeast, and certain enriched foods. Absorption occurs in the jejunum by sodium-dependent active transport. Deficiency can manifest with oral (angular cheilitis, cracked lips) and ocular (photophobia) symptoms. Riboflavin deficiency does not appear to be common in IBD, with only one study performed in 1983 documenting a modestly elevated incidence in CD patients compared with controls [63].

Niacin (Vitamin B3)

Niacin or nicotinic acid is another water-soluble member of the B complex family. It is a precursor to NAD+/NADH and NADP+/NADPH, and also is involved in both DNA repair and production of adrenal steroid hormones. Absorption of niacin occurs mainly in the jejunum, and dietary sources include chicken, beef, fish, cereal, nuts, dairy, and eggs. Severe deficiency can cause pellagra (diarrhea, dermatitis, and dementia), although dermatological and psychiatric symptoms are common in even mild deficiency [66].

A recent study found plasma vitamin B3 levels to be low in 77 % of CD patients with disease in remission [5]. However, these results need to be carefully interpreted, given that niacin status should be assessed via urinary biomarkers, as these are more reliable than plasma levels. Nevertheless, this study does suggest that niacin deficiency may be fairly prevalent in the CD population (prevalence in UC patients is not known). The recommended daily allowance of niacin is 14 mg/day for women,

16 mg/day for men, and 18 mg/day for pregnant or breast-feeding women [11]. If patients cannot meet these requirements, oral vitamin B3 at doses commonly found in standard multivitamin preparations should be encouraged.

Biotin (Vitamin B7)

Vitamin B7 (biotin) is a coenzyme in the metabolism of fatty acids and leucine, and it plays a role in gluconeogenesis. Like the other B vitamins, its absorption occurs primarily in the jejunum. Deficiency in biotin is rare and tends to present with mild symptoms. There has only been one study of biotin status in IBD patients, in which serum levels did not differ from that of healthy controls [63].

Fat-Soluble Vitamins

Vitamin A

Vitamin A actually refers to a group of related compounds which includes retinol/retinal (so-called *preformed* active forms of vitamin A that can only be found from animal sources, such as beef and eggs), retinoic acid (converted from retinal by the body), and the carotenoids (*provitamin* A compounds which are synthesized by plants and can be converted by humans into retinol). The most important of the carotenoids is β-carotene, which is found in carrots, greens, spinach, orange juice, sweet potatoes, and cantaloupe [11].

The vitamin A compound group plays an important role in vision and wound healing. Retinal is a vital structural component of the visual pigments of retinal rod and cone cells [20]. Retinoic acid plays an important role in wound healing, by augmenting the presence of macrophage and monocyte at the wound site and stimulating fibroblasts' production of collagen [20, 67]. Vitamin A also plays an important role in reproduction as well as serving as a hormone-like growth factor for epithelial cells, participating in cellular differentiation and gene regulation [20].

Following ingestion of dietary retinol and carotenoids, these compounds are solubilized by bile salts, absorbed by enterocytes throughout the small bowel, incorporated in chylomicrons, and shuttled between the liver (main storage site, 50–80 % of stores) and to tissues such as the retina and skin. The amount of vitamin A available from dietary carotenoids depends on the efficiency of absorption (can vary between 5 and 50 %, depending on the type and source of carotenoid), the digestibility of the associated protein complex, and the level of dietary fat accompanying carotenoid intake [11, 20]. Normal vitamin A metabolism is dependent on zinc, as this mineral is necessary for the synthesis of retinol binding protein (RBP), which transports retinol through the circulation and also is required for enzymatic reactions that activate retinol.

There have been several small studies in which mean vitamin A and β-carotene levels were found to be significantly lower in IBD patients [14, 21, 22]. These studies need to be interpreted carefully, as assessing vitamin A status can be quite complicated and serum testing does not accurately reflect body stores, as discussed further below. However, there have been also several cohort studies which suggest that the majority of IBD patients—between 36 and 90 %—have inadequate vitamin A intake with significantly lower dietary levels than the RDA (700 μg in women, 900 μg in men) [5, 6, 45].

Vitamin A deficiency remains more of a clinical diagnosis, as serum testing can be quite inaccurate and confusing. The tests available include serum retinol levels, serum retinal-binding protein, and serum carotene levels. Because most vitamin A is stored in the liver, serum retinol testing can underestimate deficiency, since retinol can be released by liver until very late stages of vitamin A deficiency. Conversely, serum retinol tests can be artificially low in the setting of severe protein-energy malnutrition (i.e., IBD patient who is cachectic or losing weight), partially because production of the retinol's binding protein (RBP) is decreased. Serum carotene levels can vary tremendously based on recent intake of dietary vitamin A.

Despite these limitations, serum retinol levels (levels less than 20 μg/dL or a ratio of retinol:RBP (a molar ratio <0.8)) are suggestive of vitamin A deficiency [20]. However, in high-risk patients who do not meet these laboratory criteria, one should keep a high suspicion and observe for earlier clinical signs of vitamin A deficiency. This includes dry eyes (xerophthalmia) and impaired night vision (nyctalopia) from the loss of visual pigments—both can actually occur quite quickly in the setting of vitamin A deficiency. In addition, vitamin A deficiency is also associated with skin texture changes involving follicular hyperkeratosis (phrynoderma), impaired wound healing, unexplained anemia, and impaired immunocompetence (reduced numbers and mitogenic responsiveness of T lymphocytes) [20].

Vitamin A supplementation in IBD patients has not been well studied, so currently it is suggested that, in the absence of suspected deficiency, vitamin A should not be routinely recommended because of the risk of toxicity. For patients with deficiency, particularly those with visual changes, short courses of higher-dose vitamin A is usually recommended. For example, to treat xerophthalmia, ultra-high doses of 100,000 IU (20,000 μg) have been used, but these doses should only be done in conjunction with an ophthalmologists. In general, to replete deficient IBD patients, doses should be aimed at the DRI's Tolerable Upper Limit Intake Levels (UL) of 10,000–15,000 IU (2000–3000 μg of retinol or 3000–4500 μg of carotenoid form) per day for a 1–2 week period. Once patients are started on therapy, signs of vitamin A toxicity (headache, bone pain, liver toxicity, hemorrhage) should be closely monitored [11].

In addition, another potential indication for vitamin A supplementation may be in the perioperative period after bowel surgery and/or for patients with refractory fistulas. To enhance wound healing in the acute setting, several expert groups have recommended 10,000 IU–15,000 IU/day orally or intramuscularly for 10 days [20, 68]. This may be especially beneficial for patients who are on corticosteroids or have concomitant protein malnutrition.

Vitamin D

Vitamin D is a fat-soluble vitamin that is essential for skeletal bone health and may have an important role in regulating the adaptive immune system. Several reports have demonstrated that IBD patients are at higher risk for hypovitaminosis D, with rates between 22 and 70 % for CD patients and up to 45 % in UC [68, 69]. A more detailed discussion of the vitamin D deficiency will be covered in a separate chapter.

Vitamin E

Vitamin E refers to a group of fat-soluble vitamins which play a fundamental role in protecting the body against the damaging effects of reactive oxygen species. When located in the lipid portion of cell membranes, vitamin E protects the unsaturated membrane phospholipids from oxidative degradation from highly reactive oxygen free radicals. Vitamin E includes two classes of biologically active substances: (1) the tocopherols and (2) the related but less biologically active compounds, the tocotrienols. Amongst the tocopherols, γ-tocopherol is the most common in the North American diet, found in corn oil, soybean oil, margarine, and dressings. Alpha (α-) tocopherol, the most biologically active form of vitamin E and the second most common dietary form of vitamin E, is found in sunflower and safflower oils. Vitamin E is absorbed in the duodenum via micelle-dependent diffusion. Similar to other fat-soluble vitamins, its use depends on the presence of dietary fat and sufficient biliary and pancreatic function. Vitamin E in the form of supplements is usually found in esterified forms (which can be more stable) but is absorbed only after hydrolysis by duodenal esterases [70].

In patients with evidence of fat malabsorption and/or those receiving cholestyramine treatment, risk for potential vitamin E deficiency is increased. Currently, the RDA for vitamin E is quantified in terms of α-tocopherol equivalents (α-TEs); 1 mg of α-tocopherol is defined as one α-TE. Typical recommendation for adults (both male/female) is 15 mg/day of α-tocopherol (or 15 α-TE). Clinical manifestations suggestive of vitamin E deficiency can include the neuromuscular, vascular, and reproductive systems, including impaired vibratory and position sensation, changes in balance and coordination, muscle weakness, loss of deep tendon reflexes and visual disturbances [70, 71].

There have been three studies to date looking at vitamin E status in IBD patients. The cohorts used were heterogeneous, with one only including CD patients [63] one with only UC [72] and one study which combined UC and CD patients [22]. Of these three studies, only the study of CD patients found a significantly lower serum vitamin E level, compared with controls, and this difference appeared irrespective of disease activity. Given the very scant data available on vitamin E deficiency in IBD, there are no current recommendations on monitoring and replacement of vitamin E. However, in patients with suggestive symptoms for possible deficiency, particularly CD patients with significant fat malabsorption, low-dose supplementation

(15 mg/day) for a limited period may be warranted. Regular interval monitoring of vitamin E level is recommended during supplementation in order to prevent toxicity.

Vitamin K

Vitamin K is a fat-soluble vitamin that exists in two major forms: (1) phylloquinones, which are primarily synthesized by green plants and (2) menaquinones, which are derived mainly from bacteria. Dietary phylloquinones are absorbed by an energy-dependent process in the small intestine while the menaquinones are absorbed in the small intestine and colon by passive diffusion [73]. Like the other fat-soluble vitamins, absorption depends on a minimum amount of dietary fat and on bile salts and pancreatic juices. Good dietary sources of vitamin K include green vegetables (collards, spinach, salad greens, broccoli), brussel sprouts, cabbage, plant oils, and margarine. Because of a lack of data on optimal vitamin K need, the DRI does not provide an RDA but rather than "Adequate Intake" value for vitamin K (an observed mean value of what a group of "healthy persons" was noted to consume—which is 90 µg/day (women) to 120 µg (for men)) [11].

Vitamin K serves an important function in both skeletal bone health and normal blood clotting. Vitamin K is a known cofactor for posttranslational γ-carboxylation of multiple proteins, including blood coagulation factors as well as osteocalcin (OC), a regulator of bone mineral maturation [74, 75]. Osteocalcin is produced by osteoblasts and requires γ-carboxylation in order to bind calcium. Under conditions of vitamin K deficiency, OC remains uncarboxylated and is transferred into the circulation. Serum uncarboxylated osteocalcin (percent or total) reflects vitamin K status in the bone and is often used as an indirect measure of total vitamin K stores. The other method of measuring vitamin K status is serum phylloquinone levels, although levels can be influenced by recent dietary intake and triglyceride levels [75, 76]. The lack of a single reliable and direct method of vitamin K status is a principle limitation in interpretation of studies on this vitamin's importance in bone health.

There have been several large epidemiological studies, including one that used the Nurses' Health Study cohort and another the Framingham cohort, which demonstrate that low dietary intake of vitamin K appears to be associated with osteoporotic fracture risk and low BMD [75–77]. However, studies correlating biochemical measures of vitamin K (uncarboxylated osteocalcin level or serum phylloquinone levels) with bone disease have been less consistent, with some studies showing an association while others do not [78–80]. This likely reflects either limitations of current tests of vitamin K status, or a weak association between vitamin K status and bone disease.

In the general population, vitamin K deficiency is rare, but patients with malabsorptive disorders or who have been on chronic or frequent antibiotics may be at increased risk. Within the IBD literature, there have been relatively few studies addressing vitamin K status. The earliest study utilized abnormal prothrombin antigen assay as a surrogate measure of vitamin K status, and found that in an IBD cohort (17 CD/1 UC), 31 % were vitamin K-deficient [73]. There have been two more recent studies that measured serum uncarboxylated osteocalcin levels in CD patients and found levels to be significantly lower compared with controls [81] and with UC patients [82, 83]. Although these studies were too small to perform subgroup analysis, there was a suggestion that vitamin K deficiency was more common in patients with active inflammation and more extensive small bowel involvement, suggesting malabsorption as a potential mechanism. There have been multiple studies showing that dietary intake of vitamin K is also significantly lower in IBD patients, even in patients with disease remission, compared with controls [9, 81].

While in older adults, low intake of vitamin K has been associated with increased incidence of hip fractures, currently there does not appear to be sufficient evidence to support the use of vitamin K supplements in IBD patients as a means to prevent or treat bone disease. While there have been no trials performed in the IBD population, there have been four randomized controlled trials of phylloquinone supplementation in elderly women and healthy controls. None of these showed increased BMD in >1 skeletal site [84–86]. There have been a few positive studies from Japan, in which menaquinone-4 (a different form of vitamin K, naturally present in natto, a fermented soybean product common in Japan) at doses of 45 mg/day appeared to be more effective at improving BMD and decreased fracture risk [87, 88]. However, these studies lacked sufficient sample size and many were not placebo-controlled, so further prospective studies need to be performed.

In summary, there is evidence that inadequate dietary vitamin K may increase risk of bone disease, although this may not be adequately reflected in current measurements of vitamin K. Because of malabsorption and dietary restrictions, IBD patients may be at risk for vitamin K deficiency. There is limited evidence suggesting vitamin K deficiency may contribute to bone disease, especially in those with normal vitamin D status, although currently there is insufficient evidence to recommend oral vitamin K supplements. Rather, since vitamin K is found in large amounts in green leafy vegetables (typically at levels greater than 100 µg/100 g), increased dietary intake should be encouraged in all patients to improve bone health.

Vitamin C

Vitamin C, also known as ascorbic acid or L-ascorbic acid, is an important antioxidant in multiple tissues and also serves as a cofactor in multiple enzymatic reactions, including collagen synthesis. With respect to wound healing, vitamin C is also important, as it supports angiogenesis and regulates neutrophil activity [23].

Vitamin C cannot be synthesized intrinsically due to lack of the enzyme L-gulonolactone oxidase in humans. The RDA for vitamin C intake is 75 mg for women and 90 mg for men. Fruits and vegetables are the best dietary sources of vitamin C, particularly citrus fruits, tomatoes, and potatoes. Vitamin C is absorbed from the diet in the jejunum by active transport and passive diffusion. Once absorbed, vitamin C is concentrated primarily in its oxidized form (dehydroascorbic acid) in many vital organs, including the adrenals, brain, and eye [11].

In the general population, significant vitamin C deficiency is rare. Severe vitamin C deficiencies can result in clinical scurvy, which is characterized by bleeding gums, hemarthroses, and poor wound healing. Less severe deficiency, as measured by subnormal serum vitamin C levels, have been reported to be relatively common in IBD [21, 22]. This is most likely due to low dietary intake, which has been shown in several IBD cohort studies to be quite common [5, 15].

Vitamin C status is typically assessed by measuring plasma vitamin C levels. Other measures, such as leukocyte vitamin C concentration, could be more accurate indicators of tissue vitamin C levels, but are not yet readily available in commercial laboratories [89]. Vitamin C deficiency should also be suspected in patients with easy bruising, gingival bleeding, and enlargement and hyperkeratosis of the hair follicles. In IBD patients with vitamin C deficiency, higher dose of supplementation at 100–200 mg/day may be needed. Higher-dose vitamin C may also be helpful for those with acute wound healing needs, including fistulas or recent surgery [23]. One special consideration should be made for IBD patients who are smokers. Because of the lower concentrations of ascorbic acid in this population, it has been recommended that smokers increase their intake by an additional 35 mg/day.

Macrominerals

Calcium

Calcium is the most abundant mineral in the human body, with average body stores of 1–2 kg, 99 % of which is in the skeleton and teeth. Serum calcium level is maintained within a narrow range of 8.8–10.8 mg/dL, of which the ionized calcium concentrations range from 4.4 to 5.2 mg/dL, since both hypocalcemia and hypercalcemia have significant physiologic effects. Extracellular calcium is normally regulated in a narrow range by the combined actions of calcitonin and parathyroid hormone, which in turn regulates the activity of the vitamin D system, the main inducer of active calcium absorption in the intestine [90].

Intestinal absorption of calcium primarily occurs in the duodenum and proximal jejunum. Calcium absorption occurs by two mechanisms: (1) an unregulated paracellular route, which largely depends on dietary intake and luminal calcium concentration and (2) an active intracellular route via calcium channels, the transcription of which is dependent on vitamin-1,25OH D (1,25-OHD). In addition, calcium is secreted in the distal small bowel (distal jejunum and ileum) as well as in the colon by unclear mechanisms. Intestinal calcium losses are likely aggravated by diarrhea and malabsorption, although the extent has not been well studied [90].

Surprisingly little is known about the extent to which active small bowel inflammation can directly affect calcium absorption and impact risk for osteoporosis. This is difficult to study, given that calcium absorption is interdependent on vitamin D, a micronutrient which is insufficient in a large proportion of IBD patients, as discussed elsewhere. Further, calcium malabsorption is known to be exacerbated by magnesium deficiency (can occur with diarrhea) and glucocorticoids, which causes decreased absorption of calcium from both the intestine and kidney. In addition to malabsorption, several studies have demonstrated that as many as 80–86 % of IBD patients have inadequate daily dietary calcium intake [5, 15]. This is not surprising, since avoidance of milk and other dairy products is quite common in IBD patients, due to rates of concomitant lactose intolerance of 70–90 % [90].

Adequate calcium intake is recommended in most patients with IBD, at doses of 1000–1500 mg/day (1000 mg for women age 25 until menopause and men <65 years old; 1300 mg for women between 18 and 25 years; 1500 mg for post-menopausal women, and men >65 years old). For patients unable to tolerate dairy products, dark green leafy vegetables such as kale, collards, turnip greens, and broccoli as well as almonds, sardines, and canned salmon are recommended. For IBD patients unable to meet dietary calcium goals, calcium supplements are widely available.

There have been relatively few studies evaluating the efficacy of calcium alone or combined with vitamin D supplementation. However, from two observational cohorts, it did appear that calcium at doses of 1000 mg with nontreatment doses of vitamin D may have resulted in a slight improvement in BMD after 1 year, although no change in the incidence of fractures was seen [91]. In general, however, calcium supplementation alone is probably not sufficient to prevent bone loss in IBD patients, especially those with significant glucocorticoid exposure [92, 93], so bisphosphonate medications may be needed for clinically significant bone loss.

Magnesium

Magnesium is the fourth most abundant cation in the body and plays a fundamental role in most cellular reactions, mainly as a cofactor in enzymatic reactions involving ATP. In addition, 50–60 % of the body's magnesium is incorporated in the hydroxy-apatite crystal of bone and may be important in bone cell activity. The efficiency of absorption of magnesium ranges from 35 to 45 %, typically absorbed along the length of the small intestine, particularly in the jejunum. Once in circulation, approximately half the magnesium in plasma is free; approximately one-third is bound to albumin while the rest is complexed with citrate, phosphate, or other anions. Homeostasis of magnesium homeostasis is regulated by intestinal absorption and renal excretion [94].

There have been several epidemiological studies suggesting that dietary magnesium and hypomagnesemia may be weakly associated with osteoporosis [94, 95]. The mechanisms for magnesium deficiency on bone disease are not clear. In cell culture and animal models, magnesium has a mitogenic role on osteoblasts and deficiency of this cation leads to a decrease in osteoblastic activity. Likely more important, however, is the influence that magnesium balance has on calcium homeostasis. Magnesium deficiency is known to induce hypocalcemia, via impaired parathyroid gland function and inappropriately low PTH levels, which leads to lower intestinal calcium absorption [95]. Hypokalemia is also commonly observed in hypomagnesemic patients, occurring in 40–60 % of cases [96]. This is likely due to underlying disorders that cause both magnesium and potassium loss, such as diarrhea or malabsorption.

Magnesium deficiency is a growing problem in the Western world, with 32 % of Americans failing to meet US recommended daily allowance (RDA) [97]. IBD patients appear to be at increased risk of magnesium deficiency, with rates reported in 13–88 % of patients [98, 99]. Deficiency is likely due to a combination of decreased dietary intake [9, 99], losses from chronic diarrhea and fistula output [98], and malabsorption [98]. Clinical manifestation of magnesium deficiency includes neuromuscular hyperexcitability such as tremor and weakness, cardiovascular manifestations including widening of the QRS, and other mineral and hormone imbalance hypocalcemia, hypokalemia, and hypoparathyroidism.

Magnesium status is generally assessed by random serum magnesium levels, although these levels do not accurately reflect total body stores of magnesium as they may remain constant despite a wide range of intake levels. Leukocyte magnesium content is a much more sensitive test of nutritional status. Alternatively, 24-h urinary magnesium is quite accurate in determining total body stores, though burdensome for patients to complete. Magnesium screening and supplementation should be considered in all patients with significant diarrhea (>300 g/day), while diarrheal symptoms are active [97].

For patient with minimal food restriction, good dietary sources include seeds, nuts, legumes, and milled cereal grains, as well as dark green vegetables. For IBD patient requiring supplementation, most oral magnesium formulations can exacerbate diarrhea, although magnesium heptogluconate (Magnesium-Rougier) or magnesium pyroglutamate (Mag 2) may be better tolerated, especially if mixed with oral rehydration solution and sipped throughout the day oral magnesium (Magnesium-Rougier) or magnesium pyroglutamate (Mag 2) may be better tolerated, especially if mixed with oral rehydration solution and sipped throughout the day. The total dose of elemental magnesium required to ensure normal serum magnesium varies between 5 and 20 mmol/day [100].

Iron

Iron deficiency is the leading cause of anemia in the IBD population, present in 36–90 % of patients [101, 102]. The clinical significance, diagnosis, and treatment of iron deficiency in IBD cohorts are discussed elsewhere in a separate chapter.

Trace Elements

Zinc

Zinc is an abundant trace mineral widely distributed in different organs, with high concentrations in the kidney, liver, muscle, bone, pancreas, hair, and skin. Zinc is an essential mineral, required for catalytic activity of ≈100 enzymes, including metalloproteinases, and is also important in immune function, protein and collagen synthesis, and wound healing. Zinc is absorbed along the length of the small intestine by a poorly characterized transport mechanism [103]. Typically, good dietary sources of zinc can be found in meats, poultry, and milk. In addition, since many breads and cereal-based products are currently fortified with zinc, zinc deficiency is not common in the general population.

Zinc deficiency is thought to be relatively common in patients with chronic diarrhea, malabsorption, and hypermetabolic states. In IBD patients, a number of studies have reported low plasma zinc levels in IBD patients [5, 15]. These results are difficult to interpret, given that very little zinc is present in the serum, so this is likely a poor measure of zinc status. There have been several historical studies reporting that clinical symptoms of zinc deficiency (acrodermatitis, poor taste acuity) were not uncommon especially in CD [2], although more recent assessments of the incidence of subclinical zinc deficiency among IBD cohorts are not well characterized. Clinicians should also observe for other signs of possible zinc deficiency—including mild anemia, hair and skin changes, hypogeusia, and poor wound healing [103].

The current RDA recommendation for zinc intake is 11 mg/day for men and 8 mg/day for women. It has been suggested that for patients with significant diarrhea (>300 g of stool/day), additional zinc supplementation is reasonable with 25–50 mg of elemental zinc [103]. Unless patients have severe ongoing diarrhea, such doses should not be given for longer than 2–3 weeks as excess zinc can interfere with iron and copper absorption and can lead to deficiency of these important minerals.

To enhance wound healing, zinc supplementation of 40 mg of elemental zinc (176 mg zinc sulfate) for 10 days has been suggested [23, 103]. Zinc comes in two major forms: zinc sulfate (contains 23 % elemental zinc, so that 220 mg zinc sulfate contains 50 mg elemental zinc) and zinc gluconate (contains 14.3 % elemental zinc; 10 mg zinc gluconate contains 1.43 mg elemental zinc). One must also be careful to monitor calcium and folic acid consumption with zinc, since high intake calcium or folic acid can reduce zinc absorption. Conversely, high doses of zinc can impair absorption of iron from ferrous sulfate if a patient is also concomitantly being treated for iron deficiency anemia.

Selenium

Selenium is a necessary component of vital enzymes with antioxidant function, including glutathione peroxidase and thioredoxin reductase. In animal models, selenium has been associated with reduced risk of cancer, including colorectal cancer [104, 105], although human epidemiological data are mixed [106].

A narrow dietary intake range exists for selenium; current RDA is 55 µg/day for both men and women. Seafoods and organ meats are the richest food sources of selenium. Other sources include muscle meats, cereals and other grains, and dairy products. With prolonged low intake of selenium, symptoms associated with deficiency can manifest in form of joint pain in mild disease, and cardiomyopathy when severe. Minimal dietary intake of approximately 40 µg of selenium per day seems to be necessary to maintain glutathione peroxidase (GSH-Px), an enzyme containing selenium [105].

Absorption of selenium is poorly understood, but is believed to occur most avidly in the ileum, followed by the jejunum and large intestine. There have been five studies to date, in which selenium levels were found to be significantly lower in both UC and CD patients, compared with controls [25–27]. This observation was seen irrespective of disease activity and/or location. The exact prevalence of true selenium deficiency was not obtainable from these studies, as most only reported mean selenium levels, which can vary widely without accurately reflecting true body selenium storage.

More recently, it has been suggested that selenium status may be better assessed by measuring selenium or GSH-Px in serum, platelets, and erythrocytes and/or in whole blood. Erythrocyte selenium measurement is an indicator of long-term intake. Since no studies have yet to assess these new biomarkers, currently there is no evidence to support checking for or repleting selenium deficiency in IBD patients. The exception to this is in patients on long-term total parenteral nutrition (TPN). Selenium is now routinely added to TPN, often in premixed commercial trace element concentrates (often also including zinc, copper, manganese, and chromium). Updated guidelines from the American Society of Parenteral or Enteral Nutrition (A.S.P.E.N.) recommend that 20–60 µg daily be supplemented in TPN.

Copper

Copper is a trace element that has diverse roles in biological electron transport and oxygen transportation. Because of large stores of copper in the liver, muscle, and bone, deficiency is relatively rare. Copper absorption is tightly controlled, with absorption occurring in the small intestine. Entry at the mucosal surface is by facilitated diffusion, and exit across the basolateral membrane is primarily by active transport [26].

There have been several small studies that have addressed copper status in IBD patients, with equivocal results. While a recent study of CD patients in remission reported that serum copper was found to be low in up to 84 % of patients [5], two other studies have failed to show this. In several studies of UC patients, serum copper was found to be similar to controls in one study, and elevated in UC patients in two studies [27]. However, one must be careful in interpreting these results. Since copper does not exist as a free ion in the body, 90 % of the copper in serum is incorporated into ceruloplasmin, a functional enzyme at the erythrocyte-forming cells of the bone marrow. The remaining 10 % of copper is bound loosely to albumin. This highlights the limitation of serum copper and ceruloplasmin in determining body copper stores, as both may also be acute phase reactants. Serum copper may also be falsely decreased with certain renal diseases, with prolonged inflammation, and due to increased iron or zinc intake [106].

An RDA of 900 μg/day of copper is recommended for adults of both genders. Copper is widely available in animal products, including organ and muscle meats, chocolate, nuts, and cereal grains. Fruits and vegetables contain little copper. Currently, there are no recommended screening or supplementation guidelines for copper, other than in TPN. Guidelines from A.S.P.E.N. recommend that 0.3–0.5 mg daily be supplemented in TPN. Copper is normally excreted in bile, so lower doses should be utilized in patients with cholestasis (i.e., PSC with elevated bilirubin).

Chromium

Chromium is a trace mineral with function including potentiation of insulin action and regulation of lipid and protein metabolism. Chromium potentiates insulin action and influences carbohydrate, lipid, and protein metabolism. Chromium can exist in several valency states, with trivalent chromium being the only biologically active form and an important regulator of insulin action. As with other minerals, organic and inorganic forms of chromium are absorbed differently. Less than 2 % of the trivalent chromium consumed is absorbed [11]. In animal studies, chromium absorption was shown to be increased by oxalate intake and is higher in iron-deficient animals than in animals with adequate iron, suggesting that it shares some similarities with the iron absorption pathway.

Chromium deficiency is rare and has been reported mainly in patients on long-term TPN who presented with glucose intolerance and neuropathy, both of which were reversed with addition of chromium to TPN. Currently, A.S.P.E.N. recommends 10–15 g of chromium is added daily to TPN.

Manganese

Manganese is an essential trace element required as a catalytic cofactor for multiple enzymatic reactions. Manganese is absorbed throughout the small intestine, with iron competing for common binding sites for absorption. Good food sources include whole grains, legumes, nuts, and tea [11].

There have been virtually no cases of clinically significant manganese deficiency reported in the literature, so assessing manganese status is not necessary for IBD patients. The only exception to this is in patients on long-term TPN, in which manganese toxicity is an increasingly important problem. This is especially problematic in patients with chronic liver disease and/or cholestasis, as manganese is primarily excreted in bile. Manganese toxicity is associated with liver injury as well as neurotoxicity. The 2004 guidelines put forth by A.S.P.E.N. recommended lower doses of manganese (0.04–0.1 mg) than previous guidelines. However, there have been several studies demonstrating that even at these lower doses, whole-blood manganese levels was elevated in 82–93 % of long-term TPN patients. This may be due to the fact that most TPN formulas contain high levels of manganese contaminants and commercial trace element mixtures contain excessive manganese.

Conclusions

IBD has classically been associated with malnutrition and weight loss, although this has become less common with advances in treatment and greater proportions of patients attaining clinical remission. However, micronutrient deficiencies are still relatively common, particularly in CD patients with active small bowel disease and/ or multiple resections.

Micronutrient deficiencies are associated with several important extraintestinal complications of IBD. Anemia is the most common of these complications, and can be due to iron, vitamin B12, folate, zinc, or vitamin A deficiencies. Abnormal bone metabolism, manifesting as osteopenia or osteoporosis, can be due to inadequate intake of calcium, vitamin D, magnesium, and possibly vitamin K and vitamin B12. IBD patients have an increased incidence of venous thromboembolism, which may be due at least partly to hyperhomocysteinemic states induced by folate, vitamin B12, or pyridoxine deficiencies.

The goal of advancing nutritional therapy in IBD is to recognize and treat these complications earlier, so as to decrease morbidity and prevent long-term sequelae. Unfortunately, there are no guidelines about the timing and frequency we should be assessing micronutrient status in IBD patients. Clearly, in the presence of clinical symptoms, evaluating micronutrient status and treating deficiencies is indicated (Tables 5.4 and 5.5).

In certain high-risk populations, it may make sense to empirically supplement for a specific time period, as there is some evidence that doing so can improve outcomes or prevent complications.

Some of the more common situations are listed below (Table 5.6):

Table 5.5 Clinical manifestations and workup of micronutrient deficiency [9, 16, 106]

Clinical situation	Diagnostic testing
Anemia	Iron studies (ferritin with adjusted ranges for disease status, Transferrin, % transferrin saturation)
	Folate status (RBC folate>serum folate, homocysteine)
	B12 status (serum B12, methylmalonic acid)
	Consider zinc and serum vitamin A (serum retinol and retinol binding protein) in patients with diarrhea and malabsorption
Osteopenia/osteoporosis	Vitamin D status (vitamin 25=OH level) with goal>30
	Consider vitamin K status (serum uncarboxylated osteocalcin) Dietary evaluation of sufficient calcium, magnesium, vit K intake
Thromboembolism	Homocysteine, RBC folate, serum B12
Neuropathy	B12 status (serum B12, methylmalonic acid, B6 status (Plasma Pyridoxal-5-phosphate [PLP] level))
Dermatitis	Zinc status (dietary assessment, serum zinc); B6 status (PLP level)

Table 5.6 Empiric micronutrient supplementation in high-risk groups

Clinical situation	Empiric supplementation
• All IBD patients	Calcium 1000–1500 mg/day, Vit D 600–2000 IU/day (2–3× higher in obese patients or patients on glucocorticoids) [92, 107]
• Treatment with MTX or Sulfasalazine • Pregnancy	Folate 1 mg/day for as long as on drug or until delivery [18, 46]
• Terminal ileal resection >60 cm	Vitamin B12 1000 µg IM for life [17, 43]
• Shorter TI resections, severe ileitis • Elderly IBD patients	Higher-dose oral B12 supplements of 1000–2000 µg/day [17, 43]
• Significant diarrhea (>300 g/day)	Magnesium (300–400 mg/d) [98–100]
	Zinc gluconate 20–40 mg/day
• Steatorrea, severe PSC with cholestasis	Vitamin D 20,000–40000 IU/day [107]
	Vit A 5000–10,000 IU/day [20, 22]
	B12 1000–2000 µg/day [17, 43]
• Fistulas, nonhealing wounds	Zinc sulfate 220 mg BID × 2–4 weeks [103]
• Perioperative patients on steroids	Vitamin A 10,000 IU/day × 3–5 days [20–22]
	Vitamin C 100 mg/day [23, 89]

Table 5.7 Screening for micronutrient deficiencies in asymptomatic patients [9, 106]

All IBD patients	Annual ferritin, % iron sat, RBC folate, vitamin D-25OH
Ileal CD and elderly	Annual vitamin B12

Finally, in lower-risk patients (mild disease, in remission), recommendations for nutritional screening is even less clear. However, based on the current literature it does appear that certain micronutrients may still be commonly deficient in patients in remission, we generally recommend (Table 5.7).

While nutrition is one of the most common concerns of patients with IBD, the literature remains inadequate with respect to clear guidelines for micronutrient monitoring and supplementation. The above recommendations are based on currently available data. These will likely change over time based on ongoing studies, but currently can serve as a useful tool for clinicians to apply in their practice.

References

1. Mekhjian HS, Switz DM, Melnyk CS, et al. Clinical features and natural history of Crohn's disease. Gastroenterology. 1979;77(4):898–906.
2. Harries AD, Heatley RV. Nutritional disturbances in Crohn's disease. Postgrad Med J. 1983;59:690–7.
3. Dawson AM. Nutritional disturbances in Crohn's disease. Br J Surg. 1972;59:817–9.

4. Dawson AM. Nutritional disturbances in Crohn's disease. Proc R Soc Med. 1971;64: 166–70.
5. Filippi J, Al-Jaouni R, Wiroth JB, et al. Nutritional deficiencies in patients with Crohn's disease in remission. Inflamm Bowel Dis. 2006;12:185–91.
6. Aghdassi E, Wendland BE, Stapleton M, et al. Adequacy of nutritional intake in a Canadian population of patients with Crohn's disease. J Am Diet Assoc. 2007;107:1575–80.
7. Jahnsen J, Falch JA, Mowinckel P, et al. Body composition in patients with inflammatory bowel disease: a population-based study. Am J Gastroenterol. 2003;98:1556–62.
8. Valentini L, Schaper L, Buning C, et al. Malnutrition and impaired muscle strength in patients with Crohn's disease and ulcerative colitis in remission. Nutrition. 2008;24:694–702.
9. Sousa Guerreiro C, Cravo M, Costa AR, et al. A comprehensive approach to evaluate nutritional status in Crohn's patients in the era of biologic therapy: a case-control study. Am J Gastroenterol. 2007;102:2551–6.
10. Hass DJ, Brensinger CM, Lewis JD, et al. The impact of increased body mass index on the clinical course of Crohn's disease. Clin Gastroenterol Hepatol. 2006;4:482–8.
11. Institute of Medicine of the National Academy of Sciences, Food and Nutrition Board. Dietary reference intakes: the essential guide to nutrient requirements. Washington, DC: National Academies Press; 2006. p. 542.
12. Institute of Medicine of the National Academy of Sciences, Food and Nutrition Board. Dietary reference intakes for calcium and vitamin D. Washington, DC: National Academies Press; 2006. p. 1116.
13. Wallace TC, McBurney M, Fulgoni III VL. Multivitamin/mineral supplement contribution to micronutrient intakes in the United States, 2007–2010. J Am Coll Nutr. 2014;33(2):94–102.
14. Braegger CP, MacDonald TT. Immune mechanisms in chronic inflammatory bowel disease. Ann Allergy. 1994;72(2):135–41.
15. Vagianos K, Bernstein CN. Homocysteinemia and B vitamin status among adult patients with inflammatory bowel disease: a one-year prospective follow-up study. Inflamm Bowel Dis. 2012;18(4):718–24.
16. Weiss G, Gasche C. Pathogenesis and treatment of anemia in inflammatory bowel disease. Haematologica. 2010;95:175–8.
17. Duerksen DR, Fallows G, Bernstein CN. Vitamin B12 malabsorption in patients with limited ileal resection. Nutrition. 2006;22:1210–3.
18. Hoffbrand AV, Stewart JS, Booth CC, et al. Folate deficiency in Crohn's disease: incidence, pathogenesis, and treatment. Br Med J. 1968;2:71–5.
19. Van Gossum A, Cabre E, Hebuterne X, et al. ESPEN guidelines on parenteral nutrition: gastroenterology. Clin Nutr. 2009;28:415–27.
20. D'Ambrosio DN, Clugston RD, Blaner WS. Vitamin A metabolism: an update. Nutrients. 2011;3(1):63–103.
21. D'Odorico A, Bortolan S, Cardin R, et al. Reduced plasma antioxidant concentrations and increased oxidative DNA damage in inflammatory bowel disease. Scand J Gastroenterol. 2001;36:1289–94.
22. Hengstermann S, Valentini L, Schaper L, et al. Altered status of anti-oxidant vitamins and fatty acids in patients with inactive inflammatory bowel disease. Clin Nutr. 2008;27:571–8.
23. Sinno S, Lee DS, Khachemoune A. Vitamins and cutaneous wound healing. J Wound Care. 2011;20:287–93.
24. Hodges P, Gee M, Grace M, et al. Vitamin and iron intake in patients with Crohn's disease. J Am Diet Assoc. 1984;84:52–8.
25. Sturniolo GC, Mestriner C, Lecis PE, et al. Altered plasma and mucosal concentrations of trace elements and antioxidants in active ulcerative colitis. Scand J Gastroenterol. 1998; 33:644–9.
26. Ringstad J, Kildebo S, Thomassen Y. Serum selenium, copper, and zinc concentrations in Crohn's disease and ulcerative colitis. Scand J Gastroenterol. 1993;28:605–8.
27. Fernandez-Banares F, Mingorance MD, Esteve M, et al. Serum zinc, copper, and selenium levels in inflammatory bowel disease: effect of total enteral nutrition on trace element status. Am J Gastroenterol. 1990;85:1584–9.

28. den Heijer M, Rosendaal FR, Blom HJ, et al. Hyperhomocysteinemia and venous thrombosis: a meta-analysis. Thromb Haemost. 1998;80:874–7.
29. Cleophas TJ, Hornstra N, van Hoogstraten B, et al. Homocysteine, a risk factor for coronary artery disease or not? A meta-analysis. Am J Cardiol. 2000;86:1005–9.
30. Cattaneo M, Vecchi M, Zighetti ML, et al. High prevalence of hyperchomocysteinemia in patients with inflammatory bowel disease: a pathogenic link with thromboembolic complications? Thromb Haemost. 1998;80:542–5.
31. Mahmood A, Needham J, Prosser J, et al. Prevalence of hyperhomocysteinaemia, activated protein C resistance and prothrombin gene mutation in inflammatory bowel disease. Eur J Gastroenterol Hepatol. 2005;17:739–44.
32. Papa A, De Stefano V, Danese S, et al. Hyperhomocysteinemia and prevalence of polymorphisms of homocysteine metabolism-related enzymes in patients with inflammatory bowel disease. Am J Gastroenterol. 2001;96:2677–82.
33. Romagnuolo J, Fedorak RN, Dias VC, et al. Hyperhomocysteinemia and inflammatory bowel disease: prevalence and predictors in a cross-sectional study. Am J Gastroenterol. 2001; 96:2143–9.
34. Biasco G, Zannoni U, Paganelli GM, et al. Folic acid supplementation and cell kinetics of rectal mucosa in patients with ulcerative colitis. Cancer Epidemiol Biomarkers Prev. 1997; 6(6):469–71.
35. Giovannucci E, Rimm EB, Ascherio A, et al. Alcohol, low-methionine–low-folate diets, and risk of colon cancer in men. J Natl Cancer Inst. 1995;87:265–73.
36. Konings EJ, Goldbohm RA, Brants HA, et al. Intake of dietary folate vitamins and risk of colorectal carcinoma: results from the Netherlands cohort study. Cancer. 2002;95:1421–33.
37. Meyer F, White E. Alcohol and nutrients in relation to colon cancer in middle-aged adults. Am J Epidemiol. 1993;138:225–36.
38. Su LJ, Arab L. Nutritional status of folate and colon cancer risk: evidence from NHANES I epidemiologic follow-up study. Ann Epidemiol. 2001;11:65–72.
39. Lashner BA. Red blood cell folate is associated with the development of dysplasia and cancer in ulcerative colitis. J Cancer Res Clin Oncol. 1993;119:549–54.
40. Lashner BA, Heidenreich PA, Su GL, et al. Effect of folate supplementation on the incidence of dysplasia and cancer in chronic ulcerative colitis. A case-control study. Gastroenterology. 1989;97:255–9.
41. Lashner BA, Provencher KS, Seidner DL, et al. The effect of folic acid supplementation on the risk for cancer or dysplasia in ulcerative colitis. Gastroenterology. 1997;112:29–32.
42. Honein MA, Paulozzi LJ, Mathews TJ, et al. Impact of folic acid fortification of the US food supply on the occurrence of neural tube defects. JAMA. 2001;285:2981–6.
43. Yakut M, Ustun Y, Kabacam G, et al. Serum vitamin B12 and folate status in patients with inflammatory bowel diseases. Eur J Intern Med. 2010;21:320–3.
44. Fernandez-Banares F, Abad-Lacruz A, Xiol X, et al. Vitamin status in patients with inflammatory bowel disease. Am J Gastroenterol. 1989;84:744–8.
45. Vagianos K, Bector S, McConnell J, et al. Nutrition assessment of patients with inflammatory bowel disease. JPEN J Parenter Enteral Nutr. 2007;31:311–9.
46. Lindenbaum J. Drugs and vitamin B12 and folate metabolism. Curr Concepts Nutr. 1983;12:73–87.
47. McNulty H, Scott JM. Intake and status of folate and related B-vitamins: considerations and challenges in achieving optimal status. Br J Nutr. 2008;99 Suppl 3:S48–54.
48. Tominaga M, Iida M, Aoyagi K, Kohrogi N, Matsui T, Fujishima M. Red cell folate concentrations in patients with Crohn's disease on parenteral nutrition. Postgrad Med J. 1989;65(769):818–20.
49. Schernhammer ES, Ogino S, Fuchs CS. Folate and vitamin B6 intake and risk of colon cancer in relation to p53 expression. Gastroenterology. 2008;135:770–80.
50. Baars JE, Looman CW, Steyerberg EW, et al. The risk of inflammatory bowel disease-related colorectal carcinoma is limited: results from a nationwide nested case-control study. Am J Gastroenterol. 2011;106(2):319–28.

51. Subramanian V, Logan RF. Chemoprevention of colorectal cancer in inflammatory bowel disease. Best Pract Res Clin Gastroenterol. 2011;25(4–5):593–606.
52. Dhonukshe-Rutten RA, Lips M, de Jong N, Chin A, Paw MJ. Vitamin B-12 status is associated with bone mineral content and bone mineral density in frail elderly women but not in men. J Nutr. 2003;133(3):801–7.
53. Merriman NA, Putt ME, Metz DC, Yang YX. Hip fracture risk in patients with a diagnosis of pernicious anemia. Gastroenterology. 2010;138(4):1330–7.
54. Carmel R, Lau KH, Baylink DJ, Saxena S, Singer FR. Cobalamin and osteoblast-specific proteins. N Engl J Med. 1988;319(2):70–5.
55. Carmel R. Subtle and atypical cobalamin deficiency states. Am J Hematol. 1990;34:108–14.
56. Headstrom PD, Rulyak SJ, Lee SD. Prevalence of and risk factors for vitamin B12 deficiency in patients with Crohn's disease. Inflamm Bowel Dis. 2008;14:217–23.
57. Coull DB, Tait RC, Anderson JH, et al. Vitamin B12 deficiency following restorative procto-colectomy. Colorectal Dis. 2007;9:562–6.
58. Lenz K. The effect of the site of lesion and extent of resection on duodenal bile acid concentration and vitamin B12 absorption in Crohn's disease. Scand J Gastroenterol. 1975;10:241–8.
59. Thompson WG, Wrathell E. The relation between ileal resection and vitamin B12 absorption. Can J Surg. 1977;20:461–4.
60. Vidal-Alaball J, Butler CC, Cannings-John R, et al. Oral vitamin B12 versus intramuscular vitamin B12 for vitamin B12 deficiency. Cochrane Database Syst Rev. 2005;(3):CD004655.
61. Friso S, Jacques PF, Wilson PW, Rosenberg IH, Selhub J. Low circulating vitamin B(6) is associated with elevation of the inflammation marker C-reactive protein independently of plasma homocysteine levels. Circulation. 2001;103(23):2788–91.
62. Morris MS, Picciano MF, Jacques PF, Selhub J. Plasma pyridoxal 5'-phosphate in the US population: the National Health and Nutrition Examination Survey, 2003–2004. Am J Clin Nutr. 2008;87(5):1446–54.
63. Kuroki F, Iida M, Tominaga M, et al. Multiple vitamin status in Crohn's disease. Correlation with disease activity. Dig Dis Sci. 1993;38:1614–8.
64. Saibeni S, Cattaneo M, Vecchi M, et al. Low vitamin B6 plasma levels, a risk factor for thrombosis, in inflammatory bowel disease: role of inflammation and correlation with acute phase reactants. Am J Gastroenterol. 2003;98:112–7.
65. Costantini AI, Pala MI. Thiamine and fatigue in inflammatory bowel diseases: an open-label pilot study. J Altern Complement Med. 2013;19(8):704–8.
66. Crook MA. The importance of recognizing pellagra (niacin deficiency) as it still occurs. Nutrition. 2014;30(6):729–30.
67. Anstead GM. Steroids, retinoids, and wound healing. Adv Wound Care. 1998;11:277–85.
68. Sentongo TA, Semaeo EJ, Stettler N, et al. Vitamin D status in children, adolescents, and young adults with Crohn disease. Am J Clin Nutr. 2002;76:1077–81.
69. Leslie WD, Miller N, Rogala L, et al. Vitamin D status and bone density in recently diagnosed inflammatory bowel disease: the Manitoba IBD cohort study. Am J Gastroenterol. 2008;103:1451–9.
70. Herrera E, Barbas CJ. Vitamin E: action, metabolism and perspectives. Physiol Biochem. 2001;57(1):43–56.
71. Sokol RJ. Antioxidant defenses in metal-induced liver damage. Semin Liver Dis. 1996;16(1):39–47.
72. Ramakrishna BS, Varghese R, Jayakumar S, et al. Circulating antioxidants in ulcerative colitis and their relationship to disease severity and activity. J Gastroenterol Hepatol. 1997;12:490–4.
73. Krasinski SD, Russell RM, Furie BC, et al. The prevalence of vitamin K deficiency in chronic gastrointestinal disorders. Am J Clin Nutr. 1985;41:639–43.
74. Booth SL, Broe KE, Gagnon DR, Tucker KL, Hannan MT, McLean RR, et al. Vitamin K intake and bone mineral density in women and men. Am J Clin Nutr. 2003;77:512–6.

75. Macdonald HM, McGuigan FE, Lanham-New SA, Fraser WD, Ralston SH, Reid DM. Vitamin K1 intake is associated with higher bone mineral density and reduced bone resorption in early postmenopausal Scottish women: no evidence of gene-nutrient interaction with apolipoprotein E polymorphisms. Am J Clin Nutr. 2008;87:1513–20.
76. Booth SL, Broe KE, Peterson JW, Cheng DM, Dawson-Hughes B, Gundberg CM, et al. Associations between vitamin K biochemical measures and bone mineral density in men and women. J Clin Endocrinol Metab. 2004;89:4904–9.
77. Feskanich D, Weber P, Willett WC, Rockett H, Booth SL, Colditz GA. Vitamin K intake and hip fractures in women: a prospective study. Am J Clin Nutr. 1999;69:74–9.
78. Luukinen H, Kakonen SM, Pettersson K, et al. Strong prediction of fractures among older adults by the ratio of carboxylated to total serum osteocalcin. J Bone Miner Res. 2000;15:2473–8.
79. Szulc P, Arlot M, Chapuy MC, et al. Serum undercarboxylated osteocalcin correlates with hip bone mineral density in elderly women. J Bone Miner Res. 1994;9:1591–5.
80. Kawana K, Takahashi M, Hoshino H, et al. Circulating levels of vitamin K1, menaquinone-4, and menaquinone-7 in healthy elderly Japanese women and patients with vertebral fractures and patients with hip fractures. Endocr Res. 2001;27:337–43.
81. Duggan P, O'Brien M, Kiely M, et al. Vitamin K status in patients with Crohn's disease and relationship to bone turnover. Am J Gastroenterol. 2004;99:2178–85.
82. Kuwabara A, Tanaka K, Tsugawa N, et al. High prevalence of vitamin K and D deficiency and decreased BMD in inflammatory bowel disease. Osteoporos Int. 2009;20:935–9342.
83. Nakajima S, Iijima H, Egawa S, et al. Association of vitamin K deficiency with bone metabolism and clinical disease activity in inflammatory bowel disease. Nutrition. 2011;27:1023–8.
84. Fang Y, Hu C, Tao X, et al. Effect of vitamin K on bone mineral density: a meta-analysis of randomized controlled trials. J Bone Miner Metab. 2011;30:60–8.
85. Braam LA, Knapen MH, Geusens P, et al. Vitamin K1 supplementation retards bone loss in postmenopausal women between 50 and 60 years of age. Calcif Tissue Int. 2003;73:21–6.
86. Bolton-Smith C, McMurdo ME, Paterson CR, et al. Two-year randomized controlled trial of vitamin K1 (phylloquinone) and vitamin D3 plus calcium on the bone health of older women. J Bone Miner Res. 2007;22:509–19.
87. Shiraki M, Shiraki Y, Aoki C, et al. Vitamin K2 (menatetrenone) effectively prevents fractures and sustains lumbar bone mineral density in osteoporosis. J Bone Miner Res. 2000;15:515–21.
88. Iwamoto J, Matsumoto H, Takeda T. Efficacy of menatetrenone (vitamin K2) against non-vertebral and hip fractures in patients with neurological diseases: meta-analysis of three randomized, controlled trials. Clin Drug Investig. 2009;29:471–9.
89. Jacob RA, Sotoudeh G. Vitamin C function and status in chronic disease. Nutr Clin Care. 2002;5(2):66–74.
90. Bronner F. Mechanisms of intestinal calcium absorption. J Cell Biochem. 2003;88:387–93.
91. Shea B, Wells G, Cranney A, et al. Meta-analyses of therapies for postmenopausal osteoporosis. VII. Meta-analysis of calcium supplementation for the prevention of postmenopausal osteoporosis. Endocr Rev. 2002;23:552–9.
92. Bernstein CN, Seeger LL, Anton PA, et al. A randomized, placebo-controlled trial of calcium supplementation for decreased bone density in corticosteroid-using patients with inflammatory bowel disease: a pilot study. Aliment Pharmacol Ther. 1996;10:777–86.
93. von Tirpitz C, Klaus J, Steinkamp M, et al. Therapy of osteoporosis in patients with Crohn's disease: a randomized study comparing sodium fluoride and ibandronate. Aliment Pharmacol Ther. 2003;17:807–16.
94. Reginster JY, Strause L, Deroisy R, et al. Preliminary report of decreased serum magnesium in postmenopausal osteoporosis. Magnesium. 1989;8:106–9.
95. Rude RK, Gruber HE. Magnesium deficiency and osteoporosis: animal and human observations. J Nutr Biochem. 2004;15:710–6.

96. Whang R, Ryder KW. Frequency of hypomagnesemia and hypermagnesemia. Requested vs routine. JAMA. 1990;263(22):3063–4.
97. Krebs-Smith SM, Cleveland LE, Ballard-Barbash R, et al. Characterizing food intake patterns of American adults. Am J Clin Nutr. 1997;65(4 Suppl):1264S–8.
98. Hessov I. Magnesium deficiency in Crohn's disease. Clin Nutr. 1990;9:297–8.
99. Galland L. Magnesium and inflammatory bowel disease. Magnesium. 1988;7:78–83.
100. Jeejeebhoy KN. Clinical nutrition: management of nutritional problems of patients with Crohn's disease. CMAJ. 2002;166:913–8.
101. Gasche C, Lomer MC, Cavill I, et al. Iron, anaemia, and inflammatory bowel diseases. Gut. 2004;53:1190–7.
102. Kulnigg S, Gasche C. Systematic review: managing anaemia in Crohn's disease. Aliment Pharmacol Ther. 2006;24:1507–23.
103. Lansdown AB, Mirastschijski U, Stubbs N, et al. Zinc in wound healing: theoretical, experimental, and clinical aspects. Wound Repair Regen. 2007;15:2–16.
104. Finley JW, Davis CD, Feng Y. Selenium from high selenium broccoli protects rats from colon cancer. J Nutr. 2000;130:2384–9.
105. Lane HW, Medina D, Wolfe LG. Proposed mechanisms for selenium-inhibition of mammary tumorigenesis (review). In Vivo. 1989;3:151–60.
106. Geerling BJ, Badart-Smook A, Stockbrugger RW, et al. Comprehensive nutritional status in recently diagnosed patients with inflammatory bowel disease compared with population controls. Eur J Clin Nutr. 2000;54:514–21.
107. Jackson RD, LaCroix AZ, Gass M, et al. Calcium plus vitamin D supplementation and the risk of fractures. N Engl J Med. 2006;354:669–83.

Part III
Nutritional Treatment of Inflammatory Bowel Diseases

Chapter 6
Enteral Nutrition in the Treatment of Inflammatory Bowel Disease

Athos Bousvaros

Introduction

For over 30 years, exclusive enteral nutrition (EEN) has been utilized to treat Crohn's disease both in children and in adults. However, while EEN has gained widespread acceptance in Europe, Canada, and Japan, EEN treatment is not widely utilized in the USA. A study by Levine et al. demonstrated that approximately 60 % of European pediatric gastroenterologists utilize EEN, compared to approximately 4 % of their American counterparts [1]. The chapter below will review the evidence that EEN is effective in both adult and pediatric Crohn's disease. I will discuss the impact of EEN on clinical disease activity, biomarkers, and endoscopic healing. The chapter will also provide instruction on how to implement an EEN program, as well as the challenges one may face. The advantages and disadvantages of this form of treatment in Crohn's disease are listed in Table 6.1. The chapter will focus almost exclusively on the treatment of Crohn's disease, as there is no evidence that EEN brings about a remission in ulcerative colitis. The reader is also referred to the excellent North American Society for Pediatric Gastroenterology, Hepatology and Nutrition (NASPGHAN) clinical report on use of EEN to treat pediatric Crohn's disease [2].

A. Bousvaros, M.D., M.P.H. (✉)
Division of Gastroenterology and Nutrition, Harvard Medical School, Boston Children's Hospital, 300 Longwood Avenue, Boston, MA 02115, USA
e-mail: Athos.bousvaros@childrens.harvard.edu

© Springer International Publishing Switzerland 2016
A.N. Ananthakrishnan (ed.), *Nutritional Management of Inflammatory Bowel Diseases*, DOI 10.1007/978-3-319-26890-3_6

Table 6.1 Advantages and disadvantages of enteral nutrition therapy in inflammatory bowel disease

Advantages
Reduces disease activity
Reduces biomarkers of inflammation (sedimentation rate, fecal calprotectin)
May induce remission
Promotes weight gain
Promotes linear growth (in children)
Corrects micronutrient deficiencies
Reduces intestinal permeability
Steroid-sparing
Not immunosuppressive
Extensive experience for over 30 years, especially outside the USA
Disadvantages
May be less effective than corticosteroids, especially in adults
Usually used as a short-term induction treatment (6–12 weeks)
Limited evidence to support the use of EN as a maintenance therapy
No evidence of efficacy in ulcerative colitis
Less efficacy (though still effective) in colonic Crohn disease
Refeeding syndrome may occur
May need to be administered through nasogastric tube
Most efficacious when the patient does not eat during the induction period
Insurance may not pay
Requires large multidisciplinary team to effectively implement (including physician, nurse, registered dietician, possibly psychologist or social worker)

History

The development of EEN to treat pediatric Crohn's disease was actually preceded by encouraging preliminary data regarding home parenteral nutrition in Crohn's disease. In 1979, Strobel et al. published a case series of 17 children, age 9–20 years, who were placed on home parenteral nutrition for severe symptomatic Crohn's disease. At that time, the only readily available maintenance therapies for Crohn disease were sulfasalazine and corticosteroids. All patients had disease of their small intestine and/or colon, and many of them had complications including enterocutaneous fistulae and growth failure. The patients were placed on home parenteral nutrition with a dosage of 60–80 kcal per kilo and a daily home in volume of 3–4 L/day. The duration of remission in patients ranged from 15 days to 539 days. Benefits included fistula closure, reduction of corticosteroid dose, increase in serum albumin, improved growth, and improved nutritional status. Complications of parenteral nutrition use in this cohort included dislodgement, catheter infections, and zinc deficiency dermatitis [3].

Based on the encouraging results from home parenteral nutrition studies, Morin and colleagues published a case series in 1980 of four children who received a 6 week period of continuous enteral alimentation with elemental formula, and no concomitant treatment. Children were given approximately 80 cal per kilogram of body weight. One patient developed symptoms of bowel obstruction and underwent an ileocecectomy during the period of treatment. All children gained weight and height during treatment, and also developed reductions in the Crohn disease activity index. These children gained a mean of only 1.7 cm of height in the 2 years prior to the enteral nutrition therapy. After 6 weeks of EEN, they gained a mean of approximately 5 kg in weight and 3 cm of height over the following 6 months. There was also improvement in mid-arm circumference and triceps skin fold thickness [4]. Subsequently, O'Morain and colleagues performed a randomized 4 week trial of exclusive enteral therapy with elemental formula vs. prednisolone (0.75 mg/kg/day) in 21 patients (mostly adults: age range 15–60), with active CD (mostly small and large bowel). The investigators reported comparable changes in clinical disease activity and sedimentation rate. Patients treated with steroids exhibited greater weight gain by 3 months, while those treated with elemental diet exhibited more improvement in hemoglobin and albumin [5]. Many additional open-label and randomized trials performed in the following decade continued to demonstrate efficacy of this enteral therapy. In 1995, Griffiths and colleagues performed a meta-analysis comprising 8 randomized trials, and including 413 patients. These trials included studies comparing one type of formula with another (e.g., elemental vs. polymeric), and formula compared to corticosteroids. All trials were small or medium sized, the largest being 107 patients [6]. The rates of clinical remission in the EEN groups ranged from 22 to 82 %, whereas in the corticosteroid group the rates of clinical remission ranged from 50 to 90 %. The meta-analysis concluded that enteral nutrition was inferior to corticosteroids at inducing remission (pooled odds ratio 0.35, 95 % confidence interval 0.23–0.53), but there was no difference between elemental and polymeric formula [7]. A subsequent meta-analysis suggested that EEN may be more effective in children than adults [8].

Biological Effects of Exclusive Enteral Nutrition Treatment

Reduced Intestinal Permeability

Intestinal permeability in inflammatory bowel disease can be assessed utilizing a number of assays. Most commonly, permeability is assayed by asking a patient to ingest a compound that is only partially absorbed across the epithelial barrier, and assessing absorption of that compound by measuring levels in the blood or urine. Compounds utilized to assess permeability include lactulose, polyethylene glycol, and chromium-labeled EDTA. Studies consistently demonstrate increased permeability (a.k.a. "leaky gut") in patients with active Crohn disease, but some studies also suggest increased permeability in inactive CD, as well as unaffected family members [9, 10]. In vitro, enteral nutrition may improve epithelial cell adhesion, reduce intestinal permeability to macromolecules by restoring epithelial cell continuity, and increase epithelial monolayer integrity [11, 12]. In vivo, CD patients treated with elemental diet demonstrate reduced intestinal permeability after 4 weeks of EEN [13].

Alteration of Intestinal Microbiota

Current evidence regarding the pathogenesis of inflammatory bowel disease suggests that IBD occurs when a genetically predisposed individual is exposed to potential environmental triggers, resulting in poorly controlled intestinal inflammation. Over 140 genes have been identified that either increase or decrease the risk of inflammatory bowel disease. The lack of a clear monogenic etiology in the majority of our patients suggests that environmental causes are central in the pathogenesis of IBD. Diet is an obvious environmental factor that is an ongoing and active topic of study with respect to the pathogenesis of IBD. Current studies suggest that breastfeeding may protect against the development of IBD. In addition, patients who consume greater amounts of meat fats, polyunsaturated fatty acids, and omega-6 fatty acids may have a higher incidence of inflammatory bowel disease. There are many animal models where modification of the diet may result in the development of inflammation in a genetically predisposed post [14, 15].

An underlying common pathway by which diet might affect the development of IBD in both animals and humans is via alteration of the intestinal microbiota [16]. Through high throughput sequencing methods, we are now able to analyze the microbiota of patients with chronic illness. Published data suggests that the microbial populations are significantly different in patients with and without IBD, both at the time of disease onset, and also during subsequent time periods. The microbiota can change rapidly, and alterations in diet (such as the institution of exclusive elemental nutrition) may result in the generation of a more beneficial, less inflammatory commensal flora [17]. Interestingly, one recent study suggests that EEN may actually reduce the levels of certain supposedly "protective" microbiota such as *Faecalibacterium prausnitzii* [18]. In summary, the research on how EEN affects intestinal microbiota is in its infancy. While changes in microbiota do correlate with changes in disease activity in IBD patients, it is unclear whether the microbial alterations precede the reduction of inflammation, or occur because of the reduction in inflammation.

Immunologic Effects

Enteral nutrition contains many micronutrients that may influence the development of the mucosal immune system. In particular, retinoic acid (derived from vitamin A) may play a critical role in the development of oral tolerance, and in the maintenance of the IgA mucosal barrier [19]. Vitamin D may also play a key role in the perpetuation of certain T-cell subsets that may mediate intestinal immune tolerance [19, 20]. However, given that vitamin supplementation alone does not appear to reduce IBD disease activity, there are probably other mechanisms by which EEN more directly affects the intestinal immune system. Experiments by Sanderson and colleagues suggest that EEN may both reduce antigen presentation by MHC class II cells and also reduce production of IL-6 by epithelial cell lines [21]. The precise molecular mechanisms by which EEN impacts inflammation at the cellular level have yet to be delineated.

Clinical Benefits of Exclusive Enteral Nutrition Therapy

Induction of Remission in Active Crohn Disease

Studies in both children and adults suggest that patients with active Crohn disease treated with EEN for 6–10 weeks may achieve remission from 60 to 80 % of the time [2, 22]. A Cochrane review comparing randomized trials of EEN to some other treatment (usually corticosteroids) demonstrated an odds ratio of 0.33 favoring EEN [23]. In the single most conclusive pediatric study, Borelli et al. randomized 37 children to receive either EEN therapy (exclusive polymeric diet, no other foods allowed) or a course of tapering corticosteroids for a 10 week period. Assessments performed at the beginning and the end of the trial included history, examination, assessment of clinical disease activity, blood sampling, and ileocolonoscopy. Both groups demonstrated similar improvements in the Pediatric Crohn disease activity index (from over 35 down to 10 points), C-reactive protein (from 10 to 3 mg/dL), and ESR (from 40 to 20 mm/h). However, at the end of the 10 weeks, the proportion of children with endoscopic improvement was greater in the EEN group (74 %) compared to the steroid group (33 %) [24].

Evidence suggests that EEN may not be as effective if children are allowed to eat during the induction period. In a study by Johnson and colleagues, 50 children were randomized to receive either EEN, or 50 % EN in addition to an unrestricted regular diet. While both groups reported improved well-being, 42 % of children in the EEN group entered remission, compared to only 15 % in the partial enteral nutrition group [25]. In contrast, Levine and colleagues performed an open-label intervention in 47 children and young adults consisting of 6 weeks of enteral nutrition in conjunction with a restricted diet. The restrictive diet excluded gluten, casein, and high fat foods, but allowed limited amounts of rice-based products, fresh chicken breast, carrots, tomatoes, and water. Packaged snacks, sodas, and candies were excluded. On this dietary intervention, remission rates (as measured by Harvey Bradshaw index and PCDAI) were obtained in approximately 70 % of children and adults. Between weeks 6 and 12, the diet was liberalized in a limited manner, and 80 % of the group in remission at 6 weeks was able to stay in remission. This study suggests that limited amounts of certain types of food may not impair the efficacy of EEN [26].

Maintenance of Remission in Crohn Disease

While the evidence supporting induction of remission in both children and adults with active Crohn disease is strong, the data supporting its use in maintenance therapy is far weaker. One of the limitations of using EEN as enteral treatment is the adherence to the medical recommendation. It is challenging for an adult, let alone a child, to forego eating for prolonged periods of time. For this reason, many centers utilize EEN as a steroid sparing "bridge" to some other maintenance treatment such as immunomodulators. In adults, Takagi et al. randomized 51 adult patients with CD in remission to either an unrestricted diet, or to a diet consisting of 50 % of required calories as EN + 50 % unrestricted diet. After 1 year, 64 % of patients in the unrestricted diet group had relapsed, compared to 35 % of the 50 % EN group [27].

A retrospective analysis of a protocol utilized at the Children's Hospital of Philadelphia also suggests that partial enteral nutrition may assist in maintaining remission in a subset of patients. Forty three children underwent induction with EN via nasogastric tube with continuous feedings given over 10–12 h, and for a period ranging from 8 to 12 weeks. Unlike EEN protocols, these patients were allowed to consume 10–20% of their calories as food on any given week. Clinicians utilized either polymeric, partially hydrolyzed, or elemental formulas depending on physician preference. Concomitant therapies, including immunomodulators, biologics, and aminosalicylates, were allowed. After the induction period, 65 % of patients had achieved clinical remission. Over a 6 month period, 29 children elected to continue with the nutritional therapy. Adverse effects included nausea, vomiting, diarrhea, difficulty sleeping with the nasogastric tube, and increased urination [28].

Improvement of Nutritional Status and Growth

Treatment with corticosteroids is associated with reduction of inflammation and an improved sense of well-being, but at a cost. As mentioned previously, mucosal inflammation persists despite corticosteroid treatment. Patients receiving steroids may gain weight and fat mass, but do not exhibit gains in muscle mass, bone density, and height velocity [29, 30]. For this reason, corticosteroid sparing agents (immunomodulators and biologics) are essential in the long-term treatment of most Crohn disease patients. Studies of medical therapy suggest that anti-TNF agents are most likely superior to thiopurines and methotrexate as maintenance agents, and might do a better job of promoting linear growth, acquisition of bone density and muscle mass [31, 32]. Enteral nutrition may also play a crucial role in treating growth failure, even if given periodically. In a study performed prior to the routine use of immunomodulators for treating Crohn disease, Belli et al. administered a continuous nasogastric infusion of an elemental formula to a group of adolescents with CD and growth failure. Patients were given 50 % of their caloric requirement as EN for 1 out of every 4 months for a period of 1 year. Patients grew 7 cm/year

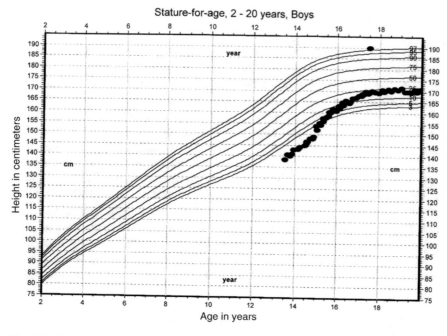

Fig. 6.1 Growth curve of a child treated with supplemental EN and biologics. The x axis represents age in years, and the y axis height in centimeters. The supplemental treatment was begun at the age of 14 years, 6 months, with increase in the patient's stature from below the third percentile to the 25 % by age 18 years

during their treatment year, compared to 2.9 cm/year in the year prior to their treatment. A comparison age matched control group only grew 1.7 cm during the period of observation [33]. Figure 6.1 demonstrates the impact of combined enteral nutrition and biologic treatment in a teenager who was not growing despite the use of immunomodulators as steroid sparing agents.

Improvement in Bone Health

Children and adults with IBD are at risk for osteopenia and osteoporosis. The causes of reduced bone density are multifactorial, and include: inflammation, reduced bone formation, increased bone resorption, hypovitaminosis D, prolonged corticosteroid therapy malnutrition, and physical inactivity [34]. Enteral nutrition therapy has been shown to improve bone formation and reduce bone resorption (as measured by C-terminal telopeptides of type 1 collagen) [35]. In addition to reducing disease activity, EN may improve bone mass by providing supplemental calcium and vitamin D [36].

Effects on Quality of Life

While the effects of EN on physical health are apparent (including reduction of inflammation, reduction of steroids dosage, and improved linear growth), the effects of quality of life in children and adults with IBD are less well studied. Quality of life is a holistic measure, encompassing not only physical but also psychological measures of well-being. Approximately 25 % of adolescents with IBD have symptoms of anxiety or depression, and may benefit from psychological interventions like cognitive behavioral therapy [37–39]. Psychological well-being has not been well studied in children receiving EN. In one study, children and adolescents receiving EEN related concerns about "feeling different" and disruption in daily activities [40]. Other studies have similarly given mixed results on the effects of EN on quality of life, with some suggesting improvement and others suggesting deterioration [41, 42]. While additional studies are needed, the current data suggests that some psychological support may be needed for children embarking on an enteral nutrition protocol. In addition, other potential contributors to reduced quality of life, such as parental stress, should be assessed before embarking on this labor-intensive treatment [43].

Infrastructure Needed for a Successful Enteral Nutrition Regimen

After a diagnosis of Crohn disease is made in a child, the physician, patient, and family typically have a meeting to plan an induction and maintenance strategy. The most common two options offered for induction of moderate disease are corticosteroids and EEN (though anti-TNF agents are increasingly being utilized earlier in the course of treatment). For the patient, the choice may initially come down to "do I take a pill once a day, or do I stop eating and have a tube down my nose for 8 weeks"? Unless the provider takes the time to explain the benefits of enteral nutrition, and has an infrastructure in place to ensure the EEN regimen is successful, prednisone becomes the default treatment. Benefits of EEN include promoting growth and controlling disease activity, while avoiding the cosmetic, immunosuppressive, and mood-altering effects of corticosteroids. While educating the family, it is also important to communicate with the patient's insurance on the benefits of treatment.

Assuming the child and family agree to proceed with EEN therapy, and the insurance approves the regimen, the next step is to meet with a registered dietician (RD). The RD can calculate the calories required by the child, and also work with the family to determine the most palatable formula. There are a number of formulas to calculate resting energy expenditure, but the Schofield equation is the one most commonly utilized [2, 44]. Some children can drink the formula by mouth, especially polymeric formulas which are more palatable. Many, however, will be unable to drink the large volumes of liquid required (often 1.5–2.5 L), and will prefer to receive a portion of the formula while asleep through a nasogastric tube. These patients often benefit from a 1 to 2 night hospitalization, so they can learn to place the tube, utilize the feeding pump, and make sure they do not develop symptoms of GE reflux of nausea. We usually start at a slow rate (75–100 mL/h, given over 10 h), then advance gradually to full volume over several days. For children who are active and can't receive all the formula overnight, there are small pumps that can be hidden in backpacks and allow administration of formula without impairment of ambulation. The choice of formula is determined by the provider and patient. The primary factor determining which formula to use is if the patient is willing to drink it. Our center has utilized both polymeric formulas (e.g. Ensure®) and partially hydrolyzed formulas (e.g. Peptomen®).

During this period, support of the patient is required in order to prevent them from abandoning the therapy. Generally speaking, phone follow-up is the main method of support, but for many patients in person visits with the nutritionist, nurse, social worker, and physician are important. In addition to optimizing the induction regiment, the physician must develop a maintenance regimen with the family. Such regimens may involve addition of a medication (immunomodulator or biologic), while others (usually in milder cases of CD) may involve some form of partial EN and dietary therapy. Whatever the maintenance regimen chosen, the efficacy of the treatment needs to be ascertained through frequent follow-up, clinical and laboratory monitoring, and possibly follow-up colonoscopy. To quote the NASPGHAN Working Group on Enteral Nutrition, "the optimal components of a successful EEN program have not been determined. …programs involving the coordinated services of a nurse and dietitian in addition to medical staff have a greater chance of success [2]".

References

1. Levine A, Milo T, Buller H, Markowitz J. Consensus and controversy in the management of pediatric Crohn disease: an international survey. J Pediatr Gastroenterol Nutr. 2003; 36:464–9.
2. Critch J, Day AS, Otley A, King-Moore C, Teitelbaum JE, Shashidhar H. Use of enteral nutrition for the control of intestinal inflammation in pediatric Crohn disease. J Pediatr Gastroenterol Nutr. 2012;54:298–305.
3. Strobel CT, Byrne WJ, Ament ME. Home parenteral nutrition in children with Crohn's disease: an effective management alternative. Gastroenterology. 1979;77:272–9.
4. Morin CL, Roulet M, Roy CC, Weber A. Continuous elemental enteral alimentation in children with Crohn's disease and growth failure. Gastroenterology. 1980;79:1205–10.
5. O'Morain C, Segal AW, Levi AJ. Elemental diet as primary treatment of acute Crohn's disease: a controlled trial. Br Med J (Clin Res Ed). 1984;288:1859–62.
6. Lochs H, Steinhardt HJ, Klaus-Wentz B, et al. Comparison of enteral nutrition and drug treatment in active Crohn's disease. Results of the European Cooperative Crohn's Disease Study. IV. Gastroenterology. 1991;101:881–8.
7. Griffiths AM, Ohlsson A, Sherman PM, Sutherland LR. Meta-analysis of enteral nutrition as a primary treatment of active Crohn's disease. Gastroenterology. 1995;108:1056–67.
8. Heuschkel RB, Menache CC, Megerian JT, Baird AE. Enteral nutrition and corticosteroids in the treatment of acute Crohn's disease in children. J Pediatr Gastroenterol Nutr. 2000;31:8–15.

9. Ainsworth M, Eriksen J, Rasmussen JW, Schaffalitzky de Muckadell OB. Intestinal permeability of 51Cr-labelled ethylenediaminetetraacetic acid in patients with Crohn's disease and their healthy relatives. Scand J Gastroenterol. 1989;24:993–8.
10. Hollander D, Vadheim CM, Brettholz E, Petersen GM, Delahunty T, Rotter JI. Increased intestinal permeability in patients with Crohn's disease and their relatives. A possible etiologic factor. Ann Intern Med. 1986;105:883–5.
11. Guzy C, Schirbel A, Paclik D, Wiedenmann B, Dignass A, Sturm A. Enteral and parenteral nutrition distinctively modulate intestinal permeability and T cell function in vitro. Eur J Nutr. 2009;48:12–21.
12. Keenan JI, Hooper EM, Tyrer PC, Day AS. Influences of enteral nutrition upon CEACAM6 expression by intestinal epithelial cells. Innate Immun. 2014;20:848–56.
13. Teahon K, Smethurst P, Pearson M, Levi AJ, Bjarnason I. The effect of elemental diet on intestinal permeability and inflammation in Crohn's disease. Gastroenterology. 1991;101:84–9.
14. Kim SC, Tonkonogy SL, Albright CA, et al. Variable phenotypes of enterocolitis in interleukin 10-deficient mice monoassociated with two different commensal bacteria. Gastroenterology. 2005;128:891–906.
15. Devkota S, Wang Y, Musch MW, et al. Dietary-fat-induced taurocholic acid promotes pathobiont expansion and colitis in Il10-/- mice. Nature. 2012;487:104–8.
16. Lee D, Albenberg L, Compher C, et al. Diet in the pathogenesis and treatment of inflammatory bowel diseases. Gastroenterology. 2015;148:1087–106.
17. Wu GD, Chen J, Hoffmann C, et al. Linking long-term dietary patterns with gut microbial enterotypes. Science. 2011;334:105–8.
18. Gerasimidis K, Bertz M, Hanske L, et al. Decline in presumptively protective gut bacterial species and metabolites are paradoxically associated with disease improvement in pediatric Crohn's disease during enteral nutrition. Inflamm Bowel Dis. 2014;20:861–71.
19. Spencer SP, Belkaid Y. Dietary and commensal derived nutrients: shaping mucosal and systemic immunity. Curr Opin Immunol. 2012;24:379–84.
20. Bruce D, Cantorna MT. Intrinsic requirement for the vitamin D receptor in the development of CD8alphaalpha-expressing T cells. J Immunol. 2011;186:2819–25.
21. Sanderson IR, Croft NM. The anti-inflammatory effects of enteral nutrition. JPEN J Parenter Enteral Nutr. 2005;29:S134–8; discussion S8–40, S84–8.
22. Wall CL, Day AS, Gearry RB. Use of exclusive enteral nutrition in adults with Crohn's disease: a review. World J Gastroenterol. 2013;19:7652–60.
23. Zachos M, Tondeur M, Griffiths AM. Enteral nutritional therapy for induction of remission in Crohn's disease. Cochrane Database Syst Rev 2007:CD000542.
24. Borrelli O, Cordischi L, Cirulli M, et al. Polymeric diet alone versus corticosteroids in the treatment of active pediatric Crohn's disease: a randomized controlled open-label trial. Clin Gastroenterol Hepatol. 2006;4:744–53.
25. Johnson T, Macdonald S, Hill SM, Thomas A, Murphy MS. Treatment of active Crohn's disease in children using partial enteral nutrition with liquid formula: a randomised controlled trial. Gut. 2006;55:356–61.
26. Sigall-Boneh R, Pfeffer-Gik T, Segal I, Zangen T, Boaz M, Levine A. Partial enteral nutrition with a Crohn's disease exclusion diet is effective for induction of remission in children and young adults with Crohn's disease. Inflamm Bowel Dis. 2014;20:1353–60.
27. Takagi S, Utsunomiya K, Kuriyama S, et al. Effectiveness of an 'half elemental diet' as maintenance therapy for Crohn's disease: a randomized-controlled trial. Aliment Pharmacol Ther. 2006;24:1333–40.
28. Gupta K, Noble A, Kachelries KE, et al. A novel enteral nutrition protocol for the treatment of pediatric Crohn's disease. Inflamm Bowel Dis. 2013;19:1374–8.
29. Tsampalieros A, Lam CK, Spencer JC, et al. Long-term inflammation and glucocorticoid therapy impair skeletal modeling during growth in childhood Crohn disease. J Clin Endocrinol Metab. 2013;98:3438–45.

30. Sylvester FA, Leopold S, Lincoln M, Hyams JS, Griffiths AM, Lerer T. A two-year longitudinal study of persistent lean tissue deficits in children with Crohn's disease. Clin Gastroenterol Hepatol. 2009;7:452–5.
31. Thayu M, Leonard MB, Hyams JS, et al. Improvement in biomarkers of bone formation during infliximab therapy in pediatric Crohn's disease: results of the REACH study. Clin Gastroenterol Hepatol. 2008;6:1378–84.
32. Dubner SE, Shults J, Baldassano RN, et al. Longitudinal assessment of bone density and structure in an incident cohort of children with Crohn's disease. Gastroenterology. 2009;136:123–30.
33. Belli DC, Seidman E, Bouthillier L, et al. Chronic intermittent elemental diet improves growth failure in children with Crohn's disease. Gastroenterology. 1988;94:603–10.
34. Pappa H, Thayu M, Sylvester F, Leonard M, Zemel B, Gordon C. Skeletal health of children and adolescents with inflammatory bowel disease. J Pediatr Gastroenterol Nutr. 2011;53:11–25.
35. Whitten KE, Leach ST, Bohane TD, Woodhead HJ, Day AS. Effect of exclusive enteral nutrition on bone turnover in children with Crohn's disease. J Gastroenterol. 2010;45:399–405.
36. Sylvester FA. Effects of exclusive enteral nutrition on bone mass, linear growth and body composition in children with Crohn's disease. Nestle Nutr Inst Workshop Ser. 2014;79:125–30.
37. Szigethy E, Levy-Warren A, Whitton S, et al. Depressive symptoms and inflammatory bowel disease in children and adolescents: a cross-sectional study. J Pediatr Gastroenterol Nutr. 2004;39:395–403.
38. Szigethy E, Bujoreanu SI, Youk AO, et al. Randomized efficacy trial of two psychotherapies for depression in youth with inflammatory bowel disease. J Am Acad Child Adolesc Psychiatry. 2014;53:726–35.
39. Mackner LM, Greenley RN, Szigethy E, Herzer M, Deer K, Hommel KA. Psychosocial issues in pediatric inflammatory bowel disease: report of the North American Society for Pediatric Gastroenterology, Hepatology, and Nutrition. J Pediatr Gastroenterol Nutr. 2013;56:449–58.
40. Gailhoustet L, Goulet O, Cachin N, Schmitz J. Study of psychological repercussions of 2 modes of treatment of adolescents with Crohn's disease. Arch Pediatr. 2002;9:110–6.
41. Afzal NA, Van Der Zaag-Loonen HJ, Arnaud-Battandier F, et al. Improvement in quality of life of children with acute Crohn's disease does not parallel mucosal healing after treatment with exclusive enteral nutrition. Aliment Pharmacol Ther. 2004;20:167–72.
42. Hill R, Lewindon P, Muir R, et al. Quality of life in children with Crohn disease. J Pediatr Gastroenterol Nutr. 2010;51:35–40.
43. Gray WN, Boyle SL, Graef DM, et al. Health-related quality of life in youth with Crohn disease: role of disease activity and parenting stress. J Pediatr Gastroenterol Nutr. 2015;60:749–53.
44. Schofield WN. Predicting basal metabolic rate, new standards and review of previous work. Hum Nutr Clin Nutr. 1985;39 Suppl 1:5–41.

Chapter 7
Elimination Diets for Inflammatory Bowel Disease

Jason K. Hou

Introduction

Questions about permissible foods are among the most common questions to health care providers from patients with Crohn's disease (CD) and ulcerative colitis (UC). Many patients are trained at a young age that "you are what you eat," and therefore often attribute dietary intake to either the cause of the inflammatory bowel disease (IBD) or to the exacerbation of symptoms from IBD. There are two competing hypotheses of how dietary intake may influence IBD activity: (1) Certain dietary components *increase* inflammation and (2) Certain dietary components *reduce* inflammation. Elimination diets—diets where specific foods or food groups are removed from the diet—are based on the first hypothesis. Advocates of the second hypothesis use dietary supplements to reduce inflammation. This chapter will focus on the first hypothesis—that certain dietary components may *drive* inflammation; therefore, elimination of the offending agent may reduce inflammation and thereby reduce IBD activity. For the purposes of focusing on the potential role of inflammation and dietary intake, the role of a low-residue diet for CD patients with an obstructing or near-obstructing stricture is not included in this chapter.

J.K. Hou, M.D., M.S. (✉)
Houston VA HSR&D Center of Excellence, Michael E. DeBakey Veterans Affairs Medical Center, Houston, TX, USA

Department of Gastroenterology and Hepatology, Baylor College of Medicine, Houston, TX, USA
e-mail: jkhou@bcm.edu

© Springer International Publishing Switzerland 2016
A.N. Ananthakrishnan (ed.), *Nutritional Management of Inflammatory Bowel Diseases*, DOI 10.1007/978-3-319-26890-3_7

Potential Mechanisms of Action: The Interactions of Diet, Microbiome, and Intestinal Inflammation

The most compelling data supporting influence of dietary intake on intestinal inflammation is in Crohn's disease. Two independent studies have demonstrated the effect of diversion of the fecal stream after ileocolonic resection, observing that inflammation recurs after ileal resection within 8 days of exposure to fecal luminal products [1, 2]. However, the fecal stream is a complex mixture of digested or partially digested food components and microbiota which also interact with each other; therefore, the actual instigating component of the fecal stream remains to be determined.

The interactions between diet, microbiome, and inflammation are a plausible link between dietary intake in either attenuating or perpetuating intestinal inflammation in IBD. Agrarian dietary patterns, as observed in certain populations from rural Africa where IBD is uncommon, have been associated with a microbiome enterotype characterized of the genera Prevotella [3, 4]. Prevotella are efficient at fermenting dietary fiber, resulting in higher concentrations of short chain fatty acids (SCFA), compounds which serve as a primary fuel source to colonocytes and may protect against intestinal inflammation [5, 6]. Conversely, high fat diets commonly encountered in Western populations with a high incidence of IBD have been linked to microbiota changes that increase bowel permeability, a hallmark of CD [7]. Hydrogen sulfide, a potentially mucosal toxic compound, is produced in the bowel from bacterial fermentation of sulfa amino acids, commonly found in high protein foods in Western diets. Furthermore, growth of populations of sulfate-reducing bacteria is fostered with diets containing milk-derived saturated fat in animal models through alteration in the bile acid composition [8, 9].

Dietary Components Associated with Risk of Developing IBD

When considering which dietary components to potentially eliminate in the treatment of IBD, it is useful to review what dietary components have been associated with an increased risk of developing IBD. Several dietary components have been implicated as the cause of IBD or intestinal inflammation associated with IBD activity; however, the majority of available studies are retrospective with small sample sizes. Dietary studies are particularly prone to recall bias which questions the validity of many of the existing retrospective studies. A systematic review of dietary components associated with an increased risk of IBD observed that (1) high diets high in fats, polyunsaturated fatty acids (PUFA), omega-6 fatty acids, and meat were associated with an increased risk of CD and UC; (2) diets high in fiber and fruit were associated with a decreased CD risk; and (3) diets high vegetable intake were associated with a decreased risk of UC [10]. The majority of studies included in the systematic review were retrospective; however, observations from the few prospective studies and subsequently published studies appear to support these general trends.

One of the first dietary components associated with causing IBD or increasing intestinal inflammation was sugar and refined carbohydrates [11–14]. These early studies were questionnaire-based, case-control studies regarding dietary patterns prior to IBD diagnosis. Subsequent studies have failed to consistently show an association with refined sugars or carbohydrates with either an increased risk of developing IBD or the exacerbation of IBD symptoms [10]. Furthermore, ecological studies evaluating temporal trends of sugar consumption and CD incidence failed to show an association between refined sugar intake and the incidence of CD [15].

Based on the most recent prospective cohort studies, the most compelling dietary components associated an increased risk of developing IBD are fatty acid and protein composition [16–19]. In a large prospective European cohort, high intake of animal protein was associated with an increased risk of developing UC (OR 3.29, 95 % CI 1.34–8.04), but not vegetable protein intake (OR 1.70, 95 % CI 0.59–4.81) [20]. A trend towards increased risk of animal protein intake and CD was observed, but it was not statistically significant (OR 2.70, 95 % CI 0.69–10.52). One of the potential explanations for the association of animal-based protein is that they result in higher intestinal concentrations of sulfate, which has been associated with endoscopic activity in UC [21]. Another potential mechanism of action for red/animal meats perpetuating intestinal inflammation may lie in the balance of PUFA. Long chain omega-3-PUFA such as docosahexonenoic acid (DHA), eicosapentaenoic acid (EPA), and docosepentaenoic acid (DPA) are metabolized into anti-inflammatory cytokines such as leukotriene B5. On the other hand, omega-6 PUFA, such as linoleic acid, are converted to arachidonic acid (AA) and its pro-inflammatory cytokines (i.e., prostaglandin E2, leukotriene B4, and thromboxane B2). The pattern of increased levels of pro-inflammatory cytokines such as prostaglandin E2 and leukotriene B4 has been observed in the colonic mucosa of patients with UC, and attenuation of prostaglandin E2 in rectal mucosa has been proposed as one of the mechanisms of action for sulfasalazine [22].

Despite the biologic plausibility of the PUFA mechanism of intestinal inflammation, therapeutic attempts to supplement omega-3 PUFA have failed to show efficacy in two large prospective randomized controlled trials in CD [23]. One potential reason the trials failed to show efficacy may be that the absolute amount of omega-3 PUFA is not as important as the relative balance of omega-3 PUFA to omega-6 PUFA. Both omega-3 and omega-6 PUFA utilize lipoxygenase and cyclooxygenase in a competitive manner, with increases in availability of omega-3 PUFA inhibiting the metabolism of omega-6 PUFA and vice versa. Therefore, supplementation of omega-3 PUFA without consideration of omega-6 PUFA may not result in adequate changes of the cytokine milieu for clinical efficacy. Furthermore, there may be genetic influences of dietary intake of PUFA on the risk of IBD and disease activity. Single nucleotide polymorphisms of tumor necrosis factor α (TNFα) 857 and interleukin-6 174 have been reported to be associated with dietary fat intake and CD activity. A dietary pattern with an increased ratio of omega-6 PUFA to omega-3 PUFA intake was associated with higher disease activity and polymorphism in 857 TNFα [24].

Management of Superimposed Maldigestion

In addition to the microbiome and mucosal cytokine modulation, elimination diets may reduce gastrointestinal symptoms among patients with IBD by treating super-imposed maldigestion. Many elimination diets include a reduction or complete exclusion of carbohydrates, gluten, and dairy products and may thus treat unrecog-nized celiac disease, lactose intolerance, or irritable bowel syndrome (IBS). The low Fermentable Oligo-, Di-, and Monosaccharides (FODMAP) diet, described in more detail later in this chapter, has been associated with improvement in symptoms of IBS [25, 26]. A randomized, crossover study of the low FODMAP diet compared to a typical Australian diet showed a reduction in overall gastrointestinal symptoms, and specifically in bloating, pain, and passage of wind among patients on the low FODMAP diet—symptoms often seen in IBD [26]. Symptoms of pain and diarrhea from IBS are particularly difficult to distinguish from symptoms of active IBD, yet are very common among patients with IBD. In a systematic review, the prevalence of IBS among patients with IBD was estimated to be 39 % (95 % CI 30–48 %) [27]. Even if elimination diets may not directly influence intestinal inflammation related to IBD, improvement of gastrointestinal symptoms of IBS may improve the overall quality of life in patients with IBD and hence remain valuable in the management of IBD.

Bowel Rest

The most extreme form of an elimination diet is total bowel rest. The early hypoth-esized reasons of the efficacy of bowel rest included reduction of mechanical trauma, intestinal secretions, and antigenic stimuli from oral dietary intake [28, 29]. Concomitant TPN with bowel rest was also evaluated to offset malnutrition due to increased requirements of protein and calories secondary to intestinal inflammation [30]. Early reports in the 1970s report the effectiveness of bowel rest of avoiding surgery in up to 70 % of hospitalizations for small bowel Crohn's disease [31]. In a case series of 100 patients with CD over a 7-year period, bowel rest was associated with clinical remission of 77 %, of which 81 % achieved remission without predni-sone [32]. The 1-year remission rate of patients who received TPN and bowel rest was reported to be 54 %. Interestingly, bowel rest failed to show efficacy in colonic disease, with 43 % of colonic CD and all patients with severe UC still requiring surgery despite bowel rest [31]. Interpretation of these findings must be taken in context of medical therapy, or lack thereof, at the time of those early reports, as well as the retrospective, observational study designs.

   In contrast to the promising data from descriptive studies, subsequent con-trolled trials of bowel rest failed to show efficacy over oral intake for UC or CD [28, 33]. One of the first controlled trials evaluating bowel rest included 36 IBD patients (27UC, 9CD) with all patients receiving oral prednisone and randomized to either bowel rest with TPN or a routine oral diet. No benefit was observed in this study, with 35 % requiring surgery in the oral diet arm and 47 % requiring surgery in the bowel rest/TPN arm [33]. Similar results were reported in a separate study of 47 patients with acute colitis, with surgery being required in 11 % of patients in the bowel rest arm and 5 % in the oral diet arm (not statistically significant) [11]. Following these studies, the use of total bowel rest as therapy for IBD has been limited primarily to patients with short bowel syndrome or high output fistulas.

Enteral Therapy

Exclusive enteral therapy (EEN), or use of prepared elemental, semi-elemental, or complete liquid nutrition as the sole source of diet, may be considered the next level of elimination diet after bowel rest with or without TPN. EEN has been studied extensively in CD and is now considered first line therapy for induction of pediatric CD in Europe [34, 35]. There have been several prospective clinical trials evaluating the efficacy of EEN in the induction and remission of CD [36–55]. Overall, response rates to EEN exceed 80 % among children with CD, although a Cochrane review of EEN found that EEN was inferior to steroids in inducing remission [56]. An additional barrier to EEN is the difficulty in maintaining EEN over long periods of time due to the poor palatability of most EEN formulations or the requirement of feeding tubes. For maintenance of remission, some studies have explored the use of non-exclusive enteral nutrition with a diet in which half of the daily calories were from an elemental supplement, with nearly 50 % reduction in CD relapse rates compared to a regular diet [57]. Interestingly, there has been no substantial evidence that the protein or fat content of EEN makes a significant difference in induction or maintenance of remission [56].

As was observed in the limited data on bowel rest, EEN has not been shown to be effective in UC, and observations from the clinical trials in CD suggest response rates are higher among those with small bowel disease [56, 58]. The reason for the lack of efficacy of EEN in ulcerative colitis or colonic Crohn's is interesting and will require further investigation.

Whole Food Restricted Diets

Whole food restricted diets refer to the elimination of specific foods with caloric and nutritional requirements met through the consumption of whole foods, as opposed to manufactured enteral or parenteral supplementation as in EEN or TPN. Several small trials of diet restriction using whole foods have demonstrated improved disease activity and prolonged time to relapse [59–64].

Food-Based Elimination Diet

In a prospective study of patients with UC, patients who reported higher levels of meat, eggs, protein, and alcohol consumption were more likely to have a relapse [64]. In this study, the association was stronger for red and processed meats compared to other forms of meat. In another small, unblinded, non-randomized study of 22 patients with CD, higher rates of clinical remission with a semi-vegetarian vs. an omnivorous diet over 2 years (94 % vs. 33 %) was observed [59]. In this study, patients with medically or surgically induced remission were included and treated with a semi-vegetarian diet—allowing for fish once weekly and meat once every 2 weeks. Limitations of this study were that patients were allowed to self-select to continue the restricted diet or resume a normal diet, which may contribute to bias. Furthermore, this study was not randomized which limits the validity of its findings.

Identifying food-specific IgG4 levels has also been evaluated as a method of selecting food groups for elimination to treat IBD. In this study, eggs and beef were the most common foods with high IgG4 antibody levels and were therefore excluded by the greatest number of patients [60]. The 29 patients on the exclusion diet experienced a significant reduction in symptoms based on a modified Crohn's Disease Activity Index and reduction in the ESR as compared to pretreatment levels. However, this study lacked a control group and this approach will require further study.

Low Fermentable Oligo-, Di-, and Monosaccharides Diet

The low FODMAP diet has been studied primarily for IBS and functional gastrointestinal disorders, but has recently been studied as a potential therapy for IBD. The underlying mechanistic theory of the FODMAP diet is that poorly absorbed carbohydrates result in bacterial overgrowth and increased intestinal permeability, resulting in penetration of food or bacterial antigens and propagating intestinal inflammation [65]. In other studies, bacterial overgrowth has been shown to increase intestinal permeability, which has also been associated with the pathogenesis of CD [66, 67].

Two small pilot studies evaluating the low FODMAP diet to treat IBD support the possibility of efficacy in IBD [68, 69]. In one study among eight patients w/UC who had undergone colectomy, the low FODMAP diet is associated with a drop in median stool frequency per day from 8 to 4 ($p=0.02$). However, no benefit was observed among five UC patients enrolled in the prospective arm of the same study [69]. In a retrospective study of 72 patients with IBD who had received education on the low FODMAP diet, 70 % of patients who self-reported adherence to the low FODMAP diet at 3 months reported improvements in pain, bloating, and diarrhea compared to those who did not remain on the low FODMAP diet ($p<0.02$) [68]. These studies are highly subject to bias due to their retrospective nature and lack objective data regarding inflammatory changes associated with dietary intervention; more rigorous, prospective studies evaluating the low FODMAP diet will be required.

Patient-Directed Elimination Diet

In contrast to eliminating food groups based on potential inflammatory responses, a patient-directed elimination diet relies on the clinical or subjective disease response to food groups in individual patients. This approach is by definition anecdotal and cannot be generalized between patients.

One of the early studies of patient-directed elimination was a small, unblinded study of 20 patients with CD in remission [61]. The ten patients in the intervention arm determined which foods they were intolerant to, and were instructed to specifically avoid them. Patients in the control group consumed a standard unrefined carbohydrate rich diet. At 6 months, 70 % of the intervention patients remained in remission compared to none of the control group.

A multicenter study of 136 patients with active CD patients induced into remission with an elemental diet and oral corticosteroids further evaluated the role of a patient-directed elimination diet [63]. Eighty-four percent of patients achieved clinical remission with an elemental diet and oral steroids and were randomized to either a steroid taper or diet treatment group. Patients randomized to the steroid group received 40 mg/day of prednisone and tapered over 12 weeks. They were provided general dietary advice on healthy eating. Patients randomized to the diet treatment group were instructed to introduce one new food daily and to exclude foods that precipitated CD symptoms. Intention-to-treat analysis showed a median length of remission of 3.8 months in the steroid arm vs. 7.5 months in the diet arm; relapse rates were 79 % vs. 62 % at 2 years in the steroid and diet arms, respectively ($p=0.048$) [63].

Defined Diets

Defined diets are dietary regimens prescribed based on an underlying "theory" of how food interacts with the body with little or no formal scientific data. Defined diets are also typically promoted in the lay literature rather than through formal medical advice. There are several defined diets promoted to reduce intestinal inflammation and related medical conditions [65, 70–73]. In this chapter, we will describe the most commonly advocated defined diet for IBD, the Specific Carbohydrate Diet (SCD).

Specific Carbohydrate Diet

Although initially promoted as a diet to treat celiac disease by Dr. Sidney Haas in 1924, the SCD was popularized for the treatment of IBD by biochemist Elaine Gottschall through her lay book *Breaking the Vicious Cycle* [70]. Her daughter was reportedly cured of UC on the SCD, and she has become a strong advocate for the SCD to treat IBD [70]. The underlying theory of the SCD is that di- and polysaccharide carbohydrates are poorly absorbed in the human intestinal tract, resulting in bacterial and yeast overgrowth and subsequent overproduction of mucus. These effects are hypothesized to result in small bowel injury thus perpetuating the cycle of carbohydrate malabsorption and intestinal injury [70]. The proposed mechanism of action for the SCD is similar to the low FODMAP diet; however, the SCD and FODMAP diets are diametrically opposed when it comes to recommendations on eliminating several food groups, such as honey and many fruits and vegetables [65]. While the SCD and low FODMAP diets are similar in with regard to unrestricted meat intake and high restrictions of cereal grains, the FODMAP diet is highly restrictive on certain fruit and vegetable intake, whereas the SCD has unrestricted fruit and vegetable intake except for potatoes and yams.

The SCD is highly restrictive on all carbohydrates except for monosaccharides (i.e., glucose, fructose, and galactose); grains are completely excluded. Fresh fruits and vegetables are acceptable with the exception of potatoes and yams. Canned fruits and vegetables are also excluded due to possible added sugars and starches. Unprocessed meats are permitted in the SCD; however, processed, canned, and most smoked meats are restricted due to possible sugars and starches used in additives. Certain legumes (i.e., lentils, split pea) are permitted, however others (i.e., chickpeas and soybeans) are not. Saccharin and honey are permitted in addition to moderate use of sorbitol and xylitol. Milk is not permitted in the SCD due to lactose content; however, certain lactose free cheeses are permitted as may be found in homemade lactose-free yogurt.

There is only one study prospectively evaluating SCD among patients with CD, which reported clinical and mucosal improvements with the SCD among pediatric CD patients [74]. However, the study only consisted of 16 patients and was uncontrolled. As described above, there are inconsistent data showing any association between dietary consumption of carbohydrates and an increased risk of IBD. Although two cohort studies showed no association between carbohydrate intake and IBD, neither study differentiated monosaccharides from other carbohydrates which could limit their applicability to the mechanism of action hypothesized in the SCD [17, 20].

Data to support the mechanism of action regarding carbohydrate malabsorption and subsequent bacterial overgrowth is difficult to interpret: detecting bacterial overgrowth using commercially available tests are fraught with misclassification. Carbohydrate intake has been associated with changes in the microbiome, including influencing the relative abundance of firmicutes within human feces [3] and the proportional abundance of Candida and the methanogen archaea Methanobrevibacter

[75]. Other microbiome changes related to carbohydrate intake, such as growth of Prevotella and Ruminococcus, can produce substrates for fermentation that can be used by Methanobrevibacter to produce CH_4 and or CO_2 [75]. The subsequent intestinal gas production may contribute to gas or bloating symptoms associated with either IBD or functional GI disorders.

While dietary intake of carbohydrates may affect the microbiome composition, how much mucosal bowel injury occurs through the production of short-chain organic acids, as proposed by the SCD, is less clear. The references in *Breaking the Viscous Cycle* only cite case studies on systemic D-lactic acidosis, not mucosal concentrations of organic acids or mucosal injury [76–78].

What to Tell Patients

There are several biologically plausible mechanisms through which dietary intake may affect intestinal inflammation in IBD; however, with the exception of EEN for CD, there is little formal scientific data to support dietary interventions as a primary treatment for IBD. Although the palatability may limit the widespread acceptance of EEN as a first line therapy, it demonstrates a crucial role of dietary intake in the management of IBD (Table 7.1).

Table 7.1 How to discuss elimination diets with patients with IBD

Acknowledge that diet may affect their GI symptoms	• May alter mucosal inflammation
	• May reduce gas/bloating from malabsorption or IBS overlap
Avoid overly restrictive diets	• May result in protein-calorie or micronutrient deficiencies
	• Consult a dietician
Diet recommendations	
Exclusive enteral nutrition	• Of dietary therapies, has the most robust data showing efficacy in IBD (primary in Crohn's disease)
	• For highly motivated patients for PO intake or willing to have a feeding tube
Food-based elimination diet	• Only small, non-randomized, uncontrolled studies
	• Low FODMAP diet may be beneficial for patients with suspected IBS overlap symptoms
Patient-directed elimination diet	• Must be individualized for each patient
	• Initially encourage a liberal diet
	• Encourage use of a food and symptom diary
Defined diets (i.e., specific carbohydrate diet, paleolithic diet)	• Very little data to show benefit or harm
	• Assess for micronutrient deficiencies
	• Encourage patient to liberalize diet if no benefit

Patients have access to a tremendous amount of information from lay literature and the Internet which is often confusing and contradictory [79]. Many patients with IBD develop strong perceptions that dietary intake influences IBD symptoms; it is a necessity for clinical providers to be able to converse with patients regarding questions involving dietary therapy or elimination diets. Although data are lacking to support any one particular dietary therapy, there is little data to show any of the described elimination dietary interventions have an adverse effect on IBD or intestinal inflammation. If patients are highly motivated, consideration of EEN may be considered. In patients who are interested in a whole food-based diet, one practical approach to dietary therapy may be to start with a patient-directed, individualized elimination diet. However, an important consideration is to work with patients and a dietician to avoid an overly restrictive diet which may result in protein-calorie malnutrition or micronutrient deficiency.

References

1. Rutgeerts P, et al. Effect of faecal stream diversion on recurrence of Crohn's disease in the neoterminal ileum. Lancet. 1991;338:771–4.
2. D'Haens GR, et al. Early lesions of recurrent Crohn's disease caused by infusion of intestinal contents in excluded ileum. Gastroenterology. 1998;114:262–7.
3. Wu GD, et al. Linking long-term dietary patterns with gut microbial enterotypes. Science. 2011;334:105–8.
4. De Filippo C, et al. Impact of diet in shaping gut microbiota revealed by a comparative study in children from Europe and rural Africa. Proc Natl Acad Sci U S A. 2010;107:14691–6.
5. Flint HJ, Bayer EA, Rincon MT, Lamed R, White BA. Polysaccharide utilization by gut bacteria: potential for new insights from genomic analysis. Nat Rev Microbiol. 2008;6:121–31.
6. Scheppach W, Weiler F. The butyrate story: old wine in new bottles? Curr Opin Clin Nutr Metab Care. 2004;7:563–7.
7. Cani PD, et al. Changes in gut microbiota control inflammation in obese mice through a mechanism involving GLP-2-driven improvement of gut permeability. Gut. 2009;58:1091–103.
8. Devkota S, et al. Dietary-fat-induced taurocholic acid promotes pathobiont expansion and colitis in Il10-/- mice. Nature. 2012;487:104–8.
9. Sartor RB. Gut microbiota: diet promotes dysbiosis and colitis in susceptible hosts. Nat Rev Gastroenterol Hepatol. 2012;9:561–2.
10. Hou JK, Abraham B, El-Serag H. Dietary intake and risk of developing inflammatory bowel disease: a systematic review of the literature. Am J Gastroenterol. 2011;106:563–73.
11. Miller B, Fervers F, Rohbeck R, Strohmeyer G. [Sugar consumption in patients with Crohn's disease]. Verhandlungen Dtsch Ges Für Inn Med. 1976;82 Pt 1:922–4.
12. James AH. Breakfast and Crohn's disease. Br Med J. 1977;1:943–5.
13. James AH. Breakfast and Crohn's disease. Br Med J. 1978;2:1715–6.
14. Mayberry JF, Rhodes J, Newcombe RG. Increased sugar consumption in Crohn's disease. Digestion. 1980;20:323–6.
15. Sonnenberg A. Geographic and temporal variations of sugar and margarine consumption in relation to Crohn's disease. Digestion. 1988;41:161–71.
16. Shoda R, Matsueda K, Yamato S, Umeda N. Epidemiologic analysis of Crohn disease in Japan: increased dietary intake of n-6 polyunsaturated fatty acids and animal protein relates to the increased incidence of Crohn disease in Japan. Am J Clin Nutr. 1996;63:741–5.

17. Hart AR, et al. Diet in the aetiology of ulcerative colitis: a European prospective cohort study. Digestion. 2008;77:57–64.
18. Ananthakrishnan AN, et al. A prospective study of long-term intake of dietary fiber and risk of Crohn's disease and ulcerative colitis. Gastroenterology. 2013;145:970–7.
19. John S, et al. Dietary n-3 polyunsaturated fatty acids and the aetiology of ulcerative colitis: a UK prospective cohort study. Eur J Gastroenterol Hepatol. 2010;22:602–6.
20. Jantchou P, Morois S, Clavel-Chapelon F, Boutron-Ruault M-C, Carbonnel F. Animal protein intake and risk of inflammatory bowel disease: the E3N prospective study. Am J Gastroenterol. 2010;105:2195–201.
21. Magee EA, et al. Associations between diet and disease activity in ulcerative colitis patients using a novel method of data analysis. Nutr J. 2005;4:7.
22. Sharon P, Ligumsky M, Rachmilewitz D, Zor U. Role of prostaglandins in ulcerative colitis. Enhanced production during active disease and inhibition by sulfasalazine. Gastroenterology. 1978;75:638–40.
23. Feagan BG, et al. Omega-3 free fatty acids for the maintenance of remission in Crohn disease: the EPIC randomized controlled trials. JAMA. 2008;299:1690–7.
24. Guerreiro CS, et al. Fatty acids, IL6, and TNFalpha polymorphisms: an example of nutrigenetics in Crohn's disease. Am J Gastroenterol. 2009;104:2241–9.
25. Rao SSC, Yu S, Fedewa A. Systematic review: dietary fibre and FODMAP-restricted diet in the management of constipation and irritable bowel syndrome. Aliment Pharmacol Ther. 2015;41(12):1256–70. doi:10.1111/apt.13167.
26. Halmos EP, Power VA, Shepherd SJ, Gibson PR, Muir JG. A diet low in FODMAPs reduces symptoms of irritable bowel syndrome. Gastroenterology. 2014;146:67–75.e5.
27. Halpin SJ, Ford AC. Prevalence of symptoms meeting criteria for irritable bowel syndrome in inflammatory bowel disease: systematic review and meta-analysis. Am J Gastroenterol. 2012;107:1474–82.
28. McIntyre PB, et al. Controlled trial of bowel rest in the treatment of severe acute colitis. Gut. 1986;27:481–5.
29. Greenberg GR, et al. Controlled trial of bowel rest and nutritional support in the management of Crohn's disease. Gut. 1988;29:1309–15.
30. Holm I. Benefits of total parenteral nutrition (TPN) in the treatment of Crohn's disease and ulcerative colitis. A clinical review. Acta Chir Scand. 1981;147:271–6.
31. Reilly J, Ryan JA, Strole W, Fischer JE. Hyperalimentation in inflammatory bowel disease. Am J Surg. 1976;131:192–200.
32. Ostro MJ, Greenberg GR, Jeejeebhoy KN. Total parenteral nutrition and complete bowel rest in the management of Crohn's disease. JPEN J Parenter Enteral Nutr. 1985;9:280–7.
33. Dickinson RJ, et al. Controlled trial of intravenous hyperalimentation and total bowel rest as an adjunct to the routine therapy of acute colitis. Gastroenterology. 1980;79:1199–204.
34. Sandhu BK, et al. Guidelines for the management of inflammatory bowel disease in children in the United Kingdom. J Pediatr Gastroenterol Nutr. 2010;50 Suppl 1:S1–13.
35. Caprilli R, et al. European evidence based consensus on the diagnosis and management of Crohn's disease: special situations. Gut. 2006;55 Suppl 1:i36–58.
36. Akobeng AK, Miller V, Stanton J, Elbadri AM, Thomas AG. Double-blind randomized controlled trial of glutamine-enriched polymeric diet in the treatment of active Crohn's disease. J Pediatr Gastroenterol Nutr. 2000;30:78–84.
37. Bamba T, et al. Dietary fat attenuates the benefits of an elemental diet in active Crohn's disease: a randomized, controlled trial. Eur J Gastroenterol Hepatol. 2003;15:151–7.
38. Gassull MA, et al. Fat composition may be a clue to explain the primary therapeutic effect of enteral nutrition in Crohn's disease: results of a double blind randomised multicentre European trial. Gut. 2002;51:164–8.
39. Giaffer MH, North G, Holdsworth CD. Controlled trial of polymeric versus elemental diet in treatment of active Crohn's disease. Lancet. 1990;335:816–9.

40. Griffiths AM, Pendley F, Issenman R, Cockram D, Jacobsen K, Kelley MJ, et al. Elemental versus polymeric nutrition as primary therapy of active Crohn's disease: a multi-centre pediatric randomized controlled trial. J Pediatr Gastroenterol Nutr. 2000;31(S75).
41. Kobayashi K, et al. [A randomized controlled study of total parenteral nutrition and enteral nutrition by elemental and polymeric diet as primary therapy in active phase of Crohn's disease]. Nihon Shokakibyo Gakkai Zasshi. 1998;95:1212–21.
42. Leiper K, et al. A randomised controlled trial of high versus low long chain triglyceride whole protein feed in active Crohn's disease. Gut. 2001;49:790–4.
43. Mansfield JC, Giaffer MH, Holdsworth CD. Controlled trial of oligopeptide versus amino acid diet in treatment of active Crohn's disease. Gut. 1995;36:60–6.
44. Middleton SJ, Rucker JT, Kirby GA, Riordan AM, Hunter JO. Long-chain triglycerides reduce the efficacy of enteral feeds in patients with active Crohn's disease. Clin Nutr. 1995;14:229–36.
45. Park RH, Galloway A, Danesh BJ, Russell RI. Double-blind controlled trial of elemental and polymeric diets as primary therapy in active Crohn's disease. Eur J Gastroenterol Hepatol. 1991;3:483–9.
46. Raouf AH, et al. Enteral feeding as sole treatment for Crohn's disease: controlled trial of whole protein v amino acid based feed and a case study of dietary challenge. Gut. 1991;32:702–7.
47. Rigaud D, et al. Controlled trial comparing two types of enteral nutrition in treatment of active Crohn's disease: elemental versus polymeric diet. Gut. 1991;32:1492–7.
48. Royall D, et al. Comparison of amino acid v peptide based enteral diets in active Crohn's disease: clinical and nutritional outcome. Gut. 1994;35:783–7.
49. Sakurai T, et al. Short-term efficacy of enteral nutrition in the treatment of active Crohn's disease: a randomized, controlled trial comparing nutrient formulas. JPEN J Parenter Enteral Nutr. 2002;26:98–103.
50. Verma S, Brown S, Kirkwood B, Giaffer MH. Polymeric versus elemental diet as primary treatment in active Crohn's disease: a randomized, double-blind trial. Am J Gastroenterol. 2000;95:735–9.
51. Borrelli O, et al. Polymeric diet alone versus corticosteroids in the treatment of active pediatric Crohn's disease: a randomized controlled open-label trial. Clin Gastroenterol Hepatol. 2006;4:744–53.
52. González-Huix F, et al. Polymeric enteral diets as primary treatment of active Crohn's disease: a prospective steroid controlled trial. Gut. 1993;34:778–82.
53. Lindor KD, Fleming CR, Burnes JU, Nelson JK, Ilstrup DM. A randomized prospective trial comparing a defined formula diet, corticosteroids, and a defined formula diet plus corticosteroids in active Crohn's disease. Mayo Clin Proc. 1992;67:328–33.
54. Lochs H, Meryn S, Marosi L, Ferenci P, Hörtnagl H. Has total bowel rest a beneficial effect in the treatment of Crohn's disease? Clin Nutr. 1983;2:61–4.
55. Malchow H, et al. Feasibility and effectiveness of a defined-formula diet regimen in treating active Crohn's disease. European Cooperative Crohn's Disease Study III. Scand J Gastroenterol. 1990;25:235–44.
56. Zachos M, Tondeur M, Griffiths AM. Enteral nutritional therapy for induction of remission in Crohn's disease. Cochrane Database Syst Rev. 2007;CD000542. doi:10.1002/14651858. CD000542.pub2.
57. Takagi S, et al. Effectiveness of an 'half elemental diet' as maintenance therapy for Crohn's disease: a randomized-controlled trial. Aliment Pharmacol Ther. 2006;24:1333–40.
58. Lochs H, et al. ESPEN guidelines on enteral nutrition: gastroenterology. Clin Nutr. 2006;25:260–74.
59. Chiba M, et al. Lifestyle-related disease in Crohn's disease: relapse prevention by a semi-vegetarian diet. World J Gastroenterol. 2010;16:2484–95.
60. Rajendran N, Kumar D. Food-specific IgG4-guided exclusion diets improve symptoms in Crohn's disease: a pilot study. Colorectal Dis. 2011;13:1009–13.
61. Jones VA, et al. Crohn's disease: maintenance of remission by diet. Lancet. 1985;2:177–80.

62. Bartel G, et al. Ingested matter affects intestinal lesions in Crohn's disease. Inflamm Bowel Dis. 2008;14:374–82.
63. Riordan AM, et al. Treatment of active Crohn's disease by exclusion diet: East Anglian multi-centre controlled trial. Lancet. 1993;342:1131–4.
64. Jowett SL, et al. Influence of dietary factors on the clinical course of ulcerative colitis: a prospective cohort study. Gut. 2004;53:1479–84.
65. Gibson PR, Shepherd SJ. Personal view: food for thought—western lifestyle and susceptibility to Crohn's disease. The FODMAP hypothesis. Aliment Pharmacol Ther. 2005;21:1399–409.
66. Teshima CW, Dieleman LA, Meddings JB. Abnormal intestinal permeability in Crohn's disease pathogenesis. Ann N Y Acad Sci. 2012;1258:159–65.
67. Hollander D, et al. Increased intestinal permeability in patients with Crohn's disease and their relatives. A possible etiologic factor. Ann Intern Med. 1986;105:883–5.
68. Gearry RB, et al. Reduction of dietary poorly absorbed short-chain carbohydrates (FODMAPs) improves abdominal symptoms in patients with inflammatory bowel disease—a pilot study. J Crohns Colitis. 2009;3:8–14.
69. Croagh C, Shepherd SJ, Berryman M, Muir JG, Gibson PR. Pilot study on the effect of reducing dietary FODMAP intake on bowel function in patients without a colon. Inflamm Bowel Dis. 2007;13:1522–8.
70. Gottschall EG. Breaking the vicious cycle: intestinal health through diet. Baltimore: The Kirkton Press; 1994.
71. Haas SV, Haas MP. The treatment of celiac disease with the specific carbohydrate diet; report on 191 additional cases. Am J Gastroenterol. 1955;23:344–60.
72. Voegtlin WL. The stone age diet: based on in-depth studies of human ecology and the diet of man. New York: Vantage Press; 1975.
73. Eaton SB, Konner M. Paleolithic nutrition. A consideration of its nature and current implications. N Engl J Med. 1985;312:283–9.
74. Cohen SA, et al. Clinical and mucosal improvement with specific carbohydrate diet in pediatric Crohn disease. J Pediatr Gastroenterol Nutr. 2014;59:516–21.
75. Hoffmann C, et al. Archaea and fungi of the human gut microbiome: correlations with diet and bacterial residents. PLoS One. 2013;8:e66019.
76. Stolberg L, et al. d-Lactic acidosis due to abnormal gut flora: diagnosis and treatment of two cases. N Engl J Med. 1982;306:1344–8.
77. Traube M, Bock JL, Boyer JL. D-Lactic acidosis after jejunoileal bypass: identification of organic anions by nuclear magnetic resonance spectroscopy. Ann Intern Med. 1983;98:171–3.
78. Oh MS, et al. D-lactic acidosis in a man with the short-bowel syndrome. N Engl J Med. 1979;301:249–52.
79. Hou JK, Lee D, Lewis J. Diet and inflammatory bowel disease: review of patient-targeted recommendations. Clin Gastroenterol Hepatol. 2013;12(10):1592–600. doi:10.1016/j.cgh.2013.09.063.

Chapter 8
Prebiotics and Probiotics in Inflammatory Bowel Disease (IBD)

Bincy P. Abraham and Eamonn M.M. Quigley

Introduction

There has been considerable interest in the potential role that the gut microbiome might play, not just in the pathogenesis of inflammatory bowel disease (IBD), but also as the source of new therapeutic approaches. The current, and most widely held, hypothesis of the pathogenesis of IBD revolves around an abnormal adaptive immune system response to the commensal intestinal microflora in a predisposed host [1]. Several lines of evidence support this hypothesis. In several animal models of IBD, inflammation develops only in the presence of commensal bacteria; germ-free animals will remain healthy [2, 3]. Animal studies also show that different bacteria can provoke inflammation in different parts of the gastrointestinal tract. For example, in the IL-10 knockout mouse model of IBD *Klebsiella* spp. cause a moderate pancolitis whereas *Bifidobacterium animalis* induces inflammation localized to the distal colon and duodenum [4, 5]. Furthermore, bacterial products have been linked to fibrotic processes, adhesions, cicatrization, and even colon carcinogenesis in animal models [6–10]. Evidence to support a role for the microbiome is not confined to animal studies. Crohn's disease patients with the NOD2/CARD15 genetic mutation demonstrate defective epithelial clearance of invasive bacteria [11] and subjects with IBD have been shown to demonstrate an altered composition of their commensal bacterial population. In IBD, in comparison to healthy control subjects and unaffected relatives, the diversity of the luminal microbiota is reduced, *Bacteroides*, *Escherichia coli*, and *Enterococci* are increased, and

B.P. Abraham, M.D., M.S., F.A.C.P. (✉)
E.M.M. Quigley, M.D., F.R.C.P., F.A.C.P., F.A.C.G., F.R.C.P.I.
Division of Gastroenterology and Hepatology, Houston Methodist Hospital and Weill Cornell Medical College, Fondren Inflammatory Bowel Disease Program, Lynda K and David M Underwood Center for Digestive Disorders, 6550 Fannin St. SM 1001, Houston, TX 77030, USA
e-mail: bpabraham@houstonmethodist.org

© Springer International Publishing Switzerland 2016
A.N. Ananthakrishnan (ed.), *Nutritional Management of Inflammatory Bowel Diseases*, DOI 10.1007/978-3-319-26890-3_8

butyrate-producing bacteria such as *Bifidobacterium* and *Lactobacillus* spp. are reduced [12–14]. Patients with pouchitis also demonstrate a reduction in the diversity of their luminal microbiota compared to those with ileal pouch-anal anastomosis (IPAA) with no pouchitis [15]. The role of the microbiome is also supported by an old observation, namely, that the restoration of the fecal stream after reanastomosis of diverting ileostomies increases the risk of clinical relapse of Crohn's disease [16]. Finally, Bacteroides species have been linked to exacerbations of colitis and early postoperative recurrence of Crohn's disease after surgical resection [17, 18].

The precise nature of the microbial, host, and environmental factors and their interactions in IBD remain to be fully elucidated [19]. However, it must also be noted that environmental triggers linked to the pathogenesis of IBD, such as cigarette smoking, consumption of a high fat diet, use of nonsteroidal anti-inflammatory drugs (NSAIDs), and early exposure to antibiotics, have also been found to modify the composition of the intestinal microbiome, suggesting that their role in the precipitation and/or exacerbation of IBD may be related to their impact on the gut microbiome [20–24].

While these observations could indicate that interventions, such as prebiotics and probiotics, that have the potential to modify the gut microbiome might beneficially alter the course of disease in IBD, it remains unclear, at a very fundamental level, whether tissue damage, in IBD, results from an abnormal immune response to a normal microbiota or from a normal immune response mounted appropriately against an abnormal microbiota. To further complicate the issue, a study that examined mucosal biopsies from IBD patients showed significant differences in microbiota composition between inflamed and noninflamed areas of the gut suggesting that observed microbial changes may be a consequence rather than a cause of the IBD process [25]. At the very least and pending further clarification, relationships between the microbiota and the host should, at this time, be considered bi-directional; a factor that must be borne in mind when contemplating studies which involve manipulating the microbiota in IBD [26]. Also, the timing of an individual's exposure to risk factors, including disruption of the microbiome, as well as of interventions such as the ingestion of dietary supplements, such as prebiotics and probiotics, may be critical. For example, exposure to antibiotics in early childhood has been identified as a risk factor for the subsequent development of IBD [27] Reducing this risk may best be achieved by early interventions, perhaps with the use of prebiotics and probiotics during or immediately after antibiotic exposure; expecting similar results when these same interventions are administered years later may be unrealistic. It may simply be too late.

Prebiotics and Probiotics: Definitions and Mechanisms of Action Relevant to IBD

Prebiotics

Prebiotics are nondigestible but fermentable ingredients that beneficially affect the host by selectively stimulating the growth and activity of one species or a limited number of species of bacteria in the colon. Prebiotics undergo fermentation by resident bacteria into short chain fatty acids (SCFAs) and lactate in the colon, thereby lowering luminal pH, and as a result, stimulating the growth and activity of *Firmicutes*, *Bifidobacteria*, and *Lactobacillus*, but impeding the proliferation of *Bacteroidetes and Clostridium difficile* [28–30]. Prebiotics have also been proposed to promote the integrity of the intestinal barrier and modulate mucosal and systemic immune responses by reducing activation of the pro-inflammatory cytokines tumor necrosis factor (TNF)-alpha, interleukin (IL)-1B, IL-17, and IP-10 [31, 32].

Examples of nondigestible dietary oligosaccharides include lactosucrose, fructo- and galacto-oligosaccharides, insulin, psyllium, bran, and germinated barley; of these, only two, inulin and oligofructose, fulfill all criteria required for classification as a prebiotic. Both are found in certain plants as storage carbohydrates [33]. Prebiotics may not be harmful but may cause gastrointestinal side effects such as nausea and abdominal pain and, as a consequence, may not be tolerated by everyone.

Probiotics

Probiotics are defined as live microbial food ingredients that alter the microflora and confer a health benefit to the host [34, 35]. Dead organisms or bioactive molecules produced by bacteria such as proteins, polysaccharides, nucleotides, or peptides, may also benefit the host but have been little studied [36].

Probiotics can ameliorate intestinal inflammation through several mechanisms. Studies show that probiotics alter the mucosal immune system through a process mediated by Toll-like receptors (TLR's) to promote T-helper1 cell differentiation, thereby, augmenting antibody production, increasing phagocytic and natural killer cell activity, inhibiting the NF-KB pathway, inducing T cell apoptosis, increasing intestinal anti-inflammatory cytokines such as IL-10 and transforming growth factor (TGF)-beta, and simultaneously reducing pro-inflammatory cytokines such as TNF-alpha, interferon(IFN)-gamma, and IL-8 [37–44].

Probiotics improve barrier function by inhibiting apoptosis of intestinal epithelial cells, promoting synthesis of proteins that are critical components of tight junctions, and increasing the mucus layer [45, 46]. Probiotics beneficially modulate the composition of the microbiota by inhibiting the growth of potentially pathogenic bacteria through the production of bacteriocins and the creation of a more acidic milieu that is toxic to more pro-inflammatory bacteria, and promotes a predominance of beneficial Lactobacillus and Bifidobacterium species [47–49]. Probiotics increase bacterial and decrease fungal diversity and can also increase production of fatty acids that have anti-inflammatory and anticarcinogenic properties [50–52].

It is critical, at this juncture, to emphasize that no two probiotics are the same, despite commercial claims to the contrary. To be effective at their likely site of action, probiotics need to be able to survive stomach acid, bile, and digestive enzymes [36]. Probiotics usually do not colonize the adult intestine and, therefore, must be taken indefinitely for continued effects. Although probiotics and prebiotics have a long safety record, there may still be risks in certain disease populations.

Particular vigilance is recommended for example, among those who suffer from immunodeficiency, those with a severe attack of acute pancreatitis, or those that have central vein lines in situ [36, 53].

Synbiotics

Synbiotics, defined as a combination of a probiotic and a prebiotic, aim to increase the survival and activity of proven probiotics in vivo, to promote or enhance the beneficial properties of both products. In vitro studies show that synbiotics exert anti-inflammatory effects and some demonstrate antiproliferative properties [54].

Prebiotics and Probiotics in the Management of IBD

Several studies have evaluated the use of prebiotics, probiotics, and synbiotics in patients with Crohn's disease, ulcerative colitis, and pouchitis.

Crohn's Disease

Prebiotics

Only two published RCTs evaluated prebiotic therapy in CD. Interestingly, the placebo-treated subjects in both studies had a better response than those who received the prebiotic. One study evaluated the response of 103 patients to fructo-oligosaccharides, which, based on CDAI scores assessed at the end of 4 weeks, was not beneficial clinically [55]. An evaluation of the microbiome of treated individuals showed no differences in fecal numbers of *Bifidobacteria* or *Faecalobacterium prausnitzii* [55]. The other trial used lactulose which also showed no clinical benefit in CD [56].

Probiotics

The data on probiotic use in CD is also both very limited and far from promising.

Induction of Remission

For induction of remission in CD, two open label studies showed improvement in CDAI scores: Together these two studies included a total of only 14 patients and used *Lactobacillus rhamnosus* GG in one study and a combination of Lactobacillus and Bifidobacterium species in the other study [57, 58]. However, a placebo-controlled trial admittedly involving only 11 patients who initially received concurrent antibiotic and steroid therapy for a week and were then randomized to placebo or Lactobacillus GG, showed no difference between the groups in regard to the time to relapse of Crohn's disease (16 vs. 12 weeks, $p=0,5$). However, only 5 out of the 11 patients completed the study [59].

Maintenance of Remission

In the maintenance of remission in Crohn's disease, a study involving the use of *Lactobacillus rhamnosus* GG in children showed no benefit over placebo, and in fact was stopped early due to these negative findings and difficulty in recruitment [60].

Overall, a Cochrane review and a more recent meta-analysis of eight randomized controlled studies showed no benefit of probiotics in the maintenance of remission in Crohn's disease based on clinical and endoscopic relapse rates [61, 62]. Most of the studies analyzed in these reviews involved *Lactobacilli*. Three studies using *S. boulardii* showed a benefit with treatment but were limited to a maximum of only 32 patients, thereby, limiting the clinical significance of this observation [63–65]. In fact, one study showed a benefit for Saccharomyces in comparison to mesalamine; a medication class that does not have strong clinical evidence of efficacy in Crohn's disease [64]. A later, larger study administered *S. boulardii* to 165 patients and failed to discern any difference in clinical relapse rates based on Crohn's Disease Activity Index (CDAI) between probiotic and placebo control groups [66]. A 1-year long study of *E. coli* Nissle 1917 compared to placebo did not show any significant difference in the time to relapse between the two groups [67].

Three low quality studies examined the efficacy of probiotics (*Lactobacillus rhamnosus* GG, *Lactobacillus johnsonii*) in preventing postoperative recurrence of Crohn's disease and showed no benefit in terms of prolonging the time interval to relapse after surgery [68, 69].

Synbiotics

A small open label trial of ten active Crohn's disease patients taking the product "Synergy" (containing oligofructose and inulin) for 21 days showed a significant decrease from baseline in disease activity, an increase of numbers of *Bifidobacteria*, and an increase in TLR expression and IL-10 secretion in mucosal dendritic cells [70]. Another small study of 25 patients, using a symbiotic preparation that combined *Bifidobacterium longum* and Synergy, showed an improvement in CDAI scores in the symbiotic group in comparison to placebo at 3 and 6 months. However, baseline CDAI scores were higher in the placebo group, thus, limiting the interpretability of the study and its translation to clinical practice [71].

A randomized controlled trial (RCT) using a synbiotic (containing lactobacilli and fermentable fibers) to maintain infliximab-induced remission of luminal Crohn's disease did not show a statistically significant difference in time to relapse between the groups given episodic infliximab with synbiotic in comparison to those who received infliximab plus a placebo [72].

Therefore, prebiotics, probiotics, and synbiotics have not been found to be useful in the induction or maintenance of remission, or in preventing postoperative recurrence in Crohn's disease. Ghouri et al., in their systematic review, suggested that these disappointing results may be due to the transmural nature of the disease, the poor design of studies to date, or both [73].

Ulcerative Colitis

Prebiotics

Although lactulose demonstrated a protective effect as a prebiotic in mouse models of colitis, human studies unfortunately have not been as positive. The lactulose trial described previously in the section on Crohn's disease also included UC patients. Fourteen patients were given standard therapy alone or in combination with 10 g lactulose daily. After 4 months, the lactulose group showed no clinical benefit based on clinical or endoscopic activity over those randomized to placebo. However, those on lactulose did have a greater improvement in quality of life [56].

Two studies evaluating a germinated barley food product and another ispaghula husk showed efficacy in getting mild to moderately active UC patients into remission [74–76]. A preparation combining oligofructose with inulin was associated with a reduction of inflammation in UC, as evidenced by lower calprotectin levels in feces [77]. These studies suggest a potential role for prebiotics in UC that should be reevaluated in larger RCTs.

Probiotics

Induction of Remission

A 2007 Cochrane review that evaluated the use of probiotics (*Saccharomyces boulardii* and VSL#3) for inducing remission in mild to moderate UC had 4 studies that met criteria totaling 244 patients concluded that probiotics in combination with conventional therapy did not increase remission rates but did provide a modest benefit in terms of reducing disease activity [78].

Two large studies that were published after the Cochrane review suggested a favorable effect of VSL#3 [79, 80]. Both studies evaluated patients using the probiotic as an adjunct to standard therapy comprising either aminosalicylates or thiopurines. In the first of these studies, VSL#3 increased remission rates, defined as a drop in Ulcerative Colitis Disease Activity Index (UCDAI) scores by more than 50 % together with mucosal healing, at 12 weeks; however, the generalizability of these results was constrained by both the short duration of the study and a large dropout rate of the placebo group [79]. The study by Tursi et al., while finding no difference in remission rates, based on the physician's global assessment and endoscopic scores, did note some clinical effects as evidenced by reductions in rectal bleeding and stool frequency scores [80].

A study in 29 newly diagnosed children with UC that added VSL#3 to standard treatment with steroids and 5-aminosalicylic acid reported a significantly higher remission rate of 93 % for the combination therapy in comparison to only 36 % for those who received standard therapy plus placebo [81].

A Japanese RCT using a Bifidobacteria-fermented milk (BFM), which contained *Bifidobacterium* strains and *L. acidophilus,* also reported a significant reduction in endoscopic and histologic scores compared to those on placebo [82].

In a relatively large study that randomized 100 patients with active UC to ciprofloxacin or placebo for 1 week followed by *E. coli* Nissle or placebo for 7 weeks as adjunctive treatments showed that fewer patients on the probiotic achieved clinical remission, and that the probiotic group experienced the largest number of withdrawals [83].

While most probiotic studies have delivered the active agent orally, rectal administration has also been studied. One study that evaluated the use of *E. coli* strain Nissle 1917, administered as an enema, in the treatment of acute proctitis or proctosigmoiditis did not show benefit over placebo [84]; in contrast, a study comparing placebo plus mesalamine to *Lactobacillus reuteri* ATCC 55730 administered as an enema plus mesalamine showed greater improvements in clinical disease severity, inflammatory markers, and endoscopic findings, based on the Mayo score, in the probiotic group [85].

Currently, there is insufficient evidence to recommend for or against the use of probiotics for the induction of remission in UC. Indeed, a meta-analysis concluded that, along with many methodological differences and significant heterogeneity of studies, probiotics do not differ significantly from placebo for efficacy and safety in achieving remission in ulcerative colitis [86].

Maintenance of Remission

Evidence from several controlled trials using several different probiotics, including *E. coli* Nissle 1917, *S. boulardii, B. breve* strain Yakult, and *B. bifidum* strain Yakult, has suggested a role for probiotics in the maintenance of remission in patients with mild to moderate ulcerative colitis with most studies showing similar efficacy and safety to standard 5-ASA regimens [87]. However, other studies using *L. acidophilus* La-5 and *Bifidobacterium animalis* subspecies *lactis* BB-12 had less favorable results [88].

Several RCTs using *E. coli* Nissle 1917 (EcN) showed that this probiotic organism was equivalent to low dose mesalamine (1.2–1.5 g/day) in maintaining remission based on either quality of life scores, endoscopy or histology [89–91].

While there were no differences in time to relapse between the treatments, one study reported relapse rates around 70 % in both arms suggesting the inclusion of a sicker UC population [89]. An open-label RCT comparing the probiotic *Lactobacillus GG* (18×10^9 viable bacteria/day) alone, mesalamine in a dose of 2.4 g/day, and the combination of *Lactobacillus* GG and mesalamine failed to show any difference in relapse rates between the three groups over a 12-month period based on UCDAI scores [92]. Adverse events such as nausea, epigastric pain, headache, flatulence, and diarrhea had been reported in these studies, but without any statistically significant differences between the probiotic vs. the mesalamine groups.

Small studies in children support the use of probiotics for maintenance of remission in UC. The addition of VSL#3 to standard therapy significantly decreased relapse rates compared to placebo (21.4 % vs. 73.3 %) when given within a year of induction of remission in 29 children with UC [81]. An open label trial of VSL#3 given in addition to standard treatment reported a remission rate of 61 % in 18 children with UC [93].

A 2011 Cochrane review that analyzed four studies containing a total of 587 patients concluded that there was insufficient data at that time to permit definitive comparisons between probiotics and any other therapy in terms of their efficacy and safety in the maintenance of remission of UC [94]. Relapses were actually numerically higher (40 %) in probiotic-treated patients in comparison to those treated with mesalazine (34 %). Rates of adverse events were similar (26 % in probiotic- and 24 % in mesalazine-treated patients). Unfortunately, all four studies had issues with either incomplete data and/or unclear methods of blinding or randomization [94].

Overall, studies of probiotics in the induction and/or maintenance of remission in UC suggest a trend toward clinical benefit. Based on the available data it is impossible to discern if a specific probiotic species, strain, or preparation is superior to others in UC; further, large, high-quality clinical trials are needed to better define the overall placement of probiotics in the management of UC and to delineate those strains which are optimal.

Synbiotics

Several synbiotic products have been evaluated in UC. In a small randomized, placebo-controlled study of 18 patients with active UC, the synbiotic, Synergy, which combines *Bifidobacterium longum* with a prebiotic mixture of inulin and oligofructose, when taken twice daily for 1 month produced a statistically significant reduction in the inflammatory markers TNF-alpha and IL-1alpha, more epithelial regeneration on mucosal biopsies, and a trend toward a reduction in endoscopically visualized levels of inflammation [95].

In a large open label study, 120 UC patients who either were in remission or had mildly active disease were randomized to receive either the probiotic *B. Longum*, a prebiotic in the form of psyllium, or a synbiotic which combined the two products [96]. After 4 weeks, while there was no improvement in health-related quality of life, as measured by the Inflammatory Bowel Disease Questionnaire, in those who received either the probiotic or prebiotic alone, subjects in the synbiotic group had a significant improvement in their quality of life. This study did not assess endoscopically defined disease activity, however. Another study that evaluated 41 patients using a synbiotic which combined a *B. breve* strain with a galacto-oligosaccharide reported an improvement in endoscopically defined levels of inflammation, based on Matt's Classification [97], in the synbiotic group compared to a placebo/standard therapy group when assessed after 1 year of follow-up [98].

There are several limitations to studies of synbiotics in UC, including substantial variability in the types and doses of probiotics used, the small size of most study populations, short duration of observation, and the lack of endoscopic assessment. These severely limit our ability to provide a firm conclusion on the efficacy of synbiotics in UC. Larger studies are warranted.

Pouchitis

Up to 60 % of UC patients with an IPAA will develop pouchitis [99]. That pouchitis can be successfully treated with antibiotics strongly suggests that the microbiome of the pouch plays a key role in the development of this inflammatory process.

Probiotics

Five RCTs evaluated the effect of probiotics in pouchitis, as assessed by the Pouchitis Disease Activity Index (PDAI); an 18-point scale incorporating symptoms, endoscopic appearances, and histological findings [100].

Induction of Remission

In a study evaluating the induction of remission in acute pouchitis, although *Lactobacillus* GG was shown to alter the pouch flora, there were no associated benefits in terms of symptoms or endoscopic findings when compared to placebo [101].

Maintenance of Remission

Four studies that evaluated the probiotic cocktail VSL#3 showed benefits in maintaining remission in patients who had developed pouchitis and had been successfully treated with antibiotics; sustained remission was observed in 40–90 % of those treated with the probiotic cocktail, in comparison to only 0–60 % in those who received a placebo [102–105].

Among asymptomatic UC patients with pouches who were monitored at 3–6 month intervals after surgery, the administration of VSL#3 had a positive impact: mucosal regulatory T cells were increased and the expression of the pro-inflammatory cytokine IL-1β mRNA in the mucosa was reduced [105].

The most recent systematic review on probiotics in pouchitis noted limitations in all five studies: small size of study populations (ranging from 15 to 40 patients), short duration of study (ranging from 3 to 12 months), and a lack of uniformity in probiotic dosing [73]. Veerappan, based on a review of several studies, suggested that probiotics may be effective in pouchitis due to positive effects on bacterial diversity in the pouch [106]. Indeed, diversity had been shown to be reduced in UC patients with ileo-anal pouches in comparison to those who had undergone the same surgical procedure for familial adenomatous polyposis (FAP) syndromes [107]. Bacterial diversity was significantly reduced in all UC patients compared to those with FAP with or without pouchitis. Diversity was lower still in those with UC and pouchitis in comparison to FAP patients who developed pouchitis.

Prebiotics

One small RCT in 21 patients with an IPAA compared the impact of 3 weeks of dietary supplementation with inulin in a dose of 24 g/day with that of placebo, on pouch morphology and physiology [108]. Inulin reduced inflammation in the pouch, as assessed endoscopically and histologically. In comparison to placebo, the inulin group demonstrated increased concentrations of butyrate, a lower pH, decreased numbers of *Bacteroides fragilis*, and diminished concentrations of secondary bile acids in feces; all of which may have contributed to its clinical benefits including improvements in endoscopic and histologic inflammation.

There have been no RCTs evaluating the use of synbiotics in pouchitis.

Safety

Prebiotics, probiotics, and synbiotics are generally regarded as safe. Furthermore, their track record in IBD, a population that may be susceptible to intestinal translocation and, thus, systemic sepsis, has been reassuring. Of concern was a case of systemic dissemination leading to sepsis in a newborn given *E. coli* strain Nissle 1917 for viral gastroenteritis [109]. Adequate longer-term maintenance studies are unavailable and needed in the evaluation of both efficacy and safety. Due to cost of some of these probiotics, a cost-effectiveness analysis would be useful in obtaining insurance coverage as well as for documenting the cost to healthcare.

Summary

Despite the undoubted role of the microbiota in IBD and the relative attractiveness of prebiotics, probiotics, and synbiotics as therapeutic interventions, the extant literature on these therapies is far from impressive and suffers from the many aforementioned limitations. Furthermore, generic issues relating to quality control continue to bedevil what is essentially a lightly regulated market. Many probiotic and symbiotic products on sale in supermarkets and pharmacies have not been adequately tested for the viability of their bacteria over the duration of their recommended shelf lives nor have their precise composition been rigorously defined. Significant confounders, such as diet and concomitant medications (including antibiotics, proton pump inhibitors, and antidiarrheals), have often not been adequately controlled for.

The net result is that, given the thin database, firm recommendations on the use of pre-, pro- and synbiotics in IBD are simply not possible at this time.

It is, therefore, abundantly clear that more randomized clinical trials involving larger patient populations and of adequate duration are needed to properly evaluate the benefits of these products and to evaluate optimal, strain, dosing, formulation, and route of administration in each of the major subtypes of IBD. Such studies should also seek to define those most likely to respond to these interventions; are responses dictated by disease location and phenotype? Could a baseline study of the microbiota predict responders or even allow one to define the optimal therapy for a given individual? Longitudinal studies of the impact of pre-, pro- and synbiotics on the microbiota would also be of great interest. Studies of the microbiota in IBD should, ideally, include detailed examination of the juxtamucosal, as well as the fecal microbiome.

Could interventions that modulate the microbiota prevent the de novo development of IBD? Long-term studies of this strategy among individuals at increased risk for the development of IBD, such as those with a strong family history or who have been exposed to known environmental risk factors such as early antibiotic use, smoking, high fat, and low fiber diet, are certainly possible. With regard to risk factors for relapse in IBD, *Clostridium difficile* has been repeatedly identified as a major culprit; could the prophylactic administration of a probiotic or prebiotic prevent the development of *C. difficile*-related infections and IBD relapses in susceptible individuals?

Conclusions

Despite their theoretical attractiveness, based on current concepts of IBD pathophysiology, available data on the benefits of prebiotics, probiotics, and synbiotics in the management of IBD is far from convincing. While there is no evidence that probiotics are of value in the treatment of Crohn's disease, there remain some grounds for optimism in UC and, especially, in pouchitis. It is to be hoped that the delineation of the role of components of the microbiota in IBD will permit the development of optimal bacteriotherapeutic strategies and that high-quality clinical trials will provide the clinician with the robust evidence of efficacy and safety that he or she seeks.

References

1. Bamias G, Nyce MR, De La Rue SA, Cominelli F. New concepts in the pathophysiology of inflammatory bowel disease. Ann Intern Med. 2005;143:895–904.
2. Onderdonk AB, Franklin ML, Cisneros RL. Production of experimental ulcerative colitis in gnotobiotic guinea pigs with simplified microflora. Infect Immun. 1981;32:225–31.
3. Sellon RK, Tonkonogy S, Schultz M, et al. Resident enteric bacteria are necessary for development of spontaneous colitis and immune system activation in interleukin-10-deficient mice. Infect Immun. 1998;66:5224–31.
4. Sartor RB. Microbial influences in inflammatory bowel disease: role in pathogenesis and clinical implications. In: Sartor RB, Snadborn WJ, editors. Kirsner's inflammatory bowel diseases. Philadelphia: Elsevier; 2004. p. 138–62.
5. Moran JP, Walter J, Tannock GW, Tonkonogy SL, Sartor RB. Bifidobacterium animalis causes extensive duodenitis and mild colonic inflammation in monoassociated interleukin-10 deficient mice. Inflamm Bowel Dis. 2009;15:1022–31.
6. Bothin C, Midtvedt T. The role of gastrointestinal microflora in postsurgical adhesion formation—a study in germfree rats. Eur Surg Res. 1992;24:309–12.
7. Mourelle M, Salas A, Guarner F, et al. Stimulation of transforming growth factor beta1 by enteric bacteria in the pathogenesis of rat intestinal fibrosis. Gastroenterology. 1998;114:519–26.
8. Van Tol EAF, Holt L, Ling Li F, et al. Bacterial cell wall polymers promote intestinal fibrosis by direct stimulation of myofibroblasts. Am J Physiol. 1999;277:G245–55.
9. Rigby RJ, Hunt MR, Scull BP, et al. A new animal model of postsurgical bowel inflammation and fibrosis: the effect of commensal microflora. Gut. 2009;58:1104–12.
10. Shanahan F. The colonic microbiota in health and disease. Curr Opin Gastroenterol. 2013;29:49–54.
11. Ogura Y, Bonen DK, Inohara N, et al. A frameshift mutation in nod2 associated with susceptibility to Crohn's disease. Nature. 2001;411:603–6.
12. Swidsinski A, Ladhoff A, Pernthaler A, et al. Mucosal flora in inflammatory bowel disease. Gastroenterology. 2002;122:44–54.
13. Seksik P, Rigottier-Gois L, Gramet G, et al. Alterations of the dominant faecal bacterial groups in patients with Crohn's disease of the colon. Gut. 2003;52:237–42.
14. Joossens M, Huys G, Cnockaert M, et al. Dysbiosis of the faecal microbiota in patients with Crohn's disease and their unaffected relatives. Gut. 2011;60:631–7.
15. Ruseler-van Embden JG, Schouten WR, van Lieshout LM. Pouchitis: result of microbial imbalance? Gut. 1994;35:658–64.
16. D'Haens GR, Geboes K, Peeters M, et al. P: early lesions of recurrent Crohn's disease caused by infusion of intestinal contents in excluded ileum. Gastroenterology. 1998;114:262–7.
17. Rath H, Ikeda J, Wilson K, Sartor R. Varying cecal bacterial loads influences colitis and gastritis in HLA-B27 transgenic rats. Gastroenterology. 1999;116:310–9.
18. Neut C, Bulois P, Desreumaux P, Membre JM, Lederman E, Gambiez L, Cortot A, Quandalle P, van Kruiningen H, Colombel JF. Changes in the bacterial flora of the neoterminal ileum after ileocolonic resection for Crohn's disease. Am J Gastroenterol. 2002;97:939–46.
19. Quigley E. Commensal bacteria: the link between IBS and IBD? Curr Opin Clin Nutr Metab Care. 2011;14:497–503.

20. Biedermann L, Zeitz J, Mwinyi J, Sutter-Minder E, Rehman A, Ott SJ, et al. Smoking cessation induces profound changes in the composition of the intestinal microbiota in humans. PLoS One. 2013;8:e59260.
21. Hildebrandt MA, Hoffmann C, Sherrill-Mix SA, Keilbaugh SA, Hamady M, Chen YY, et al. High-fat diet determines the composition of the murine gut microbiome independently of obesity. Gastroenterology. 2009;137:1716–24.
22. Murphy EF, Cotter PD, Healy S, Marques TM, O'Sullivan O, Fouhy F, et al. Composition and energy harvesting capacity of the gut microbiota: relationship to diet, obesity and time in mouse models. Gut. 2010;59:1635–42.
23. Montenegro L, Losurdo G, Licinio R, Zamparella M, Giorgio F, Ierardi E, et al. Non steroidal anti-inflammatory drug induced damage on lower gastro-intestinal tract: is there an involvement of microbiota? Curr Drug Saf. 2014;9:196–204.
24. Hviid A, Svanström H, Frisch M. Antibiotic use in inflammatory bowel diseases in childhood. Gut. 2011;60:49–54.
25. Walker AW, Sanderson JD, Churcher C, et al. High-throughput clone library analysis of the mucosa-associated microbiota reveals dysbiosis and differences between inflamed and noninflamed regions of the intestine in inflammatory bowel disease. BMC Microbiol. 2011;11:7.
26. Sartor RB. Key questions to guide a better understanding of host-commensal microbiota interactions in intestinal inflammation. Mucosal Immunol. 2011;4:127–32.
27. Ungaro R, Bernstein CN, Gearry R, Hviid A, Kolho KL, Kronman MP, et al. Antibiotics associated with increased risk of new-onset Crohn's disease but not ulcerative colitis: a meta-analysis. Am J Gastroenterol. 2014;109:1728–38.
28. Gibson GR, Roberfroid MB. Dietary modulation of the human colonic microbiota: introducing the concept of prebiotics. J Nutr. 1995;125:1401–12.
29. Walker AW, Duncan SH, McWilliam Leitch EC, Child MW, Flint HJ. pH and peptide supply can radically alter bacterial populations and short-chain fatty acid ratios within microbial communities from the human colon. Appl Environ Microbiol. 2005;71:3692–700.
30. Koleva PT, Valcheva RS, Sun X, Gänzle MG, Dieleman LA. Inulin and fructo-oligosaccharides have divergent effects on colitis and commensal microbiota in HLA-B27 transgenic rats. Br J Nutr. 2012;108(9):1633–43.
31. Looijer-van Langen MA, Dieleman LA. Prebiotics in chronic intestinal inflammation. Inflamm Bowel Dis. 2009;15:454–62.
32. Nishimura T, Andoh A, Hashimoto T, Kobori A, Tsujikawaand T, Fujiyama Y. J Clin Biochem Nutr. 2010;46:105–10.
33. Guarner F. Inulin and oligofructose: impact on intestinal diseases and disorders. Br J Nutr. 2005;93 Suppl 1:S61–5.
34. Howarth GS, Wang H. Role of endogenous microbiota, probiotics and their biological products in human health. Nutrients. 2013;5:58–81.
35. FAO/WHO. Guidelines for the evaluation of probiotics in food. Report of a joint FAO/WHO working group on drafting guidelines for the evaluation of probiotics in food. London (Ontario, Canada): World Health Organization; 2002.
36. Shanahan F, Quigley EM. Manipulation of the microbiota for treatment of IBS and IBD-challenges and controversies. Gastroenterology. 2014;146(6):1554–63.
37. Kaila M, Isolauri E, Soppi E, Virtanen E, Laine S, Arvilommi H. Enhancement of the circulating antibody secreting cell response in human diarrhea by a human Lactobacillus strain. Pediatr Res. 1992;32:141–4.
38. Ogawa T, Asai Y, Tamai R, Makimura Y, Sakamoto H, Hashikawa S, Yasuda K. Natural killer cell activities of synbiotic Lactobacillus casei ssp. casei in conjunction with dextran. Clin Exp Immunol. 2006;143:103–9.
39. Petrof EO, Kojima K, Ropeleski MJ, Musch MW, Tao Y, De Simone C, et al. Probiotics inhibit nuclear factor-kappaB and induce heat shock proteins in colonic epithelial cells through proteasome inhibition. Gastroenterology. 2004;127:1474–87.

40. Di Marzio L, Russo FP, D'Alo S, Biordi L, Ulisse S, Amico-sante S, et al. Apoptotic effects of selected strains of lactic acid bacteria on a human T leukemia cell line are associated with bacterial arginine deiminase and/or sphingomyelinase activities. Nutr Cancer. 2001;40:185–96.
41. Maassen CB, van Holten-Neelen C, Balk F, den Bak-Glashouwer MJ, Leer RJ, Laman JD, et al. Strain- dependent induction of cytokine profiles in the gut by orally administered Lactobacillus strains. Vaccine. 2000;18:2613–23.
42. Morita H, He F, Fuse T, Ouwehand AC, Hashimoto H, Hosoda M, et al. Adhesion of lactic acid bacteria to caco-2 cells and their effect on cytokine secretion. Microbiol Immunol. 2002;46:293–7.
43. Ma D, Forsythe P, Bienenstock J. Live Lactobacillus reuteri is essential for the inhibitory effect on tumor necrosis factor alpha-induced interleukin-8 expression. Infect Immun. 2004;72:5308–14.
44. West CE, Jenmalm MC, Prescott SL. The gut microbiota and its role in the development of allergic disease: a wider perspective. Clin Exp Allergy. 2015;45(1):43–53.
45. Mack DR, Ahrne S, Hyde L, Wei S, Hollingsworth MA. Extra- cellular MUC3 mucin secretion follows adherence of Lactobacillus strains to intestinal epithelial cells in vitro. Gut. 2003;52:827–33.
46. Yan F, Polk DB. Probiotic bacterium prevents cytokine-induced apoptosis in intestinal epithelial cells. J Biol Chem. 2002;277:50959–65.
47. Servin AL. Antagonistic activities of lactobacilli and bifidobacteria against microbial pathogens. FEMS Microbiol Rev. 2004;28:405–40.
48. Collado MC, Surono IS, Meriluoto J, Salminen S. Potential probiotic characteristics of lactobacillus and enterococcus strains isolated from traditional dadih fermented milk against pathogen intestinal colonization. J Food Prot. 2007;70:700–5.
49. Sartor RB. Therapeutic manipulation of the enteric microflora in inflammatory bowel diseases: antibiotics, probiotics, and prebiotics. Gastroenterology. 2004;126(6):1620–33.
50. Shiba T, Aiba Y, Ishikawa H, Ushiyama A, Takagi A, Mine T, Koga Y. The suppressive effect of bifidobacteria on Bacteroides vulgatus, a putative pathogenic microbe in inflammatory bowel disease. Microbiol Immunol. 2003;47:371–8.
51. Kuhbacher T, Ott SJ, Helwig U, Mimura T, Rizzello F, Kleessen B, Gionchetti P, Blaut M, Campieri M, Folsch UR, Kamm MA, Schreiber S. Bacterial and fungal microbiota in relation to probiotic therapy (VSL#3) in pouchitis. Gut. 2006;55:833–41.
52. Ewaschuk JB, Walker JW, Diaz H, Madsen KL. Bioproduction of conjugated linoleic acid by probiotic bacteria occurs in vitro and in vivo in mice. J Nutr. 2006;136:1483–7.
53. Whelan K, Myers CE. Safety of probiotics in patients receiving nutritional support: a systematic review of case reports, randomized controlled trials, and nonrandomized trials. Am J Clin Nutr. 2010;91(3):687–703. doi:10.3945/ajcn.2009.28759.
54. Grimoud J, Durand H, de Souza S, Monsan P, Ouarné F, Theodorou V, Roques C. In vitro screening of probiotics and synbiotics according to anti-inflammatory and anti-proliferative effects. Int J Food Microbiol. 2010;144(1):42–50.
55. Benjamin JL, Hedin CR, Koutsoumpas A, et al. Randomised, double-blind, placebo-controlled trial of fructo-oligosaccharides in active Crohn's disease. Gut. 2011;60(7):923–9.
56. Hafer A, Krämer S, Duncker S, Krüger M, Manns MP, Bischoff SC. Effect of oral lactulose on clinical and immunohistochemical parameters in patients with inflammatory bowel disease: a pilot study. BMC Gastroenterol. 2007;7:36.
57. Gupta P, Andrew H, Kirschner BS, Guandalini S. Is lactobacillus GG helpful in children with Crohn's disease? Results of a preliminary, open-label study. J Pediatr Gastroenterol Nutr. 2000;31:453–7.
58. Fujimori S, Tatsuguchi A, Gudis K, et al. High dose probiotic and prebiotic cotherapy for remission induction of active Crohn's disease. J Gastroenterol Hepatol. 2007;22:1199–204.
59. Schultz M, Timmer A, Herfarth HH, et al. Lactobacillus gg in inducing and maintaining remission of Crohn's disease. BMC Gastroenterol. 2004;4:5.
60. Bousvaros A, Guandalini S, Baldassano RN, et al. A randomized, double-blind trial of lactobacillus gg versus placebo in addition to standard maintenance therapy for children with Crohn's disease. Inflamm Bowel Dis. 2005;11:833–9.

61. Rolfe VE, Fortun PJ, Hawkey CJ, Bath-Hextall F. Probiotics for maintenance of remission in Crohn's disease. Cochrane Database Syst Rev 2006;CD004826.
62. Rahimi R, Nikfar S, Rahimi F, et al. A meta-analysis on the efficacy of probiotics for maintenance of remission and prevention of clinical and endoscopic relapse in Crohn's disease. Dig Dis Sci. 2008;53:2524–31.
63. Plein K, Hotz J. Therapeutic effects of Saccharomyces boulardii on mild residual symptoms in a stable phase of Crohn's disease with special respect to chronic diarrhea—a pilot study. Z Gastroenterol. 1993;31(2):129–34.
64. Guslandi M, Mezzi G, Sorghi M, Testoni PA. Saccharomyces boulardii in maintenance treatment of Crohn's disease. Dig Dis Sci. 2000;45(7):1462–4.
65. Garcia Vilela E, De Lourdes De Abreu Ferrari M, Oswaldo Da Gama Torres H, et al. Influence of Saccharomyces boulardii on the intestinal permeability of patients with Crohn's disease in remission. Scand J Gastroenterol. 2008;43(7):842–8.
66. Bourreille A, Cadiot G, Le Dreau G, FLORABEST Study Group, et al. Saccharomyces boulardii does not prevent relapse of Crohn's disease. Clin Gastroenterol Hepatol. 2013;11(8):982–7.
67. Malchow HA. Crohn's disease and Escherichia coli: a new approach to therapy to maintain remission of colonic Crohn's disease. J Clin Gastroenterol. 1997;25:653–8.
68. Marteau P, Lemann M, Seksik P, et al. Ineffectiveness of lactobacillus johnsonii la1 for prophylaxis of postoperative recurrence in Crohn's disease: a randomised, double blind, placebo controlled GETAID trial. Gut. 2006;55:842–7.
69. Van Gossum A, Dewit O, Louis E, et al. Multicenter randomized controlled clinical trial of probiotics (lactobacillus johnsonii, la1) on early endoscopic recurrence of Crohn's disease after Ileo-caecal resection. Inflamm Bowel Dis. 2007;13:135–42.
70. Lindsay JO, Whelan K, Stagg AJ, Gobin P, Al-Hassi HO, Rayment N, Kamm MA, Knight SC, Forbes A. Clinical, microbiological, and immunological effects of fructo-oligosaccharide in patients with Crohn's disease. Gut. 2006;55:348–55.
71. Steed H, Macfarlane GT, Blackett KL, et al. Clinical trial: the microbiological and immunological effects of synbiotic consumption—a randomized double-blind placebo-controlled study in active Crohn's disease. Aliment Pharmacol Ther. 2010;32(7):872–83.
72. Rutgeerts P, D'Haens G, Baert F, et al. Randomized placebo controlled trial of pro and prebiotics (synbiotics cocktail) for maintenance of infliximab induced remission of luminal Crohn's disease. Gastroenterology. 2004;126:A467.
73. Ghouri YA, Richards DM, Rahimi EF, Krill JT, Jelinek KA, DuPont AW. Systematic review of randomized controlled trials of probiotics, prebiotics, and synbiotics in inflammatory bowel disease. Clin Exp Gastroenterol. 2014;7:473–87.
74. Bamba T, Kanauchi O, Andoh A, Fujiyama Y. A new prebiotic from germinated barley for nutraceutical treatment of ulcerative colitis. J Gastroenterol Hepatol. 2002;17(8):818–24.
75. Kanauchi O, Suga T, Tochihara M, et al. Treatment of ulcerative colitis by feeding with germinated barley foodstuff: first report of a multicenter open control trial. J Gastroenterol. 2002;37(14):67–72.
76. Hallert C, Kaldma M, Petersson BG. Ispaghula husk may relieve gastrointestinal symptoms in ulcerative colitis in remission. Scand J Gastroenterol. 1991;26(7):747–50.
77. Casellas F, Borruel N, Torrej A, et al. Oral oligofructose enriched inulin supplementation in acute ulcerative colitis is well tolerated and associated with lowered faecal calprotectin. Aliment Pharmacol Ther. 2007;25(9):1061–7.
78. Mallon P, McKay D, Kirk S, Gardiner K. Probiotics for induction of remission in ulcerative colitis. Cochrane Database Syst Rev 2007;(4):CD005573
79. Sood A, Midha V, Makharia GK, et al. The probiotic preparation, VSL#3 induces remission in patients with mild-to-moderately active ulcerative colitis. Clin Gastroenterol Hepatol. 2009;7(11):1202–9.
80. Tursi A, Brandimarte G, Papa A, et al. Treatment of relapsing mild-to-moderate ulcerative colitis with the probiotic VSL#3 as adjunctive to a standard pharmaceutical treatment: a double-blind, randomized, placebo-controlled study. Am J Gastroenterol. 2010;105(10):2218–27.
81. Miele E, Pascarella F, Giannetti E, et al. Effect of a probiotic preparation (vsl#3) on induction and maintenance of remission in children with ulcerative colitis. Am J Gastroenterol. 2009;104:437–43.

82. Kato K, Mizuno S, Umesaki Y, et al. Randomized placebo-controlled trial assessing the effect of bifidobacteria-fermented milk on active ulcerative colitis. Aliment Pharmacol Ther. 2004;20(10):1133–41.
83. Petersen A, Mirsepasi H, Halkjaer S, et al. Ciprofloxacin and probiotic Escherichia coli Nissle add-on treatment in active ulcerative colitis: a double blind randomized placebo controlled clinical trial. J Crohns Colitis. 2014;8(11):1498–505.
84. Matthes H, Krummenerl T, Giensch M, Wolff C, Schulze J. Clinical trial: probiotic treatment of acute distal ulcerative colitis with rectally administered Escherichia coli Nissle 1917 (EcN). BMC Complement Altern Med. 2010;10:13.
85. Oliva S, Di Nardo G, Ferrari F, et al. Randomised clinical trial: the effectiveness of Lactobacillus reuteri ATCC 55730 rectal enema in children with active distal ulcerative colitis. Aliment Pharmacol Ther. 2012;35(3):327–34.
86. Zigra PI, Maipa VE, Alamanos YP. Probiotics and remission of ulcerative colitis: a systematic review. Neth J Med. 2007;65:411–8.
87. Shanahan F, Collins SM. Pharmabiotic manipulation of the microbiota in gastrointestinal disorders, from rationale to reality. Gastroenterol Clin North Am. 2010;39:721–6.
88. Wildt S, Nordgaard I, Hansen U, Brockmann E, Rumessen JJ. A randomised double-blind placebo-controlled trial with Lactobacillus acidophilus La-5 and Bifidobacterium animalis subsp. lactis BB-12 for maintenance of remission in ulcerative colitis. J Crohns Colitis. 2011;5(2):115–21. doi:10.1016/j.crohns.2010.11.004.
89. Kruis W, Schutz E, Fric P, et al. Double-blind comparison of an oral escherichia coli preparation and mesalazine in maintaining remission of ulcerative colitis. Aliment Pharmacol Ther. 1997;11:853–8.
90. Rembacken BJ, Snelling AM, Hawkey PM, Chalmers DM, Axon AT. Non-pathogenic escherichia coli versus mesalazine for the treatment of ulcerative colitis: a randomised trial. Lancet. 1999;354:635–9.
91. Kruis W, Fric P, Pokrotnieks J, et al. Maintaining remission of ulcerative colitis with the probiotic escherichia coli nissle 1917 is as effective as with standard mesalazine. Gut. 2004;53:1617–23.
92. Zocco MA, dal Verme LZ, Cremonini F, et al. Efficacy of Lactobacillus GG in maintaining remission of ulcerative colitis. Aliment Pharmacol Ther. 2006;23(11):1567–74.
93. Huynh HQ, deBruyn J, Guan L, et al. Probiotic preparation vsl#3 induces remission in children with mild to moderate acute ulcerative colitis: a pilot study. Inflamm Bowel Dis. 2009;15:760–8.
94. Naidoo K, Gordon M, Fagbemi AO, Thomas AG, Akobeng AK. Probiotics for maintenance of remission in ulcerative colitis. Cochrane Database Syst Rev. 2011;12:CD007443
95. Furrie E, Macfarlane S, Kennedy A, Cummings JH, Walsh SV, O'Neil A, Macfarlane GT. Synbiotic therapy (Bifidobacterium longum/Synergy 1) initiates resolution of inflammation in patients with active ulcerative colitis: a randomised controlled pilot trial. Gut. 2005;54:242–9.
96. Fujimori S, Gudis K, Mitsui K, et al. A randomized controlled trial on the efficacy of synbiotic versus probiotic or prebiotic treatment to improve the quality of life in patients with ulcerative colitis. Nutrition. 2009;25(5):520–5.
97. Matts SG. The value of rectal biopsy in the diagnosis of ulcerative colitis. Q J Med. 1961;30:393–407.
98. Ishikawa H, Matsumoto S, Ohashi Y, et al. Beneficial effects of probiotic bifidobacterium and galacto-oligosaccharide in patients with ulcerative colitis: a randomized controlled study. Digestion. 2011;84(2):128–33.
99. Sandborn WJ. Pouchitis following ileal pouch-anal anastomosis: definition, pathogenesis, and treatment. Gastroenterology. 1994;107:1856–60.
100. Calabrese C, Fabbri A, Gionchetti P, et al. Controlled study using wireless capsule endoscopy for the evaluation of the small intestine in chronic refractory pouchitis. Aliment Pharmacol Ther. 2007;25(11):1311–6.

101. Kuisma J, Mentula S, Jarvinen H, Kahri A, Saxelin M, Farkkila M. Effect of Lactobacillus rhamnosus GG on ileal pouch inflammation and microbial flora. Aliment Pharmacol Ther. 2003;17(4):509–15.
102. Gionchetti P, Rizzello F, Venturi A, et al. Oral bacteriotherapy as maintenance treatment in patients with chronic pouchitis: a double-blind, placebo-controlled trial. Gastroenterology. 2000;119(2):305–9.
103. Gionchetti P, Rizzello F, Helwig U, et al. Prophylaxis of pouchitis onset with probiotic therapy: a double-blind, placebo-controlled trial. Gastroenterology. 2003;124(5):1202–9.
104. Mimura T, Rizzello F, Helwig U, et al. Once daily high dose probiotic therapy (VSL#3) for maintaining remission in recurrent or refractory pouchitis. Gut. 2004;53(1):108–14.
105. Pronio A, Montesani C, Butteroni C, et al. Probiotic administration in patients with ileal pouch-anal anastomosis for ulcerative colitis is associated with expansion of mucosal regulatory cells. Inflamm Bowel Dis. 2008;14(5):662–8.
106. Veerappan GR, Betteridge J, Young PE. Probiotics for the treatment of inflammatory bowel disease. Curr Gastroenterol Rep. 2012;14:324–33.
107. McLaughlin SD, Walker AW, Churcher C, et al. The bacteriology of pouchitis: a molecular phylogenetic analysis using 16S rRNA gene cloning and sequencing. Ann Surg. 2010;252:90–8.
108. Welters CFM, Heineman E, Thunnissen FBJM, van den Bogaard AEJM, Soeters PB, Baeten CGMI. Effect of dietary inulin supplementation on inflammation of pouch mucosa in patients with an ileal pouch-anal anastomosis. Dis Colon Rectum. 2002;45:621–7.
109. Guenther K, Straube E, Pfister W, et al. Severe sepsis after probiotic treatment with Escherichia coli NISSLE 1917. Pediatr Infect Dis J. 2010;29:188–9.

Part IV
Complicated Nutritional Issues in Inflammatory Bowel Diseases

Chapter 9
Total Parenteral Nutrition and Inflammatory Bowel Disease: Indications, Long term Outcomes, and Complications

Priya Loganathan, Alyce Anderson, William Rivers, Claudia Ramos Rivers, Mahesh Gajendran, and David G. Binion

Introduction

Intestinal failure is associated with the inability to maintain protein, energy, electrolyte, fluid, or micronutrients balance while the individual is receiving a conventional diet. Total parenteral nutrition (TPN) is a life saving modality which can sustain individuals who are unable to eat with specialized, high osmolality intravenous fluids administered into a high velocity flow central vein. TPN has demonstrated an important role in sustaining individuals with life-threatening disease. Given the strong propensity for intestinal damage and dysfunction in patients with inflammatory bowel disease (IBD), a subset of IBD patients require TPN as a result of extensive small bowel injury/stricture formation and associated obstructive symptoms that prevent adequate oral intake. IBD patients also frequently report a history of extensive small bowel surgery with loss of mucosal absorptive surface. Together, obstructive disease and surgical manipulation of the gut represent the two most common IBD related complications that will require parenteral nutrition support. TPN can also be useful in the setting of perioperative nutritional support, and function to restore nutritional status in malnourished individuals who require surgery. Perioperative TPN has been shown to improve operative outcomes and assists the individual in regaining the ability to tolerate foods. Programs for intestinal rehabilitation, TPN, and new medications that function to accelerate intestinal

P. Loganathan, M.B.B.S. • A. Anderson, B.S. • W. Rivers, B.S. • C.R. Rivers, M.D.
D.G. Binion, M.D. (✉)
Division of Gastroenterology, Hepatology and Nutrition, University of Pittsburgh School of Medicine, UPMC Presbyterian Hospital, 200 Lothrop Street, Pittsburgh, PA 15143, USA
e-mail: binion@pitt.edu

M. Gajendran, M.B.B.S.
Department of Internal Medicine, University of Pittsburgh Medical Center, Pittsburgh, PA, USA

© Springer International Publishing Switzerland 2016

A.N. Ananthakrishnan (ed.), *Nutritional Management of Inflammatory Bowel Diseases*, DOI 10.1007/978-3-319-26890-3_9

151

adaptation represent important advances in the care of IBD patients suffering from intestinal failure and short bowel syndrome (SBS). In the following sections we review the history of TPN in IBD management.

Background

The Development of Total Parenteral Nutrition and Home Intravenous Fluid Support

The concept of providing nutrient and fluid support intravenously dates back to the seventeenth century, when Sir Christopher Wren and Robert Boyle experimented with the injection of animals with a variety of substances including oil and wine. Later, Wilkinson described the intravenous infusion of an electrolyte salt solution into a patient dying from cholera in 1963, which was followed by the introduction of TPN by Lawson in 1965. The use of exclusive parenteral intravenous nutrition support was demonstrated by Dudrick, Willmore, and Vars who showed that the administration of continuous hypertonic dextrose and amino acids into a central vein could provide sufficient calories, ensuring adequate nutrition and growth initially in beagle puppies, and subsequently in human infants [1].

Following these early clinical discoveries, TPN has emerged as an established modality to provide intravenous nutrition to patients with a nonfunctioning gastrointestinal (GI) tract and in patients who are unable to obtain sufficient nutrition via enteral routes. The successful implementation of TPN as a treatment modality reflects the increasing number of physicians with expertise in intestinal rehabilitation, the availability of specialty pharmacies to formulate and provide parenteral nutrition to patients for home infusion, the advent of central venous access catheters usable by patients, and finally better access to home nursing care expertise to assist patients with the initiation and routine use of TPN. In the USA between 1989 and 1992, the annual prevalence of home parenteral nutrition (HPN) use was 120 per 100,000 individuals. This number was estimated as 40,000 patients in the USA were on HPN as of 1997 [2].

TPN: Basic Principles of Administration

Routine use of TPN involves important logistic issues. These logistics include central venous access devices, specialty pharmacies capable of formulating the intravenous product, and nursing support.

Delivery of TPN to central veins as opposed to peripheral veins is essential, as the hypertonicity of this fluid would cause injury/sclerosis to low flow peripheral veins. Central veins have estimated flow rates of 1000 cm^3/h, while peripheral veins have flow rates which are typically 10 % of flow that characterizes central veins.

The optimal location for central access is the subclavian vein, as this site carries the lowest risk of infection. At the present time, ultrasound guided placement of the catheter is recommended to avoid potential complications associated with subclavian access. When TPN is anticipated for a prolonged time period, more permanent central lines are preferred. Stable central lines used in TPN administration include percutaneous intravenous central catheters (PICC) placed in the brachial vein, tunneled subclavian central catheters with a cuff serving to anchor the line and prevent infections (i.e., Hickman, Broviac, Hohn, Groshong catheters), and implanted ports (i.e., Infusaport, Mediport). The choice of venous access is dependent on a variety of factors but not limited to, patient preference, IBD complications, and frequency and necessity of access the catheter. For example, daily use of TPN favors a tunneled line or PICC line, while intermittent access may work best for a subcutaneous port. In the setting of IBD, many patients have ostomies, which further complicates TPN administration. An ostomy site increases the potential for bacterial contamination on the abdominal wall, and warrants placement of the venous access device on the contralateral side of the body. When subclavian access is no longer available due to venous damage (i.e., vanishing venous access), alternative central access sites can include tunneled PICC lines into the internal jugular vein, femoral veins, and lumbosacral veins.

TPN solution macronutrients can be formulated in either 3 in 1 or 2 in 1 solutions. The 3 in 1 solution includes a combination of protein, carbohydrate, and lipid components in a single mixture, while the 2 in 1 solution only contains amino acid and carbohydrate components. Administration of intravenous fat emulsion of greater than 3 g/kg per day has been associated with hepatic dysfunction, one of the important reasons for providing a variety of solutions for long term TPN support. Although 2 in 1 solutions may prevent long term lipid injury to the liver, adequate fat absorption from the gut will be required to prevent development of essential fatty acid deficiency over time.

TPN administration requires pharmaceutical expertise to determine optimal pH and macronutrient concentrations. This pharmaceutical expertise is essential to prevent precipitation of ingredients which has the potential to result in iatrogenic pulmonary emboli. Filters of 1.2 μm for 3 in 1 solutions and 0.22 μm for 2 in 1 solutions are mandated by the FDA to prevent accidental infusion of particulates.

Indications for TPN in IBD: Overview

IBD consists of two primary disease classifications, Crohn's disease (CD) and ulcerative colitis (UC). Worsening malnutrition has historically been the major indication for TPN in the treatment of IBD. Malnutrition was most frequently observed in the setting of small bowel inflammation in CD, as compared to UC where inflammation is typically limited to the colon. In past decades, malnutrition was commonly encountered as adult CD patients would present clinically weighing typically 10 % less than ideal body weight. More recent data suggests that CD patients under their ideal body weight are in fact rare, and the majority of CD patients will be above their ideal body weight [3]. In pediatric IBD, two-thirds of hospitalized CD patients have hypoalbuminemia, anemia, and negative nitrogen balance at presentation prior to the initiation of therapy. In addition to weight loss and protein caloric malnutrition [4] vitamin deficiency and deficiency of trace elements are hallmark features of active IBD.

There are various underlying mechanisms which contribute to nutritional deficiency in IBD, including extensive bowel disease impairing mucosal function and the ability to absorb nutrition, anatomic short bowel due to extensive surgical resection(s) with loss of absorptive surface area, anorexia, postprandial pain and food aversion due to luminal stenosis, and intermittent partial obstruction along with bacterial overgrowth. In patients who are unable to maintain nutritional needs (or regain losses) with an injured gastrointestinal tract, TPN represents an essential modality to both prevent further nutritional deficiency, restore nutritional homeostasis and prevented long term complications of nutritional deficiency.

The potential benefits of initiating TPN must also be counterbalanced by potential negative factors. Specifically, TPN high cost and potential serious complications and adverse reactions, including thrombosis, loss of venous access and infection, most commonly associated with the central venous catheter. The appropriate use of TPN in the management of IBD relies on the selection of appropriate candidates with significant nutritional deficits which cannot be corrected within a short time period using enteral approaches. Guidelines for the optimized use of TPN have been developed by the American Society for Parenteral and Enteral Nutrition (ASPEN) (Table 9.1).

Table 9.1 Guidelines for use of TPN in IBD and quality of evidence

TPN and Crohn's disease
Category A
Parenteral nutrition is not the primary treatment in intraluminal Crohn's disease
Category B
TPN is indicated in Crohn's patients who are:
Malnourished
At risk of becoming malnourished
Have inadequate or unsafe oral intake
Have a non (or poorly) functioning or perforated gut
Or gut is inaccessible (obstructed gut, a short bowel, high intestinal output, enterocutaneous fistula)
Specific deficiency like trace elements, vitamins should be corrected by appropriate supplementation
TPN and Ulcerative colitis (UC)
Category B
TPN is indicated in UC patients only when they are malnourished or at risk of being malnourished before or after surgery if they cannot tolerate food or enteral feed
No role for TPN during acute inflammatory state for enabling bowel rest
Category A suggests good research based evidence to support the recommendation
Category B suggests fair research based evidence to support the recommendation

Thus, TPN is reserved for very specific indications where the success of enteral nutrition is either impossible or poor. The following is a pragmatic list of the most common indications for the use of TPN in the management of IBD:

1. Impossible enteral nutrition.
2. To prepare the nutritionally depleted IBD patient for surgery and support through the postoperative period.
3. Post multiple major bowel resections for Crohn's disease resulting in SBS.
4. For a patient who failed to respond to maximum medical therapy and in whom surgery is to be avoided if possible.
5. In malnourished IBD patients with growth retardation.
6. Presence of intestinal fistula.
7. Avoidance of enteral nutrition.
8. Clinical features suggestive of ileus or subileus concerning the small intestine.

Specific Indications for TPN in IBD

Supportive Therapy for Short Bowel Syndrome and Life Sustaining Therapy

SBS is the term used to describe the clinical condition where the gastrointestinal tract fails to sustain nutritional and absorptive function due to the congenital or acquired loss of intestinal anatomy. SBS most commonly develops in patients who have suffered a loss of two-thirds of the length of their small intestine. However, the relationship between resection length and development of SBS and intestinal failure is highly variable between patients, and often reflects the age and underlying health of the individual, the time over which enterectomy(ies) were performed (i.e., a single massive resection will result in SBS more commonly than multiple smaller resections over multiple years), the remaining anatomic segments of bowel, motility patterns, and the capacity for the individual to undergo intestinal adaptation. In general, older individuals who suffer from oncologic and vascular insults, as well as massive single resections, are at the highest risk for developing SBS and requiring parenteral intravenous support. CD patients who are at risk for SBS are typically younger individuals, more commonly subjected to multiple, smaller resections. Historically, up to 16 % of individuals developing SBS as a complication of intestinal surgery suffered from CD [5].

SBS can lead to

Loss of absorptive surface area
Loss of site-specific transport processes
Loss of site-specific endocrine cells and gastrointestinal (GI) hormones
Loss of ileocecal valve

The major complication of extensive enterectomy is loss of absorptive surface area, but intestinal adaptation and redundancy of function will allow the majority of patients to tolerate this insult. In individuals where the adaptive process is insufficient, chronic high diarrheal output and dehydration will ensue. Evaluation of individuals suffering from this acquired SBS will require detailed dietary histories to determine the effects of specific foods and liquids on fecal output. The major goal of intestinal rehabilitation is to prevent the need for parenteral fluid support by modifying diet to maximize nutrient absorption while minimizing malabsorption, most frequently of simple carbohydrates and water which are often ingested in excess amounts by individuals suffering from SBS and chronic dehydration. Emphasis on monitoring fluid balance is essential in this early SBS physiology, as significant short and long term morbidity and mortality can be associated with volume loss, electrolyte shifts, and acute and chronic dehydration. Diarrhea in SBS originates in the vasculature prior to being pumped into the gastrointestinal lumen where it will fail to be reabsorbed in the second half of the GI tract due to anatomic loss. Diarrhea in SBS results in malabsorption of macro and micronutrients, electrolytes, and water. This malabsorption of water and electrolytes leads to voluminous diarrhea, hyponatremia, and hypokalemia [6]. The careful management and appropriate nutritional support is needed for these patients, especially in the case of parenteral nutrition. Success of interventions to manage SBS will immediately impact the daily input and output tally, and will also provide early guidance on the individual with high losses who will require intravenous support. These individuals who fail to respond adequately to oral rehydration solution and dietary modifications (separating solid foods from liquids at mealtime) will likely require either daily intravenous volume support or TPN. Permanent TPN support is needed in patients with less than 120 cm of intestine without colon in continuity and less than 60 cm with colonic continuity [7]. TPN administered as in home option not only avoids prolonged hospitalization but also delays the need for surgery [8].

Volume and Calorie Replacement

TPN can be administered either through central line or a peripherally inserted central catheter (PICC), but generally central line is preferred. Central TPN provides the patient with the majority of nutrients including carbohydrates, protein, fat, vitamin, salt, and trace elements. The subclavian vein is the usual site for catheterization. During the first few days volume can be adjusted to 30–40 mL/kg body weight/day depending on the patient hydration status [9]. The well-nourished adult patient should receive 25–30 kcal/kg BW/day via central access and for a malnourished patient it can be up titrated accordingly. For postoperative patients, 35–45 kcal/kg BW/day might be necessary. Composition of TPN is given in Table 9.2.

Amino acids in the parenteral nutrition solution are tailored to maintain a stable nitrogen balance. The amount of protein in TPN typically varies from 0.8 to 1.5 g/kg/day according to the need of the patient. In rare situations where IBD has resulted

Table 9.2 Composition of TPN

Nutritional element	Volume	Calories	Amount	Function
Amino acids	1000	340	85 g in well nourished	Stable nitrogen balance
			To 125 g in high catabolism state	
Dextrose	1000	340	100 g and adjusted according to the serum glucose level	Important source of calorie
Fat	500	550	50–70 %—linoleic acid	Source of essential fatty acid
			5–10 %—linolenic acid	
Glutamine supplementation			0.3–0.5 g/kg/day	Intestino-trophic effect, decrease IL6 production
Trace elements and vitamin			5 mL/day	Integral part of human enzymes function and for the synthesis of DNA

in a protein losing enteropathy/colopathy, higher amounts of amino acid support can be considered (i.e., 2.0 g/kg/day). Postoperative patients and individuals with an increased catabolic metabolism (i.e., extensive mucosal ulceration) require more amino acids in their TPN compared to well-nourished patients. Amino acid support in TPN includes glutamine, which is felt to be an essential amino acid for gut health, as it plays a significant role in providing energy to enterocytes [10]. Additional components of TPN support include high concentrations of dextrose, an inexpensive and important source of calories and available in varied concentration.

Use of Teduglutide in Conjunction with TPN

Teduglutide is a glucagon-like peptide 2 analogue, which was developed to promote intestinal adaptation, restoration of intestinal integrity, and ultimately decreasing the need for TPN support in patients suffering from SBS. It is a subcutaneously administered synthetic protein which differs from native GLP2 analogue by the substitution of glycine for alanine at the second position from the N-terminus. This substitution makes it resistant against dipeptidyl peptidase-4 and thereby increasing its half-life from 60–90 min (native GLP-2) to 180–330 min (Teduglutide) [11]. Studies have shown that teduglutide improves intestinal function and structural integrity through significant intestinotrophic and pro absorptive effects [12]. Repeated administration of teduglutide is thought to stimulate intestinal epithelial crypt cell growth and reducing enterocyte apoptosis which results in increased villous height, plasma Citrulline concentration, and lean body mass. Additional mechanisms attributed to teduglutide which may benefit SBS include decreased gastric acid secretion and gastric emptying and stimulating intestinal blood flow thereby increasing the intestinal barrier function, leading to improved fluid and nutrient and absorption [13]. Teduglutide was shown to be well tolerated and effective in CD patients on TPN in the pivotal trial and improved disease activity scores in 44 % of CD patients in a separate study who were not on TPN [14].

Primary Therapy: Gut Rest in Patients with Severe Illness

Primary medical therapy for CD relies on induction treatment with steroids and/or biologic anti-TNF agents, and maintenance treatment with immunomodulators and biologics (anti-TNF agents and alpha4 integrin inhibitors). Therapy with aminosalicylates and antibiotics have been used in specific subgroups of patients, but failed to show the success of immunomodulators and biologic agents. Despite the increase in available medical options, there are a subset of patients who may fail to respond to medical therapy. Surgical intervention for medically refractory inflammatory disease will often be considered in CD, but is more ominous in patients with both small and large bowel involvement as the colectomy and end ileostomy will not guarantee clinical remission. Relapse of CD will generally be followed by small bowel resection, which raises the potential for SBS in patients who have failed all medical options going on the require additional surgery [15]. In this rare, but very serious cohort of CD patients, bowel rest with TPN to provide exclusive nutritional support can achieve clinical remission in up to 77 % of individuals. The exact mechanism of a TPN/bowel rest treatment approach is not precisely known, and mechanisms have been hypothesized to include reduction in enteric flora dependent on enteral intake as a "prebiotic" substrate, decreased production of gut hormones, decreased autonomic stimulation, and simply halting the digestive process. In the setting of enterocutaneous fistula, the interruption of oral intake and digestion will typically cause a decrease in the secretion of digestive fluids (i.e., pancreatic enzymes and bile) into the lumen which can potentially track into the fistula, effectively "digesting" the wound and preventing it from healing. Maintaining an NPO status will often allow enterocutaneous fistula to demonstrate spontaneous closure. In the setting of partial small bowel obstruction, maintaining an NPO status will decrease abdominal pain. Thus TPN and bowel rest promotes resolution of CD symptoms such as diarrhea, abdominal pain, and abdominal masses; also it improves sense of well-being and improves the body weight [16]. Attempts to demonstrate and confirm the beneficial effect of TPN in the management of CD have been challenged by the heterogeneity of patients. Greenberg and colleagues at the University of Toronto led a multicenter, prospective controlled trial which failed to demonstrate an advantage of bowel rest using TPN as opposed to good enteral nutrition support. Furthermore, many studies consistently showed that TPN and bowel rest had lower remission rates for penetrating disease, colonic involvement, or ulcerative colitis. The therapeutic concept of bowel rest in the management of CD has been debated since 1980s, but appears to be limited to a small subset of patients and its clinical benefit does not appear to extend to the majority of patients.

Complications of Parenteral Nutrition

Although TPN is efficacious in malnourished patients and individuals who are not able to sustain themselves through enteral intake, this efficacy comes at the cost of potential complications. Complications of TPN are numerous including gastrointestinal, infectious, metabolic, vascular, biliary, and mechanical issues can contribute to the patient's morbidity and potentially mortality (Table 9.3).

Mechanical Complication

Parenteral nutrition requires venous access either peripherally or centrally. Cannulation of the subclavian, internal jugular, or femoral veins with advancement of the catheter to the superior or inferior vena cava achieves central venous accesses. Peripheral or midline catheter placement is considered to be peripheral access, and these access points do not have sufficient flow to allow for the high osmolality of TPN. Cannulation success depends upon the anatomic site and the operator's experience. Mechanical complication is often related to the catheter itself, but this complication can include catheter misplacement upon insertion, thrombotic occlusion, and catheter displacement or migration after it was placed.

Catheter misplacement: Improper placement of the central line may cause serious conditions like pneumothorax, vessel injury leading to hemothorax, brachial plexus injury, and even cardiac arrhythmia [17]. Malposition, arterial puncture, and subcutaneous hematoma are the other potential complications of catheter misplacement [18].

Thrombophlebitis/venous thrombosis: Intravenous catheters can cause endothelial injury and inflammation of the vessel. This can lead to disruption of the intimal layer of the vein, thrombosis, and accumulation of a fibrin sheath along the outer surface of the catheter [19]. Serious consequences can include intracardiac thrombosis and pulmonary embolus. Venous thrombosis may lead to distension of neck veins, swelling of the face and ipsilateral arm and can eventually progress to superior vena cava syndrome [20].

Nonthrombotic occlusion: Due to precipitation of various elements in TPN, nonthrombotic occlusion of the vessel lumen can occur [21]. It is both time consuming and challenging to differentiate between thrombotic and nonthrombotic occlusions.

Table 9.3 Complications of parenteral nutrition

Overview of parenteral nutrition related complication:
I. Mechanical/vascular
Catheter misplacement—organ damage
Embolization
Thrombus formation
Nonthrombotic occlusion
Thrombophlebitis
II. Infectious
Catheter related bloodstream infection (CRBSI)
Septicemia
III. Metabolic
Fluid imbalance
Electrolyte/mineral imbalance
Acid–base disturbance
Glucose intolerance
Metabolic bone disease
Refeeding syndrome
IV. Biliary
Cholestasis
Cholangitis
Cholecystitis
Cholestatic liver dysfunction
Cholelithiasis
V. Nutritional
Trace metal deficiency
Vitamin deficiency
Malnourishment leading to Immunosuppression
Fatty acid deficiency
VI. Gastrointestinal
Villous atrophy—In animal studies

Vanishing venous access: Long term TPN (administered through a central catheter) predisposes the patient to central vein stenosis or thrombosis. Repeated venous access can cause exhaustion of veins [22].

Air embolism: A rare, but serious, complication of air being inserted into the catheter while on TPN must be closely monitored [23].

Infective Complication

This is the second most common complication during parenteral nutrition treatment. Infective complications can arise from many potential sources. Microbes introduced through the catheter pose a significant risk for infection while infection through parenteral nutritional solutions is not as common.

Catheter related bloodstream infection (CRBSI) and catheter related bacteremia are characterized by positive cultures from peripheral blood and the indwelling catheter both producing positive cultures with the same microorganisms, without any other known source of infection [24]. Infection of the catheter insertion site is defined by the presence of inflammation, pus, quantitative culture of the proximal catheter segment and/or tip of the catheter with >10^3 colonies or semiquantitative culture of >15 colonies from fluid uptake from the insertion site [25] (Table 9.4).

Attempts to salvage catheters which have become contaminated have been attempted. Instilling catheters with a high concentration antibiotic solution in sufficient amounts to fill the lumen of the catheter (i.e., antibiotic lock) has proven to be successful in infective complications, most commonly with *Staphylococcus epidermidis*. Antibiotic sensitivity data from organisms isolated from blood cultures is the preferred strategy, and this approach has been most successfully used with vancomycin. There are case reports of antibiotic locks successfully rescuing catheters using amikacin, imipenem, aminoglycosides, and amphotericin, although the majority of gram negative and fungal line infections will require catheter removal [26].

Table 9.4 The wide spectrum causative organisms

Gram Positive
Staphylococcus aureus
Enterococcus durans
Streptococcus viridans
Peptostreptococcus
Propionibacterium
Gram Negative
Escherichia coli
Pseudomonas aeruginosa
Klebsiella pneumoniae
Enterobacter cloacae
Fungus
Candida albicans
Candida glabrata
Candida guilliermondii
Mycobacterium
Mycobacterium avium
Mycobacterium chelonae
Mycobacterium fortuitum

Metabolic Complications

Early metabolic complications of the TPN treatment can include fluid volume overload, hyperglycemia, hypokalemia, hypophosphatemia, hypomagnesaemia, refeeding syndrome, hypochloremic acidosis, and other electrolyte abnormalities.

Hyperglycemia/glucose intolerance: Initial hyperglycemic reactions can develop due to the bolus of TPN and potassium infusions. The patient must be closely monitored for hyperglycemia during this process. Chromium is an important micronutrient that becomes deficient in a long term TPN patient. Chromium has been shown to play a role in glucose intolerance, gestational diabetes, and type 2 diabetes mellitus. Studies have shown that 200 mcg/day of supplemental chromium improves the glucose variables, such as HbA1c, in those who are mildly glucose intolerant [27].

Refeeding syndrome: Malnourished patients who receive TPN are at an increased risk of developing refeeding syndrome [28]. Refeeding syndrome can be defined as the fatal shifts in fluids and electrolytes that may occur after receiving artificial feeding after a period of calorie deprivation/starvation (which may be as short as 5 days). This sudden intracellular shift is caused by hormonal and metabolic changes, leading to fluctuations in electrolyte levels and potentially serious clinical consequences including cardiac arrhythmias, mental status changes, coma, seizure, and cardiac failure. The hallmark electrolyte abnormalities associated with refeeding is hypokalemia, which is mechanistically believed to result from glycemia induced insulin secretion that causes potassium to shift into the cells, leading to loss of potassium in the extracellular spaces. Insulin also promotes synthesis of protein, glycogen, and fat, and this acceleration of metabolism can lead to rapid cellular uptake of magnesium, potassium, and thiamine, potentially causing an insufficiency of these nutrients. Thiamine (Vitamin B1) is an important coenzyme in carbohydrate metabolism and its rapid deficiency can result in Wernicke's encephalopathy (ocular abnormalities, ataxia, confusion state, hypothermia, and coma) or Korsakoff's syndrome (retrograde and anterograde amnesia, confabulation) [29]. Therefore customized TPN formulations which include extra thiamine, potassium, magnesium, and phosphorus are required to avoid refeeding complications during the initiation of enteral nutrition. Likewise, careful, close monitoring of these electrolytes is required to ensure no.

Fluid/electrolyte disturbance: Fluid overload is a common side effect of TPN infusion ranging from ankle edema to pulmonary congestion. Closely monitoring the fluid intake and urine output is important during the entire course of TPN treatment. Special attention to fluid and electrolyte balances should be implemented in patients with renal disease and in pregnant women [30] (Table 9.5).

Table 9.5 Electrolyte imbalance during TPN [30–32]

Problem	Symptom	Management
Hyperkalemia	Nausea, slow heart rate, confusion, restlessness, diarrhea, abdominal distention	Potassium should be withheld from TPN solution until underlying problem is resolved. If severe, treat with prescribed IV doses of bicarbonate, glucose, insulin, and calcium for cardioprotective effect
Hypokalemia	Flaccid muscles (atonia), malaise, fish mouth breathing, tachycardia, and arrhythmia	Regular monitoring of serum K+ and adjustments of potassium in TPN
Hyperosmolar, Hyperglycemic, Nonketotic coma (HHNK)	Hyperglycemia, absence of ketone bodies, confusion, eventually coma can rapidly advance to death if untreated	Stop hypertonic infusion and hydrate with large amounts of hypotonic solution, IV insulin with careful monitoring. Electrolyte abnormality has to be corrected
Hypomagnesemia	Hallucinations, vertigo, ileus, and hyperreflexia	Additional amounts of magnesium sulfate can be added to TPN solution
Hypercalcemia	Extreme thirst, increased urination, confusion	Treated on the basis of calcium level
		Mild <12 mg/dL: hydration
		Moderate 12–14 mg/dL: Hydration and Bisphosphonates
		Severe >14 mg/dL: Iv isotonic saline, Calcitonin, and Bisphosphonates
Hypocalcemia	Paresthesias, confusion, positive Chvostek's sign, tetany	Daily calcium supplement in solution
Hypermagnesemia	Headache, Loss of Deep tendon reflex, hypocalcemia	Magnesium replacement
Hyperphosphatemia	Hyperreflexia, carpopedal spasm	Limit phosphate intake, phosphate binders
Hypoglycemia	Diaphoresis, confusion, agitation	Dextrose infusion
Hypermagnesemia	Blocks neuromuscular conduction, depresses the conduction system in heart	Furosemide may increase its excretion
		Calcium gluconate antagonize the neuromuscular blocking effect
Hypophosphatemia	Mental deterioration	Additional amounts of phosphate added to daily TPN regimen based on levels
	Lethargy that may lead to coma. Hemolytic anemia may also occur	

Hepatobiliary Complication

Liver complications are common during TPN treatment (25–75 % of all TPN patients) and can occur within several days after initiating therapy with the majority of these hepatobiliary complications being mild and transient. The most severe hepatobiliary complication is TPN associated cholestasis (TPNAC). This potentially fatal condition can develop rapidly and will progress to fibrosis, cirrhosis, and portal hypertension. TPNAC has been linked to inflammatory activity and there is a case report of a CD patients resolving cholestasis following treatment initiation with the anti-TNF antibody infliximab [33]. Cholestasis and biliary sludge can lead to acalculous cholecystitis, due to a lack of gallbladder stimulation by cholecystokinin. Factors associated with liver dysfunction include deficiency of essential fatty acids, imbalances in the composition of amino acids, fat deposition in the liver, deficiency of choline, and absence of enteral nutrition intake [34].

Micronutrient Malnutrition

Micronutrient malnutrition can occur during long term TPN management. Chronic TPN can lead to deficiency of trace metals, fatty acids, and electrolytes, leading to the respective manifestation of deficiency symptoms. Table 9.6 shows the common micronutrient deficiencies seen in IBD patients and their clinical features.

Table 9.6 Micronutrient deficiencies

Nutrient	Clinical feature of its deficiency
Vitamins	
• A	Night blindness, dry skin and hair
• B1	Beriberi, Wernicke Korsakoff syndrome
• C	Anemia, bleeding gums, dry hair, easy bruising, nosebleed
• D	Muscle weakness, osteomalacia, rickets in children
• E	Defective platelet aggregation, Hemolysis
Chromium	Alopecia, T-cell disturbance, perineal acrodermatitis, Reduced serum alkaline phosphate levels
Selenium	Reduced levels of glutathione peroxidase level, myocarditis, and myalgia
Molybdenum	Color blindness, irritability, and tachycardia
Essential fatty acids	Dermatitis, lackluster skin and increased rate of trienoic: Tetraenoic plasma fatty acids
Zinc	Xerosis, acne, Eczema, alopecia, stomatitis, affects hunger sensation leading to anorexia, diarrhea
Choline	Fatty liver, hemorrhagic kidney necrosis

Gastrointestinal Complication

Long term TPN has been shown to cause intestinal villi hypoplasia in experimental rats. Studies on the human gastrointestinal tract have also shown a significant decrease in jejunal villi with TPN, although not to the same extent as in rodents [35]. Intestinal immunological cells have also been shown to express decreased homeostatic cellular activity and to decrease in number within patients on parenteral nutrition [36].

Costs of TPN and Quality of Life

Patients being treated with parenteral nutrition have been shown to benefit the most from a HPN treatment plan when comparing cost effective interventions due to its success in keeping the patient out of the hospital. Based on national data, HPN is 5 times more expensive than home enteral nutrition [2]. Direct costs for HPN includes the infusion pump, administration kits, catheter dressing kits, and nutrient solution. In 1992, Medicare allowance for HPN was estimated to be between $238 and $390 per day, or $86,000–$140,000 per year. It is important to know that these charges do not include medical visits, laboratory monitoring, home nursing support, or hospitalization for complications during parenteral nutrition. Medicare paid 80 % of these charges and remaining 20 % was provided by a secondary insurance provider or by the patient [37]. In European countries and Canada, the total cost of both home parenteral and enteral nutrition is covered by the National Health Services [2]. In order to be the most cost effective, it has been shown that following periodic reassessment for compliance, determining the appropriateness of parenteral formulation, infusion regimen, status of intestinal adaptation, and oral nutrient intake are important interventions for HPN patients [38].

As per Jeppesen et al., HPN was associated with a lower sickness impact profile overall, and is associated with a lower IBD Questionnaire score when compared with the patients not receiving HPN [39]. There is a significant improvement in quality of life when patients are transferred to HPN from hospitals [40].

Summary

The appropriate use of TPN in the treatment of IBD is limited to a small number of patients who are challenged with life-threatening complications involving malnutrition, SBS, and severe/refractory inflammation. Given the strong potential for complications and cost, TPN is reserved for situations where enteral nutrition has either failed or is contraindicated. The lack of clear data demonstrating the efficacy of parenteral nutrition and bowel rest as primary therapy for the treatment of IBD has positioned its role as adjunctive and supportive therapy. At the present time, more effective medical treatment options for IBD have decreased the need for TPN as a rescue modality. Future investigation to further develop new agents which promote intestinal adaptation may decrease the need for TPN support in IBD patients with severe and refractory illness. At present, TPN remains a "last ditch" life saving modality for extremely ill IBD patients with limited medical and surgical options, which can include multi-visceral organ transplantation.

References

1. Wilmore DW, Groff DB, Bishop HC, Dudrick SJ. Total parenteral nutrition in infants with catastrophic gastrointestinal anomalies. J Pediatr Surg. 1969;4(2):181–9.
2. Howard L, Ament M, Fleming CR, Shike M, Steiger E. Current use and clinical outcome of home parenteral and enteral nutrition therapies in the United States. Gastroenterology. 1995;109(2):355–65.
3. Seminerio JL, Koutroubakis IE, Ramos-Rivers C, Hashash JG, Dudekula A, Regueiro M, et al. Impact of obesity on the management and clinical course of patients with inflammatory bowel disease. Inflamm Bowel Dis. 2015.
4. Elson CO, Layden TJ, Nemchausky BA, Rosenberg JL, Rosenberg IH. An evaluation of total parenteral nutrition in the management of inflammatory bowel disease. Dig Dis Sci. 1980;25(1):42–8.
5. Thompson JS, DiBaise JK, Iyer KR, Yeats M, Sudan DL. Postoperative short bowel syndrome. J Am Coll Surg. 2005;201(1):85–9.
6. Andersson H, Bosaeus I, Brummer RJ, Fasth S, Hulten L, Magnusson O, et al. Nutritional and metabolic consequences of extensive bowel resection. Dig Dis. 1986;4(4):193–202.
7. Carbonnel F, Cosnes J, Chevret S, Beaugerie L, Ngo Y, Malafosse M, et al. The role of anatomic factors in nutritional autonomy after extensive small bowel resection. JPEN J Parenter Enteral Nutr. 1996;20(4):275–80.
8. Evans JP, Steinhart AH, Cohen Z, McLeod RS. Home total parenteral nutrition: an alternative to early surgery for complicated inflammatory bowel disease. J Gastrointest Surg. 2003;7(4):562–6.
9. Koretz RL, Lipman TO, Klein S, American GA. AGA technical review on parenteral nutrition. Gastroenterology. 2001;121(4):970–1001.
10. Buchman AL. Glutamine for the gut: mystical properties or an ordinary amino acid? Curr Gastroenterol Rep. 1999;1(5):417–23.
11. Drucker DJ, Shi Q, Crivici A, Sumner-Smith M, Tavares W, Hill M, et al. Regulation of the biological activity of glucagon-like peptide 2 in vivo by dipeptidyl peptidase IV. Nat Biotechnol. 1997;15(7):673–7.
12. Jeppesen PB, Gilroy R, Pertkiewicz M, Allard JP, Messing B, O'Keefe SJ. Randomised placebo-controlled trial of teduglutide in reducing parenteral nutrition and/or intravenous fluid requirements in patients with short bowel syndrome. Gut. 2011;60(7):902–14.
13. Berg JK, Kim EH, Li B, Joelsson B, Youssef NN. A randomized, double-blind, placebo-controlled, multiple-dose, parallel-group clinical trial to assess the effects of teduglutide on gastric emptying of liquids in healthy subjects. BMC Gastroenterol. 2014;14:25.
14. Buchman AL, Katz S, Fang JC, Bernstein CN, Abou-Assi SG, Teduglutide Study Group. Teduglutide, a novel mucosally active analog of glucagon-like peptide-2 (GLP-2) for the treatment of moderate to severe Crohn's disease. Inflamm Bowel Dis. 2010;16(6):962–73.
15. Shivananda S, Hordijk ML, Pena AS, Mayberry JF. Crohn's disease: risk of recurrence and reoperation in a defined population. Gut. 1989;30(7):990–5.
16. Ostro MJ, Greenberg GR, Jeejeebhoy KN. Total parenteral nutrition and complete bowel rest in the management of Crohn's disease. JPEN J Parenter Enteral Nutr. 1985;9(3):280–7.
17. Wistbacka JO, Nuutinen LS. Catheter-related complications of total parenteral nutrition (TPN): a review. Acta Anaesthesiol Scand Suppl. 1985;82:84–8.
18. Eisen LA, Narasimhan M, Berger JS, Mayo PH, Rosen MJ, Schneider RF. Mechanical complications of central venous catheters. J Intensive Care Med. 2006;21(1):40–6.

19. Buchman AL, Misra S, Moukarzel A, Ament ME. Catheter thrombosis and superior/inferior vena cava syndrome are rare complications of long term parenteral nutrition. Clin Nutr. 1994;13(6):356–60.
20. Flinterman LE, Van Der Meer FJ, Rosendaal FR, Doggen CJ. Current perspective of venous thrombosis in the upper extremity. J Thromb Haemost. 2008;6(8):1262–6.
21. Werlin SL, Lausten T, Jessen S, Toy L, Norton A, Dallman L, et al. Treatment of central venous catheter occlusions with ethanol and hydrochloric acid. JPEN J Parenter Enteral Nutr. 1995;19(5):416–8.
22. Yaacob Y, Zakaria R, Mohammad Z, Ralib AR, Muda AS. The vanishing veins: difficult venous access in a patient requiring translumbar, transhepatic, and trans collateral central catheter insertion. Malays J Med Sci. 2011;18(4):98–102.
23. Bosonnet L. Total parenteral nutrition: how to reduce the risks. Nurs Times. 2002;98(22): 40–3.
24. Reed CR, Sessler CN, Glauser FL, Phelan BA. Central venous catheter infections: concepts and controversies. Intensive Care Med. 1995;21(2):177–83.
25. Maki DG, Weise CE, Sarafin HW. A semiquantitative culture method for identifying intravenous-catheter-related infection. N Engl J Med. 1977;296(23):1305–9.
26. Mermel LA, Allon M, Bouza E, Craven DE, Flynn P, O'Grady NP, et al. Clinical practice guidelines for the diagnosis and management of intravascular catheter-related infection: 2009 update by the Infectious Diseases Society of America. Clin Infect Dis. 2009;49(1):1–45.
27. Anderson RA. Chromium, glucose intolerance and diabetes. J Am Coll Nutr. 1998;17(6): 548–55.
28. Mehanna HM, Moledina J, Travis J. Refeeding syndrome: what it is, and how to prevent and treat it. BMJ. 2008;336(7659):1495–8.
29. Reuler JB, Girard DE, Cooney TG. Current concepts. Wernicke's encephalopathy. N Engl J Med. 1985;312(16):1035–9.
30. Montalvo-Jave EE, Zarraga JL, Sarr MG. Specific topics and complications of parenteral nutrition. Langenbecks Arch Surg. 2007;392(2):119–26.
31. Grzegorzewska I, Czarnecki A. The influence of electrolytes on fat emulsions stability in total parenteral nutrition mixtures. Acta Pol Pharm. 1995;52(1):17–20.
32. Al-Jurf AS, Chapmann-Furr F. Phosphate balance and distribution during total parenteral nutrition: effect of calcium and phosphate additives. JPEN J Parenter Enteral Nutr. 1986;10(5):508–12.
33. Forrest EH, Oien KA, Dickson S, Galloway D, Mills PR. Improvement in cholestasis associated with total parenteral nutrition after treatment with an antibody against tumour necrosis factor alpha. Liver. 2002;22(4):317–20.
34. Grau T, Bonet A, Rubio M, Mateo D, Farre M, Acosta JA, et al. Liver dysfunction associated with artificial nutrition in critically ill patients. Crit Care. 2007;11(1):R10.
35. Buchman AL, Moukarzel AA, Bhuta S, Belle M, Ament ME, Eckhert CD, et al. Parenteral nutrition is associated with intestinal morphologic and functional changes in humans. JPEN J Parenter Enteral Nutr. 1995;19(6):453–60.
36. Tompkins RK, Waisman J, Watt CM, Corlin R, Keith R. Absence of mucosal atrophy in human small intestine after prolonged isolation. Gastroenterology. 1977;73(6):1406–9.
37. Howard L. Home parenteral nutrition: survival, cost, and quality of life. Gastroenterology. 2006;130(2 Suppl 1):S52–9.
38. Baptista RJ, Lahey MA, Bistrian BR, Champagne CD, Miller DG, Kelly SE, et al. Periodic reassessment for improved, cost-effective care in home total parenteral nutrition: a case report. JPEN J Parenter Enteral Nutr. 1984;8(6):708–10.
39. Jeppesen PB, Langholz E, Mortensen PB. Quality of life in patients receiving home parenteral nutrition. Gut. 1999;44(6):844–52.
40. Detsky AS, McLaughlin JR, Abrams HB, L'Abbe KA, Whitwell J, Bombardier C, et al. Quality of life of patients on long-term total parenteral nutrition at home. J Gen Intern Med. 1986;1(1):26–33.

Chapter 10
Short Bowel Syndrome: Physiologic Considerations and Nutritional Management

Renée M. Marchioni Beery and Vijay Yajnik

Abbreviations

Ca^{2+}	Calcium
CCK	Cholecystokinin
CD	Crohn's disease
EGF	Epidermal growth factor
GLP	Glucagon-like peptide
H_2O	Water
IBD	Inflammatory bowel disease
IF	Intestinal failure
IV	Intravenous
MCTs	Medium chain triglycerides
Mg^{2+}	Magnesium
NaCl	Sodium chloride
$NaHCO_3$	Sodium bicarbonate
ORS	Oral rehydration solution
PN	Parenteral nutrition
PN/IV	Parenteral nutrition and/or intravenous
QOL	Quality of life
SBS	Short bowel syndrome
SCFA	Short chain fatty acids

R.M. Marchioni Beery, D.O.
Department of Gastroenterology, Hepatology and Endoscopy, Brigham and Women's
Hospital, Harvard Medical School, Boston, MA, USA
e-mail: rmarchioni-beery@bwh.harvard.edu

V. Yajnik, M.D., Ph.D. (✉)
Massachusetts General Hospital, Crohn's and Colitis Center,
165 Cambridge Street, 9th floor, Boston, MA 02114, USA
e-mail: vyajnik@mgh.harvard.edu

© Springer International Publishing Switzerland 2016   169
A.N. Ananthakrishnan (ed.), *Nutritional Management of Inflammatory Bowel
Diseases*, DOI 10.1007/978-3-319-26890-3_10

SI   Small intestine
SIBO   Small intestinal bacterial overgrowth
TPN   Total parenteral nutrition
US   United States

Short bowel syndrome (SBS) refers to a malabsorptive state resulting from loss of intestinal structure and/or function due to congenitally absent, extensively resected, and/or diseased bowel. SBS can be divided into phases, some or all of which may require the provision of parenteral nutrition (PN) and/or intravenous (IV) support (i.e., fluids and/or electrolytes) to maintain adequate nutrition, hydration, and metabolic balance. SBS is typically defined by the presence of <200 cm of residual small intestine (SI) [1]. The SI has sufficient reserve such that lesser resections (of ~50 %) may be well tolerated, particularly if the duodenum, proximal jejunum, and distal 100 cm of ileum are preserved. The spectrum of SBS dysfunction ranges from mild dehydration with select nutritional deficiencies (i.e., limited intestinal resections) to severe dehydration with serious nutritional consequences including electrolyte derangements, debilitating diarrhea, and profound malnutrition (i.e., extensive intestinal resections). SBS is the most common cause of intestinal failure (IF), characterized by insufficient intestinal absorptive capacity and the inability to maintain macro- and micro-nutrient, fluid, or electrolyte autonomy without PN/IV supplementation [2].

The clinical consequences of intestinal loss are influenced not only by length of resected bowel but also by various other elements including extent and viability of residual bowel, preservation of anatomic landmarks (e.g., terminal ileum, ileocecal valve, and colon-in-continuity with SI), original organ length, and the compensatory process of intestinal adaptation. A retrospective review of 95 patients with SBS reported that most cases (76 %) resulted from a single massive intestinal resection rather than repeated lesser resections (24 %) [3]. Furthermore, PN requirements after 1 year were significantly greater in patients undergoing massive intestinal resection compared to multiple smaller resections (56 % vs. 23 %, respectively, $P<0.05$) [3]. As long-term PN requirements relate to the length of remnant SI, patients with short intestinal segments are at high risk [4].

Clinical management involving dietary modifications and partial or complete PN/IV support are generally necessary when approximately 75 % (~450 cm) of the SI has been structurally or functionally compromised [5]. Adults with residual jejunal length < approximately 100 cm without colon-in-continuity are typically permanently dependent on PN in the absence of such treatments as intestinal transplantation [6, 7]. Infants bearing <30 cm of residual SI are unlikely to be successfully weaned from PN, although this has been reported in an infant with just over 10 cm of remnant SI [8]. Important prognostic factors for SBS patients with a history of extensive enterectomy include residual intestinal health, medical comorbidities, and preserved splanchnic blood flow [7].

Etiology

In adults, conditions most commonly associated with SBS include recurrent Crohn's disease (CD) necessitating multiple intestinal resections; mesenteric injury resulting from arterial embolism, venous or arterial thrombosis, or midgut volvulus; massive enterectomy in the setting of abdominal trauma or extensive tumor resection; or radiation enteropathy. In the pediatric population, SBS most commonly results from gastrointestinal congenital anomalies (such as gastroschisis, intestinal atresia, aganglionosis, or malrotation) or infection (such as necrotizing enterocolitis). In addition to physical intestinal losses, SBS and IF can be associated with a variety of functional malabsorptive conditions in which the bowel length may be intact including inflammatory bowel disease (IBD), radiation enteropathy, congenital microvillus atrophy, refractory sprue, and chronic intestinal pseudo-obstruction, among others (Table 10.1).

Table 10.1   Causes of short bowel syndrome [7, 17]

Pediatric considerations	Adult considerations
Prenatal	*Postsurgical effects*
Vascular insults	Mesenteric vascular insults
Intestinal malrotation/volvulus	– Superior mesenteric artery thrombosis or embolism
Intestinal atresia	– Superior mesenteric vein thrombosis
Abdominal wall defects/gastroschisis	Volvulus
Postnatal	Crohn's disease (multiple intestinal resections)
Mesenteric vascular insults	Recurrent intestinal obstruction (repeated resections ± extensive adhesions)
– Superior mesenteric artery thrombosis or embolism	Abdominal trauma requiring intestinal resection
– Superior mesenteric vein thrombosis	Jejunoileal bypass (obesity surgery)
Necrotizing enterocolitis	Inadvertent gastrocolonic/ileal anastomosis
Intestinal obstruction (meconium ileus, intussusception)	Tumor resection (primary or secondary gastrointestinal tract involvement)
Crohn's disease (multiple intestinal resections)[a]	*Functional short bowel syndrome*[a]
Recurrent intestinal obstruction (repeated resections ± extensive adhesions)	Crohn's disease (inflammation/strictures)
Abdominal trauma requiring intestinal resection	Radiation enteropathy
Functional short bowel syndrome[a]	Refractory sprue
Crohn's disease (inflammation/strictures)	Scleroderma/mixed connective tissue disease
Extensive aganglionosis	Chronic intestinal pseudo-obstruction
Congenital microvillus atrophy	
Radiation enteropathy	

[a]Functional short bowel syndrome can occur in malabsorptive conditions with intact intestinal lengths

Epidemiology

The incidence and prevalence of SBS and IF in the United States (US) are difficult to ascertain due to limited national registry data and lack of prospective studies in defined SBS populations. Disease heterogeneity with variations in etiology, severity, and precise SBS definitions, combined with disparities in SI measurements, pose potential challenges [2, 6, 9]. Registries of patients receiving home parenteral support are limited to severe SBS cases and may underestimate true disease prevalence, not accounting for uncomplicated SBS patients weaned from PN/IV support or those who did not survive [2, 9]. Based on multinational European data from 1993 to 1997, the mean incidence and prevalence of patients enrolled in home PN programs slightly increased over time to an estimated 3 patients/million and 4 patients/million inhabitants/year, respectively [10, 11]. In both studies, SBS was the most common primary indication for initiating home PN, comprising 31–35 % of cases [10, 11]. A US study examining national registry information on 9288 Medicare patients receiving home nutritional support (1985–1992) estimated that 40,000 and 152,000 patients were using home parenteral and enteral nutrition, respectively, in 1992. Utilization of home parenteral and enteral nutrition doubled from 1989 to 1992, with a prevalence 4–10 times greater in the US than in other Western countries [12]. A French retrospective cohort study of 268 adult patients with nonmalignant SBS (remnant SI length ≤150 cm) followed over 25 years reported that approximately 47 % of patients initiated on home PN required long-term use [13]. Although 50–70 % of patients with SBS initially necessitating PN can be successfully weaned, these patients often subsequently require aggressive nutritional monitoring [7].

Intestinal Resection and Anastomotic Types in SBS

The main consequence of extensive intestinal resection is loss of absorptive surface area resulting in abnormally rapid transit of intestinal contents (diarrhea) with malabsorption of macro- and micro-nutrients and loss of water and electrolytes. Clinical manifestations and outcomes of SBS vary depending on residual intestinal anatomy and functionality (such as preservation of site-specific transport processes, endocrine cells, and absorptive capacity, among others). Three types of intestinal resection typically associated with SBS include limited ileal resection, commonly with cecectomy or right hemicolectomy (ileocolonic anastomosis); extensive ileal resection with or without partial colectomy (jejunocolonic anastomosis); and extensive small intestinal resection with total colectomy resulting in proximal jejunostomy (end-jejunostomy) [14]. Ileocolonic anastomoses are commonly seen with limited CD resections, while the other two circumstances often result from extensive intestinal resection(s) after mesenteric vascular injury or for recurrent CD. Patients with jejunoileal anastomoses are less commonly seen and infrequently require nutritional support; the approach to clinical management in such cases is generally similar to that of jejunocolonic anastomoses [15].

Relevant Anatomic and Physiologic Considerations

Small Intestine

The normal small bowel increases in length from approximately 250 cm in full-term newborns to up to 6–8 m in adults [1, 16]. In adults, the jejunum refers to the proximal two-fifths (~240 cm) of the SI, and the ileum refers to the distal three-fifths (~360 cm) [17]. Normal digestion and absorption reflect gradual gastric emptying of partially digested nutrients into the duodenum, where nutrient mixing with bile and pancreatic enzymes occurs. Contents are subsequently rapidly digested and absorbed, beginning in the proximal SI. Most macronutrient absorption (of fats, carbohydrates, and nitrogen) in healthy adults is primarily achieved within the proximal 100–150 cm of SI [7].

Macroscopic inspection of the SI reveals that the plicae circulares (mucosal folds on the luminal surface) appear more numerous in the proximal jejunum, decreasing in the distal SI to eventual absence in the terminal ileum. Although small intestinal enterocytes appear grossly uniform, a functional and morphologic proximal-to-distal gradient exists from the duodenum to the ileocecal valve, such that the duodenum and proximal jejunum bear greater absorptive surface area relative to the ileum. The jejunal mucosa is characterized by taller villi and deeper crypts compared to the ileum. Jejunal mucosa has "leaky" intercellular junctions, so the osmolality of its luminal contents is similar to that of plasma. Ileal mucosa is comprised of relatively impermeable, tight intercellular junctions, resulting in less water/sodium flux and the concentration of luminal contents. The ileum provides an essential site of active transport for both nutrients and non-nutrients; microvillus enzyme activity and nutrient absorptive capacity per unit length of intestine are several-fold higher in the proximal over the distal SI [14].

Overall, massive proximal jejunal resections are more favorable than equivalent massive distal intestinal resections, reflecting the adaptive ability of the ileum to compensate for absorptive processes lost with extensive jejunal resections (such as calcium (Ca^{2+}), folate, and iron absorption). Residual jejunum cannot completely compensate for massive ileal losses, particularly because it is unable to adopt specialized terminal ileal functions of bile salt and vitamin B_{12} absorption [7].

Jejunum

The intact jejunum provides a site of substantial water and nutrient absorption (Table 10.2). Despite this, limited jejunal resections may be somewhat well tolerated due to the ability of the residual ileum to adapt and compensate for lost jejunal absorption of free water, electrolytes, and macronutrients. Massive jejunal resection, however, results in rapid intestinal transit and impaired absorption of fluids, nutrients, and intestinal secretions. High jejunostomy patients exhibit substantial stomal losses due to rapid, early gastric emptying of liquids and loss of the colonic

Table 10.2 Intestinal locations with absorptive characteristics [7]

Intestinal location	Dietary constituent and nutrient absorption
Proximal small intestine	Fats
	Sugars
	Peptides and amino acids
	Iron
	Folate
	Calcium
	Water and electrolytes
Middle small intestine	Sugars
	Peptides and amino acids
	Calcium
	Water and electrolytes
Distal small intestine	Vitamin B12
	Bile salts
	Water and electrolytes
Large intestine	Amino acids
	Medium chain triglycerides
	Water and electrolytes

brake effect [18, 19]. Loss of glucagon-like peptide (GLP)-1, peptide YY, and neurotensin following intestinal and colonic resection contribute to disinhibited gastric emptying and rapid intestinal transit (as seen in jejunostomy patients lacking a colon) [20, 21]. A resultant decrease in nutrient-to-enterocyte contact time hinders nutrient absorption. Significant postprandial fluid loss is typically seen in patients bearing <100 cm of residual jejunum [19].

Gastric acid hypersecretion occurs as a result of jejunal resection due to the loss of gastric inhibitory peptide, cholecystokinin (CCK), and vasoactive intestinal peptide that are typically predominantly distributed in the jejunum. Gastric hypersecretion and serum hypergastrinemia in this setting are likely related to resected bowel length [17]. Decreased secretion of CCK and secretin are additional consequences of jejunal resection that reduce biliary and exocrine pancreatic secretions, and further impair nutrient absorption.

Ileum

The intact ileum plays a critical role in gastrointestinal motility by slowing intestinal transit, thus increasing nutrient-enterocyte contact time [16, 17]. The ileum is also the primary site for the absorption of bile acids and vitamin B_{12}-intrinsic factor complexes, uptaken by specialized transport proteins located in ileal enterocytes. Ileal resection markedly decreases intestinal transit time and significantly influences nutritional autonomy in SBS, which is highly influenced by the preservation of the ileocecal valve. The ileocecal valve provides an intestinal "brake," mediated by peptide YY, an enteric hormone that delays gastric emptying and intestinal transit. The valve structure also provides a barrier to retrograde flow and prevents migration of colonic bacteria into the small bowel. Absence of the ileocecal valve yields more rapid gastric and intestinal transit times and therefore leaves less time for nutrient, fluid, and electrolyte absorption. Small bowel bacterial colonization can predispose to small intestinal bacterial overgrowth (SIBO) and bile salt deconjugation with decreased reabsorption and increased fecal losses of bile. Depletion of the bile salt pool and diminished luminal bile salt content both lead to decreased micelle concentrations that contribute to fat malabsorption and steatorrhea [17]. SIBO can also contribute to vitamin B_{12} deficiency, as bacterial B_{12} utilization reduces that available for host absorption.

The ileum is the major intestinal site of active bile acid absorption, while only small amounts of bile acids are absorbed via passive diffusion in the jejunum and colon [17]. Ileal resections >100 cm generally impair active bile acid absorption and quickly overwhelm the passive absorptive capacity of the remaining intestine. Consequently, bile acids remaining in the SI lumen proceed to the colon, where they are deconjugated by colonic bacteria. Conjugated bile acids directly stimulate the colonic secretion of fluid and electrolytes and lead to secretory diarrhea through a variety of mechanisms [17]. Although compensation for lost bile acids ensues during the process of intestinal adaptation (with up to an eightfold increase in hepatic bile acid synthesis), massive ileal resections can exceed this compensatory effort. The resultant reduced bile acid pool hinders lipid solubilization, leading to fat malabsorption and steatorrhea. Fat present in the colon is hydroxylated to hydroxy fatty acids that stimulate net secretion by enhancing mucosal permeability, shifting net absorption to net secretion, and increasing propulsive motor movements [17].

The terminal ileum is the principal site for vitamin B_{12} absorption, a highly specialized and localized function. Residual ileum and jejunum appear unable to recruit specialized receptors necessary for vitamin B_{12} absorption and are thus unable to compensate for extensive distal ileal loss. Vitamin B_{12} malabsorption reflects the extent of ileal resection and generally manifests with ileal losses over 60 cm. In addition to vitamin B_{12} malabsorption, extensive distal ileal resections may also affect proximal intestinal functions including the absorption of jejunal calcium as demonstrated in a rat model [22].

Colon

The presence of the colon in SBS has important functional and structural implications, including water and nutrient absorption, energy salvage, and extended available surface area for the storage of luminal contents. The most crucial of these functions is water and electrolyte (e.g., Ca^{2+} and magnesium (Mg^{2+})) absorption, although some nutrients unabsorbed in the SI are also reclaimed in the colon. Intestinal motility is slowest in the colon to allow for such properties [17]. On average, 1–2 L of colonic fluid are resorbed daily, typically with only 100 mL of fecal fluid loss. The structural presence of the colon provides additional intestinal surface area (length ~150 cm), stimulates small intestinal hyperplasia, and exerts a braking effect on early gastric emptying, thus prolonging transit time, increasing luminal contact, and facilitating nutrient absorption [7, 19, 23]. SI-to-colonic anastomosis should be reestablished early if possible.

The colon serves as an important digestive organ for SBS patients and can salvage upwards of 1000 kcal of energy/day [7, 24]. Bacterial fermentation by native colonic flora converts unabsorbed complex carbohydrates into short chain fatty acids (SCFAs), including acetate, butyrate, and propionate, that are readily absorbed and used by colonocytes. SCFAs also serve as an intestinal trophic factor. Amino acids and medium chain triglycerides (MCTs) may also be modestly absorbed in the colon.

Assessments of Intestinal Length

Despite unique structural and functional distinctions, there is no clear anatomic delineation between jejunum and ileum. Such may preclude exact measurements of residual SI length. Anatomic and functional considerations in the assessment of the remnant intestine are described below.

Anatomic

Potential discrepancies may exist among autopsy, radiologic, and operative measurements of residual SI length. Autopsy studies report SI lengths as measured from the pylorus to the ileocecal valve. Alternatively, operative measurements often report SI lengths from the ligament of Treitz to the ileocecal valve [17]. Some studies report that barium follow-through studies (using opisometer measurements) can provide an accurate assessment of small bowel length in patients with residual intestinal lengths <200–250 cm [25, 26]. However, barium follow-through studies impose radiation exposure and can yield inherently limited SI measurements. Magnification effect occurs on radiographic projections that may result in a 5–10 % measurement discrepancy from actual length, depending on magnification. Furthermore, intestinal segments oriented in the anterior-posterior plane can appear foreshortened on two-dimensional radiographic imaging; this precludes accurate measurements, particularly with longer bowel lengths, that can potentially be underestimated due to looping and closely arranged intestinal segments in the pelvis [27]. A recent study of 31 IBD patients undergoing elective laparotomy for CD reported that magnetic resonance enterography images and intraoperative surgical measurements of SI length (measured in standard fashion from duodenojejunal flexure to ileocecal junction or ileocolic anastomosis) had a significant positive correlation ($P<0.001$) irrespective of bowel length. Although larger studies are needed, this technique may provide a noninvasive option guiding surgical and nutritional interventions, particularly for patients with significantly compromised bowel lengths [27].

The length of residual small bowel in continuity along the antimesenteric border measured intraoperatively is perhaps the most precise but may vary based on the degree of intestinal stretch at the time of surgery. As residual SI length reflects available postoperative absorptive surface area, documentation of this measurement appears more important than length of the resected small bowel [1].

Functional

Citrulline is a nonessential amino acid synthesized from glutamine and derived from enterocytes. Plasma citrulline concentration, as a reflection of enterocyte mass and functional absorptive bowel length, appears significantly correlated to remnant SI length ($P < 0.0001$) [28]. A postabsorptive plasma citrulline concentration threshold of 20 μmol/L was shown to be an independent indicator distinguishing transient from permanent IF in SBS patients (sensitivity 92 %; specificity 90 %) [28].

Intestinal Adaptation

Intestinal adaptation refers to the structural and metabolic responses to intestinal loss that attempt to restore absorptive capacity for water and nutrients. Sparse human data on the process and mechanisms of intestinal adaptation exist, and a majority of studies have been performed in animal models [29]. It appears that this compensatory process does occur in humans, primarily in the initial 6–12 months following massive intestinal resection and continuing over 1–2 years (or more) to reach maximal development [2, 30–32]. Structural changes that increase available absorptive surface area include cellular hypertrophy (villus elongation and crypt deepening) and increased enterocyte number along a given villus length. The intestine may lengthen in gross form but more notably increases in diameter. Functional adaptations include accelerated differentiation of crypt cells, enhanced absorptive capacity with increased microvillus enzyme activity and nutrient transporter expression, and delayed intestinal (particularly ileal) transit time [7, 14]. Intraluminal nutrients (particularly glucose and amino acids) obtained via enteral feedings and/or oral hyperphagia provoke intestinal absorptive adaptation through three major mechanisms: direct epithelial cell contact; stimulation of gastrointestinal/pancreaticobiliary secretions; and stimulation of trophic gastrointestinal hormone secretions [14, 33]. Other intestinal trophic factors include hormones, peptide growth factors, pancreaticobiliary secretions, and cytokines, among others (Table 10.3).

Remnant intestinal site appears to have an important influence on adaptive response and subsequent functional outcome. Adaptation is overall more pronounced in the ileum compared to the jejunum [7, 34, 35]. Functional jejunal adaptation generally requires the presence of some ileum and colon. Structural and functional adaptation may be limited in jejunostomy patients as a result of low

Table 10.3 Intestinal trophic factors involved in enterocyte and colonocyte proliferation [1, 7, 17]

Nutritional factors	Short-chain fatty acids (SCFAs)
	Fiber
	Glutamine
	Lecithins
	Polyamines
	Arginine
Hormones and peptide growth factors	Glucagon-like peptide-2 (GLP-2)
	Epidermal growth factor (EGF)
	Human recombinant growth hormone
	Insulin-like growth factor-1 (IGF-1)
	Vascular endothelial growth factor (VEGF)
	Peptide YY
	Leptin
	Neurotensin
	Hepatocyte growth factor
	Cholecystokinin (CCK)
	Gastrin
	Glutamine
	Enteroglucagon
	Somatostatin
	Prostaglandins
Secretions	Pancreatic
	Biliary
Cytokines	Interleukins [3, 11, 15]

circulating hormone levels including GLP-2 and peptide YY [20, 21]. Patients bearing a jejunocolic anastomosis have not demonstrated strong structural intestinal adaptation either although have shown elevated GLP-2 levels [36–38]. Functional adaptation manifests as delayed gastric emptying delayed gastric emptying and small bowel transit in the presence of high circulating peptide YY levels [20]. Elements of colonic adaptation include SI mucosal hyperplasia and alterations in colonic bacterial flora (such as increased bacterial mass and capacity for carbohydrate metabolism), leading to an increased absorption of glucose and amino acids with an amplified capacity for fluid and electrolyte absorption [7, 23].

The extent to which malabsorption improves with time depends on a variety of factors including site and length of intestinal remnant, provision of luminal nutrients, status of other digestive organs, and intestinotrophic factors [23, 29]. The degree of intestinal adaptation also appears to be dependent on type and complexity of administered nutrients [39, 40]. For instance, disaccharides appear to stimulate intestinal adaptation more than monosaccharides [40]. Highly unsaturated fats appear to more effectively stimulate intestinal adaptation over less saturated fats [41]. Some animal models have illustrated a significant degree of mucosal atrophy with exclusive use of PN [42, 43]. However, this has been debated based on data from human studies reporting that exclusive use of PN was not associated with significant intestinal atrophy, bacterial translocation, or immune dysfunction [43–46]. Although complete absence of enteral nutrition has been associated with villus hypoplasia, the actual villi remain apparently normal [44].

Clinical Presentation

As aforementioned, SBS is a heterogeneous disorder with variations in symptoms and malabsorptive severity based on extent and location of intestinal resection, presence of ileocecal valve and colon, intestinal adaptation ability, and viability of residual intestine. Diarrhea (particularly postprandial) with fluid losses predispose to significant electrolyte abnormalities, renal insufficiency, and varying degrees of acid–base disturbances. Malabsorption is a main consequence of SBS that can lead to weight loss, protein-calorie malnutrition, and a variety of nutrient deficiencies.

Details of prior surgical intervention and residual bowel length can be used to predict long-term fluid and nutritional requirements. Generally, patients with greater SI length and colon-in-continuity have more favorable clinical improvements and therapeutic outcomes. Patients with limited segmental resections may remain asymptomatic without clinically significant malabsorptive effects. High-risk nutritional categories include duodenostomy or jejunoileal anastomosis with <35 cm of residual SI; ileocolic or jejunocolic anastomosis with <60 cm of residual SI; and end-jejunostomy with <115 cm of residual SI [5]. Fecal energy loss may help to define IF but does not necessarily correlate with residual SI length [24]. As fecal energy loss reflects both energy intake and absorption, this may vary greatly among individuals [1].

Complications of SBS

Complications of SBS include dehydration with hypovolemia and renal dysfunction, electrolyte derangements, nutrient deficiencies, and generalized malnutrition. Patients with extensive SI resection and colon-in-continuity are predisposed to the formation of calcium oxalate renal stones, although uric acid stones may also develop. Cholelithiasis can occur, particularly with residual ileum <120 cm, terminal ileal resection, or total parenteral nutrition (TPN) use. Given that the incidence of gallstones appears to increase (threefold to fivefold) following ileal resection, prophylactic cholecystectomy may be considered, especially in SBS patients having undergone massive intestinal resection for mesenteric vascular disease who are at high risk for early biliary complications [17, 47, 48]. In addition, patients requiring long-term PN are at risk for hepatic steatosis and cholestatic liver disease that can result in cirrhosis and liver failure, cholecystitis (acalculous or calculous), nephropathy, central venous catheter-related complications (e.g., infection, thrombotic or non-thrombotic occlusion, pneumothorax), and metabolic bone disease [7]. D-Lactic acidosis (ataxia, visual changes, slurred speech, behavioral changes, confusion) is a rare but serious neurologic manifestation of SBS, precipitated by the increased oral intake of refined carbohydrates, that can occur in the setting of a preserved colon and may progress to coma and death [7, 49].

SBS Stages and Management Considerations

Nutritional management of SBS may be divided into three postoperative phases that reflect gradual intestinal adaptation. The first stage is characterized by massive diarrhea with resultant fluid and electrolyte losses that lasts for 1-2 weeks following intestinal resection. Both PN and IV supportive care measures are essential during this initial postoperative period. Aggressive replacement of fluid and electrolytes (e.g., potassium, Ca^{2+}, and Mg^{2+}) is paramount. Fecal output may be up to several liters per day but typically improves gradually over 1–3 months. Patients may remain on bowel rest for 5-10 days after extensive ileal resection to measure baseline water and electrolyte losses and to allow for a second operative look (assessment of anastomotic healing). Of note, oral intake can aggravate fluid losses, particularly in the early postoperative phase; gastric acid hypersecretion, parietal cell hyperplasia, and hypergastrinemia alter duodenal pH and inactivate pancreatic lipase, thus potentiating steatorrhea and fat malabsorption.

The second stage of intestinal adaptation may last from several months to over a year or more. Nutritional therapy should be introduced once fluid and electrolyte balances are adequately achieved, hemodynamic stability and intestinal blood flow are restored, and postoperative ileus has resolved. TPN is generally required within the first 7–10 days following massive enteral resection. Enteral tube feedings are generally started in the late postoperative period and should be initiated as early as possible to encourage intestinal adaptation. Standard enteral formula is generally recommended following enteral resection, with gradual advancement as tolerated to goal [1]. Oral feedings should be increased over time, with attempts to wean from IV hydration and gradually reduce the volume of enteral or parenteral nutrition. Enhanced digestion and absorption of carbohydrates and proteins are anticipated during this time.

In the third stage, maximum intestinal adaptation is reached, as reflected by adequate oral nutrition and weight maintenance. Such may occur within 1–2 years or may extend beyond this timeframe. Although some patients eventually achieve adequate nutrition with oral or enteral feeding, others may become partially or completely dependent on TPN and/or IV support (fluid and electrolytes).

As a myriad of management strategies exist, individualized approaches are required including careful attention to hydration status, tailored dietary support with provision of macro- and micro-nutrients, and correction of electrolyte and metabolic derangements [5]. Mucosal integrity of the remnant intestine must be addressed and treated accordingly, such as in cases of active CD. Additional factors for consideration in SBS management include gastrointestinal dysmotility, gastric acid hypersecretion, bile acid depletion, and altered neuroendocrine signaling pathways, among others. Optimization of pharmacotherapy, encouragement of intestinal adaptation, and prevention/treatment of complications are important considerations in SBS. Health status and quality of life (QOL) assessments are also critical in minimizing SBS morbidity and mortality.

Nutritional Management

Nutritional management of SBS is a dynamic and individualized process that may ultimately result in a variety of outcomes. While some patients obtain complete nutritional autonomy with a normal or modified diet, others require maintenance with various combinations of supplemental enteral formulas, electrolyte and fluid replacement, and PN. Most patients with <100 cm of remnant small bowel consuming an oral diet absorb only about 50–60 % of oral energy intake and must therefore be adequately supplemented. Caloric intake should be increased slowly over time to a goal of about 32 kcal/kg/day (based on ideal body weight) to compensate for malabsorptive losses [17].

Restoration of intestinal continuity via reanastomosis of SI to colon should be attempted as soon as possible once patient stability is achieved. This generally bears low morbidity and mortality risks and may allow for the discontinuation of TPN [5]. Patients exhibiting substantially preserved (≥50 %) colonic function and sufficient SI absorptive length (>100 cm) rarely require home PN. Those with preserved colon and remnant SI <100 cm have demonstrated significantly reduced home PN energy requirements compared to patients with remnant SI <100 cm and no colon [50].

Parenteral Nutrition and Fluid Requirements

Most patients with SBS initially require TPN, supplied at 25–35 kcal/kg/day (based on ideal body weight) for normally nourished adult patients [1]. Infants and children may require higher levels of support per kg [1]. Protein (as free amino acids) should be supplied at 1.0–1.5 g/kg/day (based on ideal body weight), with essential amino acids comprising 25–30 % of the total protein intake. Carbohydrate in the form of dextrose (monohydrate) is provided at approximately 3.4 kcal/mL, and the maximal infusion rate should be 5–7 mg/kg/min. Daily blood sugar measurements should range from <180–200 mg/dL. Regular insulin may be added to the TPN (initial dose 0.1 units/g dextrose) with subsequent adjustments as needed. IV lipid emulsion (1.1 kcal/mL for 10 % form and 2.0 kcal/mL for 20 % form) usually comprises 20–30 % of total calories but should generally not exceed 1 g/kg/day. A greater lipid percentage may be used in cases of difficult fluid management or glucose intolerance (using decreased dextrose calories if the supplemental insulin requirement is >0.2 units/g dextrose). Approximately 1–2 % of total calories should come from linoleic acid and 0.5 % from α-linoleic acid to prevent essential fatty acid deficiency [51]. Serum triglycerides should be monitored and kept at an optimal level of <400 mg/dL. Added PN components include electrolytes, vitamins, minerals, and trace elements, and frequent blood chemistry monitoring is required to maintain appropriate balance.

Baseline fluid requirements are about 1 mL/kcal, with additional replacement to account for gastrointestinal losses. Initial fluid type is generally 0.5 % normal saline IV. In the absence of renal insufficiency, urine output can be used to assess volume status, and additional fluid should be administered urine output measurements below the goal of 1.0-1.2 L/day. There is often a correlation between fecal and urine output. Volume status, weight, and electrolytes (particularly sodium, potassium, bicarbonate, and Mg^{2+}) should be closely monitored to maintain metabolic acid–base balance. Additionally, oral rehydration solution (ORS) should be encouraged as tolerated. Pharmacotherapeutic approaches should be optimized to reduce fluid losses (see next chapter).

The components and administration of PN and IV fluids are tailored and adjusted based on individual course and progression. TPN is initially infused continuously as immediate postoperative issues are addressed. Appropriate attempts at PN weaning should be undertaken as intestinal adaptation progresses over the course of 2 years or more. Home TPN infusion goals should be set (e.g., 1.5, 2.0, 2.5, or 3.0 L for adults; less for pediatrics), and the total volume infused should be gradually compressed (typically by 2–4 h increments) over shorter time periods toward a goal of overnight administration (10 h with additional 30–60 min taper). As the half-life of insulin is longer than that of dextrose, patients receiving significant amounts of PN-insulin may require a longer (1 h) taper. PN should be decreased as intestinal adaptation advances and fluid/nutritional balances become established, but care should be taken to avoid drastic appetite suppression with the provision of supplemental calories. PN reduction with dietary advancements require attention to laboratory data, clinical volume status and output measures (urine and fecal losses), and nutritional parameters. Acid–base disturbances may be overcome with PN solution adjustments of the chloride:acetate ratio and control of diarrheal bicarbonate loss. Visceral protein status (prealbumin), total lymphocyte count, and nitrogen balance should be routinely monitored throughout the course.

Enteral Feeding

Enteral feeding via nasogastric, nasoduodenal, or nasojejunal tube may be used to provide continual nutrition temporarily for up to 6 weeks. In a randomized crossover study of 15 postoperative SBS patients, enteral nutrition via continuous tube feeding (either exclusively or in combination with oral feeding) significantly increased the net absorption of proteins, lipids, and energy compared with oral feeding alone [52]. If a chemically defined enteral formula is used, the rate of infusion should be controlled to match osmotic inflow and osmolar absorption. Infusion rates for full-strength formulas typically start at 25 cc/h and are gradually increased to 125 cc/h, with adjustments based on demonstrated SI tolerance [17].

Placement of nasogastric tubes should be limited to 6 weeks before alternating nostrils. Percutaneous endoscopic gastrostomy tubes are not routinely recommended in typical SBS settings. Although limited published data exist to this end, gastrostomy tubes have been inserted in attempts to maximize enteral intake during PN weaning. Gastrostomy placement may be technically limited by altered postsurgical anatomy and/or the presence of abdominal adhesions following intestinal resection. Lack of data exist regarding the use of percutaneous endoscopic jejunostomy tubes in SBS. Caution is advised in this circumstance, as colonic loops may overlie dilated SI loops as frequently seen in SBS [53].

Enteral feeding not only improves intestinal adaptation and segmental absorption but may also increase transit time [30, 37, 53]. Epidermal growth factor (EGF), found in salivary glands, Brunner's glands, and pancreaticobiliary secretions, is released in response to oral intake and enhances intestinal adaptation [54]. EGF has been shown to promote enterocyte proliferation, increase sodium-glucose transport, upregulate intestinal amino acid transport, and attenuate enterocyte apoptosis during intestinal adaptation [53, 55]. Enteral feeding also helps to reduce SBS-related gallstone development. A lack of enteral stimulus for the production of CCK, the hormone essential for stimulating intrahepatic bile flow and gallbladder contraction, can predispose to cholestasis in SBS [56]. Enteral feeding also stimulates the release of GLP-2 from intestinal L cells of the distal ileum and right colon, thus promoting gallbladder contraction and decreasing biliary stone/sludge formation. Improvements in SBS-related liver dysfunction have been demonstrated with enteral feeding, particularly when PN is withdrawn [57].

Dietary Macronutrient Recommendations: General Considerations

Dietary macronutrient recommendations in SBS vary depending on the presence or absence of colon in continuity with the SI (Table 10.4). The goal is to provide about 25–35 kcal/kg/day and 1.0–1.5 kg/day of protein, depending on whether the patient requires support for weight maintenance or correction of malnutrition [1, 51]. Children, particularly neonates and infants, generally require additional energy and protein. Permissive hyperphagia (oral energy intake equivalent ≥1.5–2 times the pre-resection or pre-conditional oral intake) should be advocated, with aggressive attempts to promote nutritional autonomy. This intake appears to be profoundly important in reducing PN requirements [7]. Patients should be encouraged to eat small frequent meals throughout the day, consuming as much as tolerated based on underlying disease state, gastrointestinal symptoms, and fecal losses. This may mean consuming upwards of 4000–6000 kcal and 150 g of nitrogen daily. Complete assimilation of this intake may not be achieved based on such factors as absorptive intestinal capacity and remnant anatomy.

Table 10.4 Nutritional recommendations in short bowel syndrome based on remnant anatomy

Dietary constituent	Remnant anatomy	
	Colon-in-continuity	Jejunostomy/ileostomy
Protein	1.0–1.5 g/kg/day	1.0–1.5 g/kg/day
	Intact protein	Intact protein
	±Peptide-based formula	±Peptide-based formula
Carbohydrate	30–35 kcal/kg/day	30–35 kcal/kg/day
	Complex carbohydrates/starches	Variable types
	Soluble fiber	Soluble fiber
	– Bulks stool	– Bulks ostomy output
	– Substrate for SCFA production in colon	
Fat	20–30 % of daily energy intake	20–30 % of daily energy intake
	Medium- and long-chain triglycerides	Long-chain triglycerides
	±Low fat/high fat	±Low fat/high fat
Oxalate	Low oxalate diet (ensure adequate urine output)	No restriction needed
Oral Fluids	ORS and/or hypotonic solution	ORS
Sodium	–	Increased dietary sodium intake

Due to SBS as a malabsorptive condition, actual energy needs may be greater than those listed. Nutritional status must be adequately assessed and intake appropriately supplemented to maintain metabolic demands
ORS oral rehydration solution, *SCFA* short chain fatty acid

Proteins should comprise about 20 % of dietary intake. Small studies have evaluated the use of peptide-based diets in SBS with mixed results [58–60]. However, as nitrogen is the macronutrient least affected by decreased intestinal absorptive surface area, peptide-based diets are not routinely recommended [1, 5]. Fats should comprise 20–30 % of caloric intake and contain a high concentration of essential fatty acids to prevent deficiency. In general, complex carbohydrate intake should be encouraged, with the avoidance of simple sugars and high osmotic loads (caused by disaccharides) that can exacerbate diarrhea and increase ostomy output. In addition to hypertonic fluids, patients should also avoid caffeine, osmotically active medications, and artificial sweeteners (e.g., sorbitol) that can increase fluid secretion, stimulate intestinal motility, and further intensify rapid transit. There appears to be no clear benefit to separating liquid and solid food intake [1, 5, 7]. Lactose-containing products need not be restricted except in cases of confirmed lactase deficiency or following significant proximal jejunal resections [61, 62].

Traditionally, high-carbohydrate and low-fat diets (typically with MCTs) have been advocated in SBS. This has been based upon the central ideas that dietary fats encourage gastrointestinal hormone secretion; steatorrhea adversely influences fluid absorption; and carbohydrates pass unabsorbed through the SI to the colon, where they are fermented to SCFAs to provide energy-salvage [17]. High-fat enteral diets in animal models have been shown to enhance villus growth and accelerate intestinal adaptation following massive small bowel resection and may also be beneficial in the retention of lean body mass [63–66]. Alternatively, early low-fat diets in the rat model appear to impede post-resection intestinal adaptation in SBS by significantly decreasing ileal cell proliferation, jejunal crypt depth, ileal villus height, and ileal mucosal weight [67].

A small study in SBS patients (clinically stable for at least 6 months after intestinal resection) reported no difference in stool or ostomy volume, total calories absorbed or excreted, urine output, or electrolyte excretion when comparing high fat/low carbohydrate (60 % fat/20 % carbohydrate) and low fat/high carbohydrate (20 % fat/60 % carbohydrate) diets [68]. A subsequent study of 8 SBS patients (clinically stable for at least 12 months after intestinal resection) tolerating oral, lactose-free, low-fiber diets (22 % protein/32 % carbohydrate/46 % fat) did not support the need for dietary fat restriction. Additionally, an increase in oral caloric intake to 35–40 kcal/kg/day (based on ideal body weight) was encouraged to maintain positive nitrogen balance [69]. A study of five metabolically stable, SBS jejunostomy patients on home PN revealed that increasing dietary fat percentage led to increased amounts of steatorrhea, although the increased intake of fat over carbohydrate calories did not significantly alter ostomy volume [70]. Furthermore, high-fat diet type (based on polyunsaturated/saturated fatty acid ratio) did not seem to affect fat absorption, nor did the type or amount of dietary fat consistently impact jejunostomy output volume [70]. In this study, high fat intake did not affect monovalent cation loss (i.e., sodium and potassium) but was associated with a significant net secretion of divalent cations (i.e., Ca^{2+}, Mg^{2+}, copper, and zinc) [70]. In some reports, high-fat diets (although high in energy) have been linked to colonic water secretion, delayed gastric emptying, and early satiety [7]. Overall, it appears that the concept of net absorption generally takes precedence over high dietary fat content [17, 68]. An additional consideration is that restricting fat as a calorically concentrated energy form (containing 9 kcal/L compared to 4 kcal/L for carbohydrate) can predispose to decreased oral energy intake.

Dietary Considerations After Limited Ileal Resection/Colon-in-Continuity

Response to solid food in the late postoperative phase following limited ileal resection (<100cm) is dictated primarily by the length of resection and presence of the right colon. Patients frequently develop secretory diarrhea (without steatorrhea) with consumption of a regular diet. Treatment with a bile acid-binding resin (e.g., colestipol 1–2 g with meals or cholestyramine 2–4 g with meals) may ameliorate symptoms relating to bile acid malabsorption. Some patients with limited ileal resection and right hemicolectomy do not respond to these agents, presumably due to the loss of intestinal absorptive capacity for sodium chloride [7]. Bile salt replacement therapy with ox bile or cholylsarcosine (synthetic conjugated bile acid) is infrequently employed; although documented in some studies to increase fat absorption, fecal volume appears to remain unaltered or even increased [71–74]. Limiting oral fat intake (<40 g/day) may be clinically beneficial for reducing steatorrhea in settings of documented fat malabsorption such as in patients with limited terminal ileal resection and colon-in-continuity. This dietary modification can also improve fat-soluble vitamin absorption and net absorption of Mg^{2+}, Ca^{2+}, and zinc [7].

Complex carbohydrates, including starch, soluble fiber, and nonstarch polysaccharides, should be encouraged for SBS patients with colon-in-continuity. These substances are not absorbed by the SI and pass undigested into the colon, where they are metabolized to SCFAs by anaerobic colonic bacteria. SCFAs, particularly butyrate, are the preferred fuel for colonocytes, stimulating sodium and water absorption, and providing colonic energy salvage of up to 525–1170 kcal/day [7, 24, 75, 76]. The amount of energy absorbed in this manner is proportional to the amount of residual colon and can increase over time as intestinal adaptation takes place [7]. In addition to providing substrate for the production of SCFAs, soluble fiber can bulk stool and increase colonic transit time [77, 78]. Insoluble fiber (such as wheat bran) also appears to increase fecal weight but decreases transit time [79].

Water soluble MCTs (C8–C10 triglycerides) do not require micellar solubilization and are absorbed independently of bile salts in the colon. MCTs may supply additional energy as fat calories for patients with colon-in-continuity but appear to be of little benefit for other SBS patients such as those with an end-jejunostomy [5, 7]. For patients with remnant colon, the addition of MCTs to long-chain triglycerides can significantly improve fat and overall energy absorption compared to similar diets containing only long-chain triglycerides [80]. However, MCTs do not provide essential fatty acids and can lead to adverse effects, including nausea, vomiting, and ketosis, at high doses.

Patients with ileal resections >100 cm and colon-in-continuity are at increased risk for oxalate nephrolithiasis and should thus maintain a low oxalate diet. Calcium precipitation with free fatty acids in the colon leaves oxalate unbound and subject to systemic absorption through the colonic mucosa. Additionally, the presence of bile acids can increase colonic permeability to oxalate directly. Free oxalates in the bloodstream can precipitate in the kidney, leading to renal stones [76]. Some of the vitamin C contained in PN solutions can be converted to oxalate and result in hyperoxaluria. Dehydration and high-oxalate substances (e.g., coffee, tea, cola, chocolate, spinach, carrots, and celery) should be avoided. Increased calcium intake should be encouraged to decrease colonic oxalate absorption through formation of insoluble salts. Cholestyramine, typically dosed to reduce bile acid-induced diarrhea with terminal ileal resections <100cm, can also bind to intraluminal oxalate to further reduce oxalate absorption. Patients without a colon are theoretically not at increased risk for oxalate nephrolithiasis [5].

Dietary Considerations After Extensive Intestinal Resection

A significant amount of calories should be obtained from complex carbohydrates in SBS patients with a jejunostomy or an ileostomy. Jejunostomy patients, bearing no colon, have similar energy absorption for low-carbohydrate/high-fat and high-carbohydrate/low-fat diets and can generally consume more liberal, energy-rich diets as tolerated [7]. Although increases in the percentage of dietary fat consumption may contribute to steatorrhea, the type (polyunsaturated or saturated) and amount of dietary fat intake has not demonstrated a significant influence on jejunostomy output volume [70]. MCT supplementation does not appear to increase overall energy absorption in patients without a colon and appears to decrease carbohydrate and protein absorption [80]. Soluble fiber may be used to thicken ostomy output [51]. Patients without a colon are unable to ferment complex carbohydrates to SCFAs but should generally avoid simple carbohydrates and high osmolar loads. Such patients also require more aggressive hydration in the setting of increased stool volume [2, 23].

Fluid and Electrolyte Recommendations

Water and sodium deficiencies are most commonly seen in SBS patients with proximal jejunostomies who are unable to overcome stomal fluid losses with oral intake alone. Obligatory electrolyte losses (sodium, potassium, and Mg^{2+}) may occur in the setting of considerable stomal effluents (upwards of 3 L/day). The high volume output is primarily due to the loss of normal daily secretions (0.5 L salivary, 2 L gastric, 1.5 L pancreaticobiliary) that are further stimulated in response to food and drink [18]. Stomal effluent generally contains 90–100 mmol/L of sodium and relatively little potassium (10–20 mmol/L), along with Ca^{2+}, Mg^{2+}, zinc, copper, and iron [7].

Jejunostomy patients with net sodium absorption ("net absorbers") generally bear >100 cm residual jejunum (stomal output about 2 kg/24 h) and absorb more water and sodium than they consume orally [81]. Text management includes sodium and water supplementation, and parenteral support is typically not needed. Net sodium secretors ("net secretors") are high-output ostomy patients who generally bear <100 cm residual jejunum (stomal output 4–8 kg/24 h) and lose more water and sodium via stoma than consumed orally. "Secretor" output typically increases markedly in the daytime in response to food and decreases at night [18]. These high-output "secretor" jejunostomy patients are often persistently in negative sodium balance and generally require parenteral IV fluid for the provision of adequate water and sodium [82]. The goal is compression to overnight infusion, although additional IV fluid hydration may also be required throughout the day.

Patients with stomal losses of <1200 mL/day can typically maintain sodium balance with the addition of dietary sodium. High-output jejunostomy patients should be counseled to restrict oral hypotonic fluid intake and to consume glucose-polymer-based ORS containing 90–120 mEq/L sodium chloride (NaCl) to reduce dehydration and TPN fluid needs. ORS takes advantage of the sodium-glucose co-transporter to maintain hydration. A simply formulated ORS developed by the World Health Organization can be created by mixing NaCl (2.5 g, table salt), sodium bicarbonate ($NaHCO_3$; 2.5 g), potassium chloride (KCl; 1.5 g, prescription required), and sucrose (20 g, table sugar) in 1 L water (H_2O). Commercial ORS types are also available [17]. Patients should be advised to choose ORS as their drink of choice over H_2O when thirsty. Hypertonic fluids, such as juices and soda, present an osmotic load and should be avoided. Along with these approaches, other dietary modifications and pharmacotherapeutic options, such as antidiarrheal and antisecretory agents, can be prescribed to reduce ostomy output (see section on Dietary Macronutrient Recommendations and subsequent chapter on SBS Pharmacotherapy). For patients with residual ileum who lack jejunum, the ORS-glucose component is not crucial, as ileal water resorption is not glucose-dependent [83]. ORS may benefit patients with colon-in-continuity, although the ORS-sodium component may not be as critical provided sufficient dietary sodium is ingested. This group of patients readily absorbs sodium and water via a sharp electrochemical gradient. Slow, continuous liquid intake should be encouraged throughout the day to avoid gastric dumping [51].

Vitamin and Micronutrient Assessment and Supplementation

Micronutrients, including fat-soluble vitamins (A, D, E, K), water-soluble vitamins (e.g., B_1, B_2, B_3, B_6), and trace elements (e.g., zinc, selenium, copper) should be monitored and often require supplementation, particularly as patients are weaned from enteral or parenteral solutions that customarily contain such substances (Table 10.5). Vitamin deficiencies may develop due to a combination of malabsorption and inadequate intake (such as in patients restricting intake to prevent postprandial diarrhea). Vitamin and mineral levels must be routinely monitored and repleted on an individual basis to ensure adequate supplementation and to prevent toxicity (particularly with the fat-soluble vitamins). Supplement doses superseding those of the standard dietary reference intake may be required in SBS patients due to impaired absorption. Liquid preparations are generally preferable, as solid pills may not be properly dissolved or absorbed in the setting of rapid intestinal transit. Patients undergoing TPN weaning and those receiving <75 % of their nutritional needs parenterally should have vitamin and trace mineral levels checked approximately 2–3 times yearly or more frequently if clinically warranted.

Fat-Soluble Vitamins

Fat-soluble vitamin deficiencies are frequently detected in SBS as a consequence of fat maldigestion and malabsorption. Vitamin A, vitamin D, and vitamin E levels, in particular, should be carefully monitored to ensure adequacy of supplementation and to avoid toxicity. Vitamin A deficiency should prompt cautious repletion, as oversupplementation can lead to hepatotoxicity and liver failure. 25-Dihydroxyvitamin D levels should be monitored. SBS patients may require a wide range of supplemental vitamin D doses (from 50,000 units twice weekly to 100,000 units daily) of the parent vitamin D compound based on individual degrees of malabsorption. Serum vitamin E levels can vary based on total serum lipid concentrations, so the two values should be measured simultaneously and assessed as a ratio (vitamin E: total serum lipids). Vitamin K supplementation is rarely needed in patients with colon-in-continuity, as enteric bacteria synthesize a majority of the

Table 10.5 Vitamin, mineral, and trace element supplementation in selected patients with short bowel syndrome [7]

Micronutrient	Baseline dose requirement	Distinct considerations
Vitamin A	10,000–50,000 units orally or parenterally daily	– Caution advised with supplementation, particularly in patients with underlying liver disease, as overdosing can lead to hepatotoxicity and liver failure
Vitamin D	50,000 units 1,25(OH)$_2$D$_3$ twice weekly to twice daily	–
Vitamin E	30 International Units orally daily	–
Vitamin K	10 mg orally weekly	– Deficiency frequent in patients without residual colon and in those taking broad-spectrum antibiotics
Vitamin B$_{12}$	1000 µg injected subcutaneously monthly	– Active terminal ileal disease or resection of >60 cm of terminal ileum generally require lifelong supplementation
Vitamin C	200–500 mg orally daily	–
Bicarbonate	Supplement as needed	–
Biotin	See text	– Deficiency rarely reported
		– Consumption of raw eggs should be avoided
Calcium	1000–1500 mg orally daily	– Higher doses for patients with intact colon and hyperoxaluria to precipitate dietary oxalate
Chromium	–	– Deficiency rarely reported in association with long-term parenteral nutrition
Copper	–	– Deficiency rarely reported
Folate	1 mg orally day	– Proximal jejunal resection or disease
Iron	Supplementation based on need	– Chronic gastrointestinal blood loss (i.e., active Crohn's disease)
		– Duodenal resection or disease
Magnesium	See text	–
Multivitamin	See text	–
Phosphorous	See text	– Deficiency rarely reported
		– Close monitoring for refeeding syndrome in settings of severe malnutrition
Selenium	60–150 µg orally daily	–
Zinc	220–440 mg orally daily (gluconate or sulfate form)	–

Note: Table lists general guidelines for vitamin, mineral, and trace element supplementation. As relative absorption and dosing requirements may vary, regular monitoring with tailored repletion should occur as clinically appropriate on an individual basis.

daily vitamin K requirement (1 mg/day). The remainder of the vitamin K requirement is generally obtained through dietary means. Decreased oral intake, broad-spectrum antibiotics, and loss of residual colon predispose to vitamin K deficiency. Vitamin K is present in IV lipid emulsions but is not a component of all PN multivitamin preparations; prothrombin time should thus be monitored with vitamin K repletion when appropriate.

Water-Soluble Vitamins

Most water-soluble vitamins are absorbed in the proximal jejunum, so these deficiencies are less common in SBS patients without PN requirements, except after duodenal or proximal jejunal resection. Patients not receiving PN should generally be advised to consume one or two B-complex vitamins along with vitamin C (200–500 mg/day) on a daily basis. Niacin, pyridoxine, and riboflavin are found in multivitamin and B-complex supplements and are basically nontoxic. Caution should be exercised with vitamin C consumption, however, as excessive use can predispose to calcium oxalate nephrolithiasis. Vitamin B_{12} should be administered intramuscularly (usually 1 mg dose) on a monthly basis, particularly in patients with active terminal ileal disease or prior resection of >60 cm of terminal ileum who require lifelong supplementation. The diagnosis of B_{12} malabsorption can be made with a Schilling test, and the adequacy of B_{12} supplementation can be assessed by measuring serum methylmalonic acid concentrations. Folate deficiency may develop in patients with proximal jejunal resections and should be supplemented accordingly. Thiamine deficiency can present in the form of beriberi or Wernicke-Korsakoff syndrome and can be detected with measurement of erythrocyte thiamine transketolase activity or serum thiamin concentration. Thiamine should be parenterally repleted in settings of deficiency. Biotin deficiency has been rarely reported in SBS, particularly in patients receiving PN; the consumption of raw eggs can contribute. Biotin replacement doses have been debated, and a low dose (intramuscular 150–300 µg/day) has been suggested. However, parenteral biotin is not commercially available [1, 7, 17].

Minerals and Trace Metals

Magnesium and zinc can be rapidly depleted with diarrhea or increased ostomy output. As magnesium is normally absorbed in the distal SI and colon, deficiency is particularly common in jejunostomy patients with high stomal output. Most magnesium is present in the intracellular space, with <1 % in the extracellular space, so deficiency may occur despite normal serum concentrations. Measurement of 24-h urinary Mg^{2+} should be followed as a more sensitive indicator of Mg^{2+} levels compared to serum or plasma Mg^{2+} measurements. Urine Mg^{2+} concentrations >70 mg/24 h suggest adequate stores. Mg^{2+} repletion generally requires IV infusion. Oral magnesium is a cathartic and may exacerbate diarrhea [5]. Zinc supplements are routinely dosed due to substantial losses in small intestinal fluid (12 mg/L) and stool (16 mg/L). Standard PN formulas supply 2 mg zinc/day, and oral doses range from 220 to 440 mg/day. Plasma and leukocyte zinc concentrations do not correlate with tissue concentrations of zinc and may decline with acute and chronic inflammation; thus, erythrocyte zinc concentration may be used to assess levels. Zinc binds to albumin, but there is currently no standard conversion to account for hypoalbuminemia. Selenium can be measured with plasma concentrations and supplemented as needed at a dose of 60–150 μg/day. Copper deficiency is uncommon, as most is excreted via biliary route. Chromium deficiency has been rarely reported in association with long-term PN. Routine supplementation is not advocated, as high doses in humans have been linked with nephrotoxicity.

Most SBS patients are in a state of negative calcium balance. Oral calcium is recommended at a dose of 1000–1500 mg/day, and adequate supplementation in combination with vitamin D is particularly important for maintaining bone health. Larger calcium doses (e.g., ~2–4 g/day) may decrease diarrhea by binding to fatty acids in the colonic lumen and may also decrease the risk of calcium oxalate stones. Bone mineral density should be routinely monitored, as SBS patients are at increased risk for metabolic bone disease in the setting of malabsorption. Iron absorption is achieved in the duodenum and is not routinely supplemented in SBS patients. Supplemental iron may be required in patients with prior duodenal resection, active CD disease leading to ongoing blood loss, or other types of gastrointestinal hemorrhage. Serum ferritin should be monitored and may become elevated as an acute phase reactant or in chronic disease states. Phosphorous deficiency is rare and uncommonly requires supplementation [5]. However, close monitoring for refeeding syndrome should generally be undertaken in settings of severe malnutrition; the establishment of electrolyte replacement protocols may help to minimize risks for electrolyte imbalance associated with feeding initiation [84–87].

Maintenance Parenteral Nutrition

Despite efforts to optimize SBS therapy using a combination of nutrition and pharmacotherapy, a substantial group of patients require PN/IV support on a continual or intermittent basis. Continuous home PN requires appropriate patient selection and a multidisciplinary maintenance approach with provision of intense patient education and competent nursing care.

Catheter Considerations and Maintenance of Care

TPN should be administered through a single-lumen catheter (with tip in superior vena cava or inferior vena cava) to decrease risks of thrombosis and infection. Home TPN is usually administered via implantable port or tunneled catheter, with percutaneously inserted central catheters reserved for anticipated short-term use of <6 months [7].

The line should be used exclusively for PN and fluids; routine blood draws should be obtained from peripheral sites. Patients should be instructed in the principles of catheter care (including handwashing plus meticulous cleaning of the line with each connection/disconnection, dressing changes, etc.) and should be trained to promptly recognize signs/symptoms of catheter-related infection (i.e., erythema, tenderness, or exudate at exit site suggesting cuff infection; erythema over site of subcutaneous tunnel tract suggesting tunnel infection; fever, possibly only with PN infusions or chills with catheter flushes suggesting catheter sepsis). Of note, the absence of exit site erythema or exudative drainage does not exclude catheter sepsis. Patients should also understand their indications for TPN use and basic instructions for TPN preparation and care (i.e., TPN component mixing, catheter flushing, and IV pump function). Home environments should be evaluated to identify a clean space for TPN set-up; a small refrigerator designated only for TPN storage is recommended. Home care nurses are crucial in the initial education and maintenance efforts for home TPN use. Patients should be encouraged to explore offerings for home TPN resources, outreach organizations, and supportive care groups.

After hospital discharge, medical office appointments and laboratory monitoring for home PN patients should initially be more frequent, while stable and reliable SBS patients may have outpatient visits and laboratory testing approximately every 4 months. The catheter/port site, dressing, and surrounding skin/tissues should be closely examined at each visit to assess for signs of infection. Questions pertaining to catheter care and function should also be addressed. Appropriately maintained catheters may remain in place for several years after insertion [5].

Home PN: Complications, Economic Impact, and Quality of Life

Home PN dependence may be classified as transient or permanent (deemed irreversible). Home PN dependence appears significantly decreased with remnant SI length >75 cm, presence of >57 % (4/7) remnant colon, and early (<6 months) plasma citrulline concentration >20 μmol/L. Among 124 patients with nonmalignant SBS who became home PN independent, 26.5 % achieved this status greater than 2 years after SBS constitution [13].

Home PN is a life-sustaining therapy for SBS patients who would have otherwise died as a result of dehydration or malnutrition [88]. Stable nutritional parameters can be maintained in a majority of long-term PN patients [6]. However, home PN is a high-expenditure therapy that has been associated with various complications including catheter-related bloodstream infections, venous thrombosis, renal disease, hepatobiliary disease, and metabolic bone disease, among others [88]. The most common of these complications, line sepsis, may be recompensed with vigilant instruction and improved catheter care techniques [6]. Liver failure is the home PN-related complication associated with the greatest risk of death [89].

Home PN appears to be a significantly increased risk factor for death (5.6-fold higher, $P=0.013$) when comparing PN-dependent and enterally independent patients [90]. The morbidity risk with home PN appears increased in the absence of a specialist team and during the early treatment period [89]. Long-term outcome reports in adults suggest that most home PN-related morbidity reflects the underlying disease rather than complications from home PN itself [91]. Reduced survival probability has been demonstrated with the presence of a stoma or very short bowel remnant, age >40 or <2 years, initiation of home PN at age >45 years, and certain pathologic conditions (i.e., radiation enteritis, congenital mucosal diseases, and necrotizing enterocolitis, among others) [89, 90]. Long-term outcomes and complications of TPN are discussed in further detail in a separate chapter.

QOL measures are lower among patients requiring home PN compared to healthy individuals and to patients with other intestinal diseases not necessitating home PN [88]. Home PN-dependent patients report fears of home PN-associated adverse events as well as daytime fatigue and impaired sleep due to nocturia, pump noises, and equipment alarms [88, 92]. In a survey of 48 patients on long-term home PN, QOL was significantly correlated with depression, anxiety, fatigue, disordered sleep, and social impairment [93]. SBS-related diarrhea, food intolerance, and home PN dependency can impact travel, leisure, and recreational activities [88, 94, 95]. Families and caregivers may encounter economic challenges as a result of reduced employment rates and medical expenses (i.e., insurance premiums, copayments, pharmaceuticals, medical supplies) along with psychosocial burdens including decreased social activities, depression, and disrupted social relationships [88]. Interventions that may improve clinical outcomes and QOL among home PN patients and their caregivers include patient education initiatives, connections with support groups, and treatment of concomitant symptoms including depression and fatigue [88]. Continued efforts toward PN weaning with optimization of nutritional and pharmacotherapeutic strategies should be advocated [88].

Conclusion

SBS as a malabsorptive condition results from compromised intestinal structure and/or function due to congenitally absent, extensively resected, and/or diseased bowel. The severity of SBS is influenced by the extent and viability of residual bowel, preservation of anatomic landmarks (e.g., terminal ileum, ileocecal valve, and colon-in-continuity with SI), original organ length, and the compensatory process of intestinal adaptation. Nutritional consequences range from mild dehydration with select nutritional deficiencies (as in limited intestinal resections) to profound dehydration with serious nutritional consequences including electrolyte derangements, debilitating diarrhea, and malnutrition (as in extensive intestinal resections). PN/IV support is generally required to maintain adequate nutrition, hydration, and metabolic balance in the initial SBS management phases (e.g., postoperatively). Enteral nutrition should be encouraged as early as possible. Patients with SBS require specialized dietary modifications based on remnant anatomy including the presence of residual colon. Patients with SBS are prone to macro- and micronutrient and essential fatty acid deficiencies as well as a variety of disease-related complications. Despite efforts to optimize SBS therapy using a combination of nutrition and pharmacotherapy, a substantial group of patients require continual or intermittent PN/IV support. SBS is associated with multiple complications, high utilization of healthcare resources, decreased QOL, and substantial morbidity and mortality. A multidisciplinary approach, involving nutritional, pharmacotherapeutic, psychological, and surgical facets, is paramount in the care of SBS patients. Healthcare maintenance goals include restoring nutritional autonomy, preventing complications, and enhancing QOL. Pharmacotherapeutic options to mitigate clinical symptoms and enhance intestinal rehabilitation in SBS are discussed in the subsequent chapter.

References

1. Buchman AL, Scolapio J, Fryer J. AGA technical review on short bowel syndrome and intestinal transplantation. Gastroenterology. 2003;124(4):1111–34.
2. O'Keefe SJ, Buchman AL, Fishbein TM, Jeejeebhoy KN, Jeppesen PB, Shaffer J. Short bowel syndrome and intestinal failure: consensus definitions and overview. Clin Gastroenterol Hepatol. 2006;4(1):6–10.
3. Thompson JS. Comparison of massive vs. repeated resection leading to short bowel syndrome. J Gastrointest Surg. 2000;4(1):101–4.
4. Thompson JS, DiBaise JK, Iyer KR, Yeats M, Sudan DL. Postoperative short bowel syndrome. J Am Coll Surg. 2005;201(1):85–9.
5. American Gastroenterological Association. American Gastroenterological Association medical position statement: short bowel syndrome and intestinal transplantation. Gastroenterology. 2003;124(4):1105–10.
6. Messing B, Crenn P, Beau P, Boutron-Ruault MC, Rambaud JC, Matuchansky C. Long-term survival and parenteral nutrition dependence in adult patients with the short bowel syndrome. Gastroenterology. 1999;117(5):1043–50.
7. Buchman A. Short bowel syndrome. In: Feldman M, Friedman LS, Brandt LJ, editors. Sleisenger and Fordtran's gastrointestinal and liver disease: pathophysiology, diagnosis, management. 9th ed. Philadelphia: Elsevier; 2010. p. 1779–95.
8. Surana R, Quinn FM, Puri P. Short-gut syndrome: intestinal adaptation in a patient with 12 cm of jejunum. J Pediatr Gastroenterol Nutr. 1994;19(2):246–9.
9. Pironi L, Arends J, Baxter J, Bozzetti F, Pelaez RB, Cuerda C, et al. ESPEN endorsed recommendations. Definition and classification of intestinal failure in adults. Clin Nutr. 2014;34:171–80.
10. ESPEN—Home Artificial Nutrition Working Group, Van Gossum A, Bakker H, De Francesco A, Ladefoged K, Leon-Sanz M, Messing B, et al. Home parenteral nutrition in adults: a multicentre survey in Europe in 1993. Clin Nutr. 1996;15(2):53–9.
11. Van Gossum A, Bakker H, Bozzetti F, Staun M, Leon-Sanz M, Hebuterne Z, et al. Home parenteral nutrition in adults: a European multicentre survey in 1997. Clin Nutr. 1999;18(3):135–40.
12. Howard L, Ament M, Fleming CR, Shike M, Steiger E. Current use and clinical outcome of home parenteral and enteral nutrition therapies in the United States. Gastroenterology. 1995;109(2):355–65.

13. Amiot A, Messing B, Corcos O, Panis Y, Joly F. Determinants of home parenteral nutrition dependence and survival of 268 patients with non-malignant short bowel syndrome. Clin Nutr. 2013;32(3):368–74.
14. Tappenden KA. Pathophysiology of short bowel syndrome: considerations of resected and residual anatomy. JPEN J Parenter Enteral Nutr. 2014;38(1 Suppl):14S–22.
15. Nightingale J, Woodward JM, Small Bowel and Nutrition Committee of the British Society of Gastroenterology. Guidelines for management of patients with a short bowel. Gut. 2006;55 Suppl 4:iv1–12.
16. Kahn E, Daum F. Anatomy, histology, embryology, and developmental anomalies of the small and large intestine. In: Feldman M, Friedman LS, Brandt LJ, editors. Sleisenger and Fordtran's gastrointestinal and liver disease: pathophysiology, diagnosis, management. 9th ed. Philadelphia: Elsevier; 2010. p. 1615–40.
17. Fedorak RN, Bistritz L. Short bowel syndrome. In: Yamada T, editor. Textbook of gastroenterology. 5th ed. Oxford: Blackwell; 2009. p. 1295–321.
18. Nightingale JM, Lennard-Jones JE, Walker ER, Farthing MJ. Jejunal efflux in short bowel syndrome. Lancet. 1990;336(8718):765–8.
19. Nightingale JM, Kamm MA, van der Sijp JR, Morris GP, Walker ER, Mather SJ, et al. Disturbed gastric emptying in the short bowel syndrome. Evidence for a "colonic brake". Gut. 1993;34(9):1171–6.
20. Nightingale JM, Kamm MA, van der Sijp JR, Ghatei MA, Bloom SR, Lennard-Jones JE. Gastrointestinal hormones in short bowel syndrome. Peptide YY may be the "colonic brake" to gastric emptying. Gut. 1996;39(2):267–72.
21. Savage AP, Adrian TE, Carolan G, Chatterjee VK, Bloom SR. Effects of peptide YY (PYY) on mouth to caecum intestinal transit time and on the rate of gastric emptying in healthy volunteers. Gut. 1987;28(2):166–70.
22. Campos MS, Christensen KK, Clark ED, Schedl HP. Brush border calcium uptake in short-bowel syndrome in rats. Am J Clin Nutr. 1993;57(1):54–8.
23. Miazza BM, Al-Mukhtar MY, Salmeron M, Ghatei MA, Felce-Dachez M, Filali A, et al. Hyperenteroglucagonaemia and small intestinal mucosal growth after colonic perfusion of glucose in rats. Gut. 1985;26(5):518–24.
24. Nordgaard I, Hansen BS, Mortensen PB. Importance of colonic support for energy absorption as small-bowel failure proceeds. Am J Clin Nutr. 1996;64(2):222–31.
25. Nightingale JM, Bartram CI, Lennard-Jones JE. Length of residual small bowel after partial resection: correlation between radiographic and surgical measurements. Gastrointest Radiol. 1991;16(4):305–6.
26. Shatari T, Clark MA, Lee JR, Keighley MR. Reliability of radiographic measurement of small intestinal length. Colorectal Dis. 2004;6(5):327–9.
27. Sinha R, Trivedi D, Murphy PD, Fallis S. Small-intestinal length measurement on MR enterography: comparison with in vivo surgical measurement. AJR Am J Roentgenol. 2014;203(3):W274–9.
28. Crenn P, Coudray-Lucas C, Thuillier F, Cynober L, Messing B. Postabsorptive plasma citrulline concentration is a marker of absorptive enterocyte mass and intestinal failure in humans. Gastroenterology. 2000;119(6):1496–505.
29. Tappenden KA. Intestinal adaptation following resection. JPEN J Parenter Enteral Nutr. 2014;38(1 Suppl):23S–31.
30. Dowling RH, Booth CC. Functional compensation after small-bowel resection in man. Demonstration by direct measurement. Lancet. 1966;2(7455):146–7.
31. Perry M. Intestinal absorption following small-bowel resection. Ann R Coll Surg Engl. 1975;57(3):139–47.
32. Tilson MD. Pathophysiology and treatment of short bowel syndrome. Surg Clin North Am. 1980;60(5):1273–84.
33. Crenn P, Morin MC, Joly F, Penven S, Thuillier F, Messing B. Net digestive absorption and adaptive hyperphagia in adult short bowel patients. Gut. 2004;53(9):1279–86.

34. Hill GL, Mair WS, Goligher JC. Impairment of 'ileostomy adaptation' in patients after ileal resection. Gut. 1974;15(12):982–7.
35. Vegge A, Thymann T, Lund P, Stoll B, Bering SB, Hartmann B, et al. Glucagon-like peptide-2 induces rapid digestive adaptation following intestinal resection in preterm neonates. Am J Physiol Gastrointest Liver Physiol. 2013;305(4):G277–85.
36. De Francesco A, Malfi G, Delsedime L, David E, Pera A, Serra R, et al. Histological findings regarding jejunal mucosa in short bowel syndrome. Transplant Proc. 1994;26(3):1455–6.
37. Porus RL. Epithelial hyperplasia following massive small bowel resection in man. Gastroenterology. 1965;48:753–7.
38. Jeppesen PB, Hartmann B, Thulesen J, Hansen BS, Holst JJ, Poulsen SS, et al. Elevated plasma glucagon-like peptide 1 and 2 concentrations in ileum resected short bowel patients with a preserved colon. Gut. 2000;47(3):370–6.
39. Weser E, Babbitt J, Hoban M, Vandeventer A. Intestinal adaptation. Different growth responses to disaccharides compared with monosaccharides in rat small bowel. Gastroenterology. 1986;91(6):1521–7.
40. Lai HS, Chen WJ, Chen KM, Lee YN. Effects of monomeric and polymeric diets on small intestine following massive resection. Taiwan Yi Xue Hui Za Zhi. 1989;88(10):982–8.
41. Vanderhoof JA, Park JH, Herrington MK, Adrian TE. Effects of dietary menhaden oil on mucosal adaptation after small bowel resection in rats. Gastroenterology. 1994;106(1):94–9.
42. Williamson RC. Intestinal adaptation: factors that influence morphology. Scand J Gastroenterol Suppl. 1982;74:21–9.
43. Feldman EJ, Dowling RH, McNaughton J, Peters TJ. Effects of oral versus intravenous nutrition on intestinal adaptation after small bowel resection in the dog. Gastroenterology. 1976;70(5 Pt.1):712–9.
44. Buchman AL, Moukarzel AA, Bhuta S, Belle M, Ament ME, Eckhert CD, et al. Parenteral nutrition is associated with intestinal morphologic and functional changes in humans. JPEN J Parenter Enteral Nutr. 1995;19(6):453–60.
45. Buchman AL, Mestecky J, Moukarzel A, Ament ME. Intestinal immune function is unaffected by parenteral nutrition in man. J Am Coll Nutr. 1995;14(6):656–61.
46. Sedman PC, MacFie J, Palmer MD, Mitchell CJ, Sagar PM. Preoperative total parenteral nutrition is not associated with mucosal atrophy or bacterial translocation in humans. Br J Surg. 1995;82(12):1663–7.
47. Heaton KW, Read AE. Gall stones in patients with disorders of the terminal ileum and disturbed bile salt metabolism. Br Med J. 1969;3(5669):494–6.
48. Thompson JS. The role of prophylactic cholecystectomy in the short-bowel syndrome. Arch Surg. 1996;131(5):556–9; discussion 559–60.
49. The colon, the rumen, and D-lactic acidosis. Lancet 1990;336(8715):599–600.
50. Jeppesen PB, Mortensen PB. Significance of a preserved colon for parenteral energy requirements in patients receiving home parenteral nutrition. Scand J Gastroenterol. 1998;33(11):1175–9.
51. Matarese LE. Nutrition and fluid optimization for patients with short bowel syndrome. JPEN J Parenter Enteral Nutr. 2013;37(2):161–70.
52. Joly F, Dray X, Corcos O, Barbot L, Kapel N, Messing B. Tube feeding improves intestinal absorption in short bowel syndrome patients. Gastroenterology. 2009;136(3):824–31.
53. Buchman AL. Use of percutaneous endoscopic gastrostomy or percutaneous endoscopic jejunostomy in short bowel syndrome. Gastrointest Endosc Clin N Am. 2007;17(4):787–94.
54. Chaet MS, Arya G, Ziegler MM, Warner BW. Epidermal growth factor enhances intestinal adaptation after massive small bowel resection. J Pediatr Surg. 1994;29(8):1035–8; discussion 1038–9.
55. Helmrath MA, Shin CE, Erwin CR, Warner BW. The EGF\EGF-receptor axis modulates enterocyte apoptosis during intestinal adaptation. J Surg Res. 1998;77(1):17–22.
56. Mashako MN, Cezard JP, Boige N, Chayvialle JA, Bernard C, Navarro J. The effect of artificial feeding on cholestasis, gallbladder sludge and lithiasis in infants: correlation with plasma cholecystokinin levels. Clin Nutr. 1991;10(6):320–7.

57. Javid PJ, Collier S, Richardson D, Iglesias J, Gura K, Lo C, et al. The role of enteral nutrition in the reversal of parenteral nutrition-associated liver dysfunction in infants. J Pediatr Surg. 2005;40(6):1015–8.
58. Cosnes J, Evard D, Beaugerie L, Gendre JP, Le Quintrec Y. Improvement in protein absorption with a small-peptide-based diet in patients with high jejunostomy. Nutrition. 1992;8(6):406–11.
59. McIntyre PB, Fitchew M, Lennard-Jones JE. Patients with a high jejunostomy do not need a special diet. Gastroenterology. 1986;91(1):25–33.
60. Ksiazyk J, Piena M, Kierkus J, Lyszkowska M. Hydrolyzed versus nonhydrolyzed protein diet in short bowel syndrome in children. J Pediatr Gastroenterol Nutr. 2002;35(5):615–8.
61. Torp N, Rossi M, Troelsen JT, Olsen J, Danielsen EM. Lactase-phlorizin hydrolase and aminopeptidase N are differentially regulated in the small intestine of the pig. Biochem J. 1993;295(Pt 1):177–82.
62. Estrada G, Krasinski SD, Montgomery RK, Grand RJ, Garcia-Valero J, Lopez-Tejero MD. Quantitative analysis of lactase-phlorizin hydrolase expression in the absorptive enterocytes of newborn rat small intestine. J Cell Physiol. 1996;167(2):341–8.
63. Sukhotnik I, Gork AS, Chen M, Drongowski RA, Coran AG, Harmon CM. Effect of a high fat diet on lipid absorption and fatty acid transport in a rat model of short bowel syndrome. Pediatr Surg Int. 2003;19(5):385–90.
64. Sukhotnik I, Mor-Vaknin N, Drongowski RA, Miselevich I, Coran AG, Harmon CM. Effect of dietary fat on early morphological intestinal adaptation in a rat with short bowel syndrome. Pediatr Surg Int. 2004;20(6):419–24.
65. Choi PM, Sun RC, Guo J, Erwin CR, Warner BW. High-fat diet enhances villus growth during the adaptation response to massive proximal small bowel resection. J Gastrointest Surg. 2014;18(2):286–94; discussion 294.
66. Choi PM, Sun RC, Sommovilla J, Diaz-Miron J, Khil J, Erwin CR, et al. The role of enteral fat as a modulator of body composition after small bowel resection. Surgery. 2014;156(2):412–8.
67. Sukhotnik I, Shiloni E, Krausz MM, Yakirevich E, Sabo E, Mogilner J, et al. Low-fat diet impairs postresection intestinal adaptation in a rat model of short bowel syndrome. J Pediatr Surg. 2003;38(8):1182–7.
68. Woolf GM, Miller C, Kurian R, Jeejeebhoy KN. Diet for patients with a short bowel: high fat or high carbohydrate? Gastroenterology. 1983;84(4):823–8.
69. Woolf GM, Miller C, Kurian R, Jeejeebhoy KN. Nutritional absorption in short bowel syndrome. Evaluation of fluid, calorie, and divalent cation requirements. Dig Dis Sci. 1987;32(1):8–15.
70. Ovesen L, Chu R, Howard L. The influence of dietary fat on jejunostomy output in patients with severe short bowel syndrome. Am J Clin Nutr. 1983;38(2):270–7.
71. Furst T, Bott C, Stein J, Dressman JB. Enteric-coated cholylsarcosine microgranules for the treatment of short bowel syndrome. J Pharm Pharmacol. 2005;57(1):53–60.
72. Heydorn S, Jeppesen PB, Mortensen PB. Bile acid replacement therapy with cholylsarcosine for short-bowel syndrome. Scand J Gastroenterol. 1999;34(8):818–23.
73. Gruy-Kapral C, Little KH, Fordtran JS, Meziere TL, Hagey LR, Hofmann AF. Conjugated bile acid replacement therapy for short-bowel syndrome. Gastroenterology. 1999;116(1):15–21.
74. Kapral C, Wewalka F, Praxmarer V, Lenz K, Hofmann AF. Conjugated bile acid replacement therapy in short bowel syndrome patients with a residual colon. Z Gastroenterol. 2004;42(7):583–9.
75. Nordgaard I. Colon as a digestive organ: the importance of colonic support for energy absorption as small bowel failure proceeds. Dan Med Bull. 1998;45(2):135–56.
76. Nightingale JM, Lennard-Jones JE, Gertner DJ, Wood SR, Bartram CI. Colonic preservation reduces need for parenteral therapy, increases incidence of renal stones, but does not change high prevalence of gall stones in patients with a short bowel. Gut. 1992;33(11):1493–7.
77. Atia A, Girard-Pipau F, Hebuterne X, Spies WG, Guardiola A, Ahn CW, et al. Macronutrient absorption characteristics in humans with short bowel syndrome and jejunocolonic anastomosis: starch is the most important carbohydrate substrate, although pectin supplementation may

modestly enhance short chain fatty acid production and fluid absorption. JPEN J Parenter Enteral Nutr. 2011;35(2):229–40.

78. Meier R, Beglinger C, Schneider H, Rowedder A, Gyr K. Effect of a liquid diet with and without soluble fiber supplementation on intestinal transit and cholecystokinin release in volunteers. JPEN J Parenter Enteral Nutr. 1993;17(3):231–5.

79. Otsuka M, Satchithanandam S, Calvert RJ. Influence of meal distribution of wheat bran on fecal bulk, gastrointestinal transit time and colonic thymidine kinase activity in the rat. J Nutr. 1989;119(4):566–72.

80. Jeppesen PB, Mortensen PB. The influence of a preserved colon on the absorption of medium chain fat in patients with small bowel resection. Gut. 1998;43(4):478–83.

81. O'Keefe SJ, Peterson ME, Fleming CR. Octreotide as an adjunct to home parenteral nutrition in the management of permanent end-jejunostomy syndrome. JPEN J Parenter Enteral Nutr. 1994;18(1):26–34.

82. Lennard-Jones JE. Oral rehydration solutions in short bowel syndrome. Clin Ther. 1990;12(Suppl A):129–37; discussion 138.

83. Davis GR, Santa Ana CA, Morawski SG, Fordtran JS. Permeability characteristics of human jejunum, ileum, proximal colon and distal colon: results of potential difference measurements and unidirectional fluxes. Gastroenterology. 1982;83(4):844–50.

84. Afzal NA, Addai S, Fagbemi A, Murch S, Thomson M, Heuschkel R. Refeeding syndrome with enteral nutrition in children: a case report, literature review and clinical guidelines. Clin Nutr. 2002;21(6):515–20.

85. Brooks MJ, Melnik G. The refeeding syndrome: an approach to understanding its complications and preventing its occurrence. Pharmacotherapy. 1995;15(6):713–26.

86. Hernandez-Aranda JC, Gallo-Chico B, Luna-Cruz ML, Rayon-Gonzalez MI, Flores-Ramirez LA, Ramos Munoz R, et al. Malnutrition and total parenteral nutrition: a cohort study to determine the incidence of refeeding syndrome. Rev Gastroenterol Mex. 1997;62(4):260–5.

87. Flesher ME, Archer KA, Leslie BD, McCollom RA, Martinka GP. Assessing the metabolic and clinical consequences of early enteral feeding in the malnourished patient. JPEN J Parenter Enteral Nutr. 2005;29(2):108–17.

88. Winkler MF, Smith CE. Clinical, social, and economic impacts of home parenteral nutrition dependence in short bowel syndrome. JPEN J Parenter Enteral Nutr. 2014;38(1 Suppl):32S–7.

89. Pironi L, Goulet O, Buchman A, Messing B, Gabe S, Candusso M, et al. Outcome on home parenteral nutrition for benign intestinal failure: a review of the literature and benchmarking with the European prospective survey of ESPEN. Clin Nutr. 2012;31(6):831–45.

90. Vantini I, Benini L, Bonfante F, Talamini G, Sembenini C, Chiarioni G, et al. Survival rate and prognostic factors in patients with intestinal failure. Dig Liver Dis. 2004;36(1):46–55.

91. Lloyd DA, Vega R, Bassett P, Forbes A, Gabe SM. Survival and dependence on home parenteral nutrition: experience over a 25-year period in a UK referral centre. Aliment Pharmacol Ther. 2006;24(8):1231–40.

92. Winkler MF. Quality of life in adult home parenteral nutrition patients. JPEN J Parenter Enteral Nutr. 2005;29(3):162–70.

93. Persoon A, Huisman-de Waal G, Naber TA, Schoonhoven L, Tas T, Sauerwein H, et al. Impact of long-term HPN on daily life in adults. Clin Nutr. 2005;24(2):304–13.

94. Winkler MF, Ross VM, Piamjariyakul U, Gajewski B, Smith CE. Technology dependence in home care: impact on patients and their family caregivers. Nutr Clin Pract. 2006;21(6):544–56.

95. Winkler MF, Wetle T, Smith C, Hagan E, O'Sullivan Maillet J, Touger-Decker R. The meaning of food and eating among home parenteral nutrition-dependent adults with intestinal failure: a qualitative inquiry. J Am Diet Assoc. 2010;110(11):1676–83.

Chapter 11
Short Bowel Syndrome: Pharmacotherapy

Renée M. Marchioni Beery and Vijay Yajnik

Abbreviations

CD	Crohn's disease
FDA	Food and Drug Administration
GLP	Glucagon-like peptide
H_2	Histamine-2
IF	Intestinal failure
IT	Intestinal transplantation
IV	Intravenous
LILT	Longitudinal intestinal lengthening and tailoring
PN	Parenteral nutrition
PN/IV	Parenteral nutrition and/or intravenous
PPIs	Proton pump inhibitors
QOL	Quality of life
r-hGH	Recombinant human growth hormone
SBS	Short bowel syndrome
SI	Small intestine
SIBO	Small intestinal bacterial overgrowth
STEP	Serial transverse enteroplasty
US	United States

R.M. Marchioni Beery, D.O.
Department of Gastroenterology, Hepatology and Endoscopy, Brigham and Women's
Hospital, Harvard Medical School, Boston, MA, USA
e-mail: rmarchioni-beery@bwh.harvard.edu

V. Yajnik, M.D., Ph.D. (✉)
Massachusetts General Hospital, Crohn's and Colitis Center,
165 Cambridge Street, 9th floor, Boston, MA 02114, USA
e-mail: vyajnik@mgh.harvard.edu

© Springer International Publishing Switzerland 2016   199
A.N. Ananthakrishnan (ed.), *Nutritional Management of Inflammatory Bowel
Diseases*, DOI 10.1007/978-3-319-26890-3_11

Short bowel syndrome (SBS) refers to a malabsorptive state resulting from loss of intestinal structure and/or function due to congenitally absent, extensively resected, and/or diseased bowel. SBS is typically defined by the presence of <200 cm of residual small intestine (SI) [1]. The spectrum of SBS dysfunction ranges from mild dehydration with select nutritional deficiencies (i.e., limited intestinal resections) to severe dehydration with serious nutritional consequences including electrolyte derangements, debilitating diarrhea, and profound malnutrition (i.e., extensive intestinal resections). Parenteral nutrition (PN) and/or intravenous (IV) (i.e., fluid and/or electrolyte) support are generally required to maintain adequate nutrition, hydration, and metabolic balance. The physiologic considerations and nutritional management of SBS have been described in detail in the previous chapter.

Pharmacotherapy is generally required in SBS and tailored to mitigate clinical symptoms. In healthy subjects, several medications are absorbed in the jejunum. However, because medication malabsorption may exist in SBS, higher drug doses or alternate delivery routes (sublingual or IV) may be required to achieve adequate clinical responses. Factors influencing medication efficacy include available absorptive surface area, remnant anatomy, intestinal transit and mucosal contact time, and acid/alkaline environment, among others. Oral or enteral medication formulations are preferred given the potential risk of catheter-related infections with multiple line manipulations for IV dosing [1]. Pharmacologic therapies in SBS are outlined in Table 11.1.

Pharmacologic Management of Diarrhea

The etiology of diarrhea in SBS may be complex and multifactorial. Management strategies can be organized mechanistically (described below). As significant overlap may exist, a comprehensive approach with consideration of multiple treatment options is required.

Rapid Intestinal Transit

Antidiarrheal agents can be used to slow intestinal motility and allow for increased nutrient contact time. Opioid receptor agonists can decrease diarrhea by inhibiting small intestinal contractions. First-line agents include loperamide hydrochloride and diphenoxylate–atropine. Loperamide is a centrally acting μ-opioid agonist lacking potential for adverse central nervous system side effects (i.e., euphoria, sedation, or addiction) [2–4]. Diphenoxylate is a centrally acting opioid agonist, and its abuse potential may be limited by anticholinergic effects at high doses (i.e., tachycardia, mydriasis, or xerostomia, among others) [3]. Second-line agents include such agents as codeine or tincture of opium. In a double-blind crossover study, both loperamide hydrochloride (4 mg three times daily) and codeine (60 mg three times daily)

Table 11.1 Pharmacologic management in short bowel syndrome[a] [3]

Class	Medication	Dose
Antimotility agents	Diphenoxylate	2.5–7.5 mg orally up to four times daily (maximum dose 20–25 mg/day)
	Loperamide	2–6 mg orally up to four times daily (maximum dose 16 mg/day)
	Codeine	15–60 mg orally four times daily
	Morphine	2–20 mg orally up to four times daily
	Opium tincture (deodorized tincture of opium; laudanum)[c]	0.3–1 mL orally up to four times daily
Proton pump inhibitors[b]	Esomeprazole	20–40 mg orally or IV twice daily
	Omeprazole	20–40 mg orally twice daily
	Lansoprazole	15–30 mg orally twice daily
	Pantoprazole	20–40 mg orally twice daily
Histamine (H[2]) receptor blockers[b]	Cimetidine	200–400 mg orally or IV four times daily
	Famotidine	20–40 mg orally or IV twice daily
	Ranitidine	150–300 mg orally or IV twice daily
α_2-Adrenergic receptor blocker	Clonidine	0.1–0.3 mg orally up to three times daily 0.1–0.3 mg transcutaneously/week
Somatostatin analog	Octreotide	50–250 μg subcutaneously three to four times daily
Pancreatic enzyme replacement	Pancrelipase	500 lipase units/kg/meal (maximum dose 2,500 lipase units/kg/meal or 10,000 lipase units/kg/day)
Bile acid binding resin	Cholestyramine[d]	2–4 g orally up to four times daily
Antibiotics (for small bowel bacterial overgrowth)	Metronidazole	250 mg orally three times daily for 7–14 days
	Ciprofloxacin	500 mg orally twice daily for 7–14 days
	Augmentin	500 mg orally twice daily for 7–14 days
	Tetracycline	250–500 mg orally four times daily for 7–14 days
	Rifaximin	200–500 mg orally three times daily for 7–14 days
	Doxycycline	100 mg orally twice daily for 7–14 days
	Neomycin	500 mg orally twice daily for 7–14 days
Recombinant human growth hormone (r-hGH)	Somatropin	0.1 mg/kg injected subcutaneously daily (for duration of 4 weeks)
Glucagon-like peptide-2 (GLP-2) Analog	Teduglutide (recombinant)	0.05 mg/kg subcutaneously daily (treatment duration not restricted)

IV intravenous

[a]Doses exceeding maximum doses may be necessary in short bowel syndrome to overcome medication malabsorption

[b]Gastric acid hypersecretion generally improves after 6 postoperative months

[c]Opiates must be prescribed and dosed with care, particularly with opium tincture and paregoric. Opium tincture (deodorized tincture of opium): liquid 10 mg anhydrous morphine equivalent/mL. Paregoric (camphorated tincture of opium): liquid 2 mg anhydrous morphine equivalent/5 mL; dosed at 5–10 mg orally 1–4 times daily. Opium tincture is 25-fold more concentrated than paregoric and is thus dosed in drops (or fractions of a mL). Abbreviations should not be used when prescribing these agents to avoid medication errors. As it appears safer to dose in mL, the use of medicine droppers should be avoided [55]. Conversions: 1 mL of opium tincture = 25 mL paregoric = 65 mg codeine = 10 mg morphine

[d]Not for use with presence of <100 cm terminal ileum

significantly decreased daily volume and water content of ileostomy output, resulting in a 27 % reduction in wet weight of the ostomy effluent. Loperamide treatment was associated with fewer side effects and decreased daily losses of sodium and potassium compared to codeine [5]. Antidiarrheal agents appear to be most effective when administered 30–60 min before meals and snacks [6, 7]. As antidiarrheal effects may diminish with use over time, appropriate symptom monitoring and medication adjustments may be required [6].

Gastric Acid Hypersecretion

Hypergastrinemia leading to transient gastric acid hypersecretion can contribute to fluid and electrolyte losses, particularly in the first 6–12 postoperative months following massive intestinal resection [8]. Other consequences of gastric acid hypersecretion include compromised intestinal absorption (due to pancreatic enzyme and bile salt denaturation in the duodenum) and peptic ulcer disease [7–9]. Gastric acid hypersecretion appears to be proportional to the length of resected intestine and is influenced by the loss of various enterogastrones such as cholecystokinin, peptide YY, glucagon-like peptide (GLP)-1, secretin, and neurotensin [9, 10]. Proton pump inhibitors (PPIs; first-line agents) and histamine-2 (H_2) blockers (second-line agents), absorbed in the proximal jejunum, can be used to reduce jejunal fluid and potassium losses during this postoperative period. In a randomized, double-blind, crossover study of SBS patients (median SI length of 100 cm; fecal weight >1.5 kg/day), omeprazole 40 mg IV twice daily significantly increased median wet weight absorption by 0.78 kg/day to a total median of 2.01 kg/day compared to ranitidine 150 mg IV twice daily and no treatment [11].

Transdermal or oral administration of clonidine, an α2-adrenergic receptor agonist, can mediate several gastrointestinal functions by acting on enteric neurons. These include inhibition of gastric acid secretion, reduction of intestinal fluid secretion, stimulation of small intestinal absorption, and delay of gastrointestinal motility (gastric, small intestinal, and colonic), among others. Clonidine may also be used to facilitate colonic chloride absorption [12]. Although data in SBS is limited, a small controlled study of 8 PN-dependent, high-output proximal jejunostomy patients found that transdermal clonidine was associated with a clinically significant decrease in fecal weight ($P=0.05$) along with a significantly decreased loss of fecal sodium ($P=0.036$) [13]. The use of oral clonidine (dosed at 0.1 and 0.2 mg orally twice daily) successfully reduced fecal output by 2.5–3.0 L/day when used in 2 high-output SBS patients otherwise refractory to conventional SBS medical therapy [14]. Hypotension may be a limiting factor for clonidine use.

Octreotide, a long-acting somatostatin analog, is considered a third-line agent that may be particularly useful in high-output jejunostomy cases. This drug may influence diarrheal output via multiple mechanisms, including inhibition of gastrin and other gastrointestinal hormones. Inactivation of adenylate cyclase by octreotide inhibits the movement of ions across intestinal epithelium, thus decreasing fecal output [15, 16]. Octreotide has been shown to prolong intestinal transit time in SBS. In a 15-week, prospective, open-label trial involving 8 SBS patients, intramuscular sandostatin (20 mg dosed at weeks 0, 3, 7, and 11) significantly increased small intestinal transit time ($P = 0.03$) [15]. The use of octreotide may be limited by its subcutaneous administration route, high associated cost, and association with adverse events including malabsorption, pancreatic insufficiency, cholelithiasis, and subacute intestinal obstruction, among others [17]. Some studies have suggested that octreotide may inhibit intestinal adaptation, while other studies have not shown such an association [18, 19].

Fat Malabsorption

Several mechanisms may lead to steatorrhea in SBS including inactivation of pancreatic enzymes (particularly lipase) and depletion of the bile salt pool leading to insufficient micelle formation (particularly after ileal resection). In some situations, the absorptive environment may be optimized with pancreatic enzyme repletion to enhance fat absorption, particularly during the period of postoperative gastric acid hypersecretion [3]. This treatment should be initiated after acid suppressive and antimotility therapies have been optimized. Elemental calcium at high oral doses (2.4–3.6 g/day) may decrease diarrhea, likely by binding to fatty acids. Supplemental bile acids should only be considered with a normal gastric pH given the potential for precipitation in settings of gastric acid hypersecretion [20]. As aforementioned, cholestyramine can be used to reduce bile acid diarrhea after partial ileal resection (<100 cm of terminal ileum resected) in patients with colon-in-continuity, although this may exacerbate diarrhea in patients with a small amount of remaining ileum and intact colon by establishing a relative bile salt deficiency. Cholestyramine may predispose to fat-soluble vitamin deficiency and may worsen steatorrhea in patients with >100 cm ileal resection by binding to dietary lipids. Cholestyramine can also bind to several medications such as antibiotics, beta-blockers, oral hypoglycemic agents, and warfarin, among others [4].

Small Intestinal Bacterial Overgrowth

Postsurgical anatomic changes, including ileocecal valve resection, intestinal adhesions or strictures, and altered intestinal motility can predispose to small intestinal bacterial overgrowth (SIBO), a condition manifesting primarily as diarrhea with gas and bloating. Excess bacteria in the SI contribute to vitamin B_{12} deficiency related to bacterial consumption and fat malabsorption due to bacterial bile acid deconjugation. Rapid intestinal transit in the shortened bowel may make it difficult to differentiate between SI and colonic hydrogen production and can yield false-positive hydrogen breath test results for SIBO diagnosis. Thus, if clinical suspicion for SIBO is high, a course of antibiotic therapy (e.g., with fluoroquinolone, metronidazole, tetracycline, or rifaximin) may be beneficial. Rotating antibiotics and including drug-free intervals (for instance, cycling antibiotic courses over the initial 7-10 days of each month) may decrease the development of resistant bacterial strains [6]. However, caution must be exercised, as the use of broad-spectrum antibiotics can contribute to diarrheal symptoms and may also predispose to *Clostridium difficile* infection.

Pharmacologic Therapy for Intestinal Rehabilitation

The primary goals of intestinal rehabilitation are to achieve nutritional autonomy and improve quality of life (QOL). Promoting intestinal adaptation and optimizing hydration and enteral nutrition needs can help to wean (and ideally eliminate) long-term PN and/or IV (PN/IV) requirements [6, 21]. Growth factors may be recommended in settings of suboptimal SBS control despite maximum medical and nutritional care measures. There are currently two pharmacologic options available for the short-term treatment of SBS in patients receiving PN/IV support. Somatropin, a recombinant form of human growth hormone (r-hGH), and Teduglutide, a GLP-2 analog, are progressive pharmacologic extensions of tailored fluid, nutritional, and standard medication management strategies in SBS.

Recombinant Human Growth Hormone: Somatropin

Somatropin (Zorbtive®; EMD Serono Inc, Rockland, MA) is a type of r-hGH that was approved by the Food and Drug Administration (FDA) in 2003 for the short-term treatment of SBS in patients receiving nutritional support [22]. The recommended dose is 0.1 mg/kg injected subcutaneously for a 4-week period. Early-phase studies involving small patient samples and different doses of growth hormone in conjunction with glutamine demonstrated variable effects on intestinal absorption [23–29]. The largest included 61 patients prospectively studied using a combination of growth hormone (mean dose 0.09 mg/kg/day for 4–6 weeks), oral glutamine (30 g/day), patient education, and optimized diet. Results demonstrated that 20 of 49 (41 %) SBS patients (residual SI ≤200 cm) who initially required PN/IV support became PN/IV-independent at 1-year follow-up, and another 25 (51 %) demonstrated decreased PN/IV requirements. A majority of the subjects experienced the drug's adverse side effect of peripheral edema [25].

The phase III clinical trial was a 4-week, inpatient (dual center), double-blind, randomized, placebo-controlled, parallel-group design involving 41 PN/IV-dependent

SBS patients. The study investigated the effect of somatropin and optimized, gluta-mine-supplemented (30 g/day) diet on PN/IV requirements. Its primary endpoint was a change in weekly PN/IV requirements (collective measure of PN volume, supplemental lipid emulsion, and IV fluids). A significantly greater reduction from baseline in total parenteral volume was achieved in 16 patients receiving subcutane-ous somatropin (0.1 mg/kg/day) plus glutamine-supplemented diet (−7.7 L/week, $P<0.001$) and in 16 patients receiving somatropin plus optimized non-glutamine-supplemented diet (−5.9 L/week, $P<0.05$) compared to 9 patients receiving gluta-mine-supplemented diet alone (−3.8 L/week). Somatropin reduced weekly PN/IV frequency to 4 days (somatropin plus glutamine-supplemented diet) and 3 days (somatropin plus optimized non-glutamine-supplemented diet) compared with 2 days in the glutamine-supplemented diet only group. Optimized oral diet was continued through an observation period. Significantly greater mean reductions in the TPN-derived calorie requirement were achieved in the somatropin plus gluta-mine-supplemented diet group (−5751 kcal/week, $P<0.001$) and in the somatro-pin plus optimized non-glutamine-supplemented diet group (−4338 kcal/week, $P<0.01$) compared with glutamine-supplemented diet alone (−2633 kcal/week). At 3-month follow-up, only subjects who had received the somatropin plus gluta-mine-supplemented diet maintained significant reductions in total PN volume requirement compared to subjects who had received the glutamine-supplemented diet alone (−7.2 vs. −4.7 L/week, $P<0.005$) [30].

The most common adverse events observed with somatropin were peripheral edema (94 % vs. 44 % controls) and musculoskeletal-related events such as arthralgias (44 % vs. 1 % controls) [30]. The use of r-hGH in various dosages has also been associated with carpal tunnel syndrome, glucose intolerance and type 2 diabetes mellitus, acute pancreatitis, and unmasking of latent central hypothy-roidism, among others. Somatropin is contraindicated in patients with active malignancy or recurrent cancer, newly diagnosed SBS, active proliferative or severe non-proliferative diabetic retinopathy, and sepsis or critical illness. Patients with remnant colon should be screened for colon cancer prior to starting r-hGH. Somatropin has been associated with the development of intracranial hypertension, usually presenting within the first 8 weeks of medication initiation. Fundoscopic examination should be performed routinely before starting therapy to exclude preexisting papilledema and should be repeated periodically through-out the treatment course. If papilledema is observed, somatropin should be stopped. All reported signs and symptoms of intracranial hypertension appear to rapidly resolve with drug cessation or dose reduction [22].

Somatropin is expensive, with an approximate cost of United States (US)$20,000 for a 4-week treatment [31]. Although the drug is currently FDA approved for a single course of therapy over 1 month, patients may need re-treat-ment. Further studies are needed to determine long-term effects of r-hGH and details of therapy such as optimal dosing/administration, duration, and mainte-nance of treatment.

Glucagon-Like Peptide-2 Analog: Teduglutide

GLP-2 is a neuroendocrine peptide secreted by intestinal L cells (of the terminal ileum and colon) with targeted intestinotrophic effects. The hormone is released in response to food and plays a role in the promotion of normal intestinal growth and the proliferation of mucosal epithelium and enterocytes [32–35]. GLP-2 has been demonstrated to delay gastric motility, reduce secretions, and increase intestinal absorption [34, 36, 37]. In a study of 8 SBS patients (with resected terminal ileum and colon and no postprandial GLP-2 release), administration of GLP-2 (400 µg injected subcutaneously twice daily for 35 days) significantly improved intestinal absorption of energy, nitrogen, and wet weight (all $P = 0.04$). Body weight increased by an average of 1.2 kg ($P = 0.01$), with a significant decrease in fat mass ($P = 0.007$) and increase in lean body mass ($P = 0.004$). Solid gastric emptying was also significantly slowed ($P < 0.05$) [38].

Teduglutide (Gattex®; NPS Pharmaceuticals, Inc, Bedminster, NJ) is a recombinant human GLP-2 analog (with a longer half-life than native GLP-2) that was FDA approved in 2012 for the treatment of PN-dependent SBS [39]. Recommended dosing is 0.05 mg/kg injected subcutaneously daily. Preclinical models of SI resection suggested that teduglutide functioned similarly to native GLP-2 in enhancing intestinal barrier function and absorption [40, 41]. Teduglutide has been shown to induce structural intestinal adaptation (increased villus height and crypt depth), enhance intestinal fluid absorption, and increase plasma citrulline concentrations in SBS patients [42–46]. In a study of 16 SBS patients (with and without colon-in-continuity), subcutaneous teduglutide (given at 3 dose levels for 21 days) appeared safe and well-tolerated, with significantly increased absolute and relative wet weight absorption, urine sodium excretion, and urine weight (all $P < 0.001$). Reduction in fecal weight was also detected ($P = 0.001$) [42]. SBS patients with an end jejunostomy who received teduglutide demonstrated significantly increased villus height, crypt depth, and mitotic index. Improvements in intestinal absorption and fecal excretion reversed, however, after the drug-free follow-up period. Stomal nipple enlargement and lower extremity edema were the most common adverse effects [42]. Interestingly, treatment with teduglutide led to an almost twofold improvement in wet weight absorption compared to the pilot study involving treatment with native GLP-2, performed over 35 days in SBS subjects with similar baseline wet weight absorption [38]. This distinction may be attributed to the longer half-life of teduglutide or dose variations of GLP-2.

Two double-blind, placebo-controlled, international, phase III trials randomized 169 SBS patients who were followed over 24 weeks [43, 45]. All participants were dependent on nutritional support at baseline and required PN/IV support at least 3 times/week for a minimum of 1 year before study entry. PN/IV optimization and stabilization were undertaken in all cases (prior to randomization) to ensure consistent baseline parenteral requirements producing a urine output of 1–2 L/day. After randomization and treatment initiation, PN/IV volumes were reduced, as tolerated, if 48-h urine volumes increased at least 10 % from baseline [43, 45].

The first phase III study was a randomized, double-blind, placebo-controlled, multicenter, outpatient design ($n=83$) comparing teduglutide (0.05 or 0.10 mg/kg/day) with placebo for SBS-intestinal failure (IF). The leading causes of SI resection were Crohn's disease (CD, 36 %) and vascular disease (30 %). Results demonstrated that 46 % of the 35 patients receiving teduglutide (0.05 mg/kg/day, the FDA-approved dose) achieved ≥20 % reduction of PN/IV requirements by 20 weeks that was maintained at 24 weeks compared to placebo (6 % of 16 patients, $P<0.01$). At 24 weeks, the treatment group achieved greater reductions in PN/IV volume (−2.5 L/week from 9.6 L at baseline compared to −0.9 L/week from 10.7 L/week at baseline in placebo group). Average reduction in the provision of parenteral support from baseline to week 24 was statistically significant (912 ± 1333 kJ/day, $P=0.001$). Two patients in the treatment group (0.05 mg/kg/day) achieved complete PN/IV independence by week 24. Patients in the teduglutide treatment arm demonstrated increased villus height, crypt depth, and plasma citrulline concentrations as well as increased body weight compared to placebo ($P<0.05$) [43].

The SBS-IF patients treated with 24 weeks of teduglutide (0.05 or 0.10 mg/kg/day) were subsequently followed in a 28-week double-blind, open-label extension study in which 52 patients continued teduglutide therapy at equivalent dosing. At 1 year, clinical efficacy (defined as a clinically meaningful, ≥20 % reduction in weekly PN volume from baseline) was achieved in 68 % (0.05 mg/kg/day group; −4.9 L/week) and 52 % (0.10 mg/kg/day group) of patients. Furthermore, both groups decreased PN-dependency by 1 or more days (68 % and 37 %, respectively). Four patients became completely PN-independent [46].

The second phase III trial was a 24-week study comparing the use of subcutaneous teduglutide (0.05 mg/kg/day; $n=43$) to placebo ($n=43$) in SBS-IF [45]. The leading causes of SBS were vascular disease (34 %) and CD (21 %) [45]. The primary efficacy end point of this prospective study was the number of responders who achieved >20 % reduction in parenteral support volume from baseline at weeks 20 and 24. This study involved a more aggressive (10–30 % vs. 10 %) and earlier (2 vs. 4 week) PN/IV weaning protocol than the earlier phase III study. Decreases in parenteral support were undertaken if 48-h urine volumes surpassed baseline values by ≥10 %. Results demonstrated significantly more responders in the teduglutide group (27/43 [63 %]) compared to the placebo group (13/43 [30 %]; $P=0.002$). At week 24, there was a significantly greater average reduction in PN/IV support volume in the teduglutide group (−4.4 L/week from baseline 12.9 L/week) compared to placebo (−2.3 L/week from baseline 13.2 L/week; $P<0.001$). Additionally, reduction (of at least 1 day) in the weekly need for PN/IV support was greater in the teduglutide group (21/39 [54 %]) than in the placebo group (9/39 [23 %]; $P=0.005$). Patients appeared to maintain their body weight from baseline through week 24 [45].

Eighty-eight patients were enrolled to receive teduglutide (0.05 mg/kg/day) in an open-label, 2-year extension of the second phase III study [47]. Sixty-five patients (74 %) finished the study to completion. Of 30 patients who received teduglutide (0.05 mg/kg/day) over 30 months, 28 (93 %) achieved clinically meaningful responses, defined as a 20–100 % PN/IV volume reduction (mean −7.6 L/week). One or greater PN/IV infusion days were eliminated in 21 (71 %) patients [47].

Assessment of both phase III trials and their long-term extension studies revealed that 11 % of patients treated with teduglutide (0.05 mg/kg/day) achieved PN/IV independence [48]. Although baseline demographics and SBS characteristics varied greatly, it appeared that most patients who became PN/IV independent had colon-in-continuity and/or lower PN/IV requirements at baseline [48]. Statistical analysis for predictive factors of PN/IV independence was limited by the small patient numbers [48].

Overall, treatment was generally well tolerated, and treatment-emergent adverse events causing study discontinuation were similar between groups (teduglutide, $n=2$; placebo, $n=3$) [45]. The most common adverse effects of teduglutide reported in the phase III studies involved the gastrointestinal tract (abdominal pain and distension, nausea, stomal complications). The incidence of these effects was greatest in the initial treatment period when PN/IV reductions were seen. Concerning risks associated with teduglutide include accelerated neoplastic growth, including colon polyps. Teduglutide should not be used in patients with active malignancy. Patients should have a colonoscopy prior to drug initiation and should have periodic colonoscopy surveillance [39]. Additional precautions should be taken in patients with a history of intestinal obstruction or pancreatic, gallbladder, or biliary disease. Teduglutide use is associated with the potential risks of fluid overload and increased intestinal absorption of oral medications. Therefore, close monitoring should be undertaken in settings of cardiovascular disease or when using medications with a narrow therapeutic index, respectively.

The average wholesale cost for teduglutide is about US$295,000 yearly per individual patient. The duration of this treatment is not restricted [39]. Despite its cost, teduglutide may yield substantial healthcare savings compared to the financial burdens of PN/IV therapy and its associated complications including hospitalizations. QOL gains attributable to reduced PN/IV time and/or volume must also be considered. Individual costs related to the use of teduglutide may be quite reasonable due to broad insurance drug coverage and patient support groups that offer funding for out-of-pocket expenses [49].

As pharmacologic treatments for intestinal rehabilitation vary broadly, management plans must be individualized based on factors such as patient anatomy, functional status, comorbid conditions, symptoms, and response to therapy. Progressive studies with larger patient numbers and long-term data will guide further knowledge pertaining to the use of these relatively novel agents in clinical practice.

Surgical Management and Intestinal Transplantation

Among the most important surgical procedures for consideration in SBS is the reanastomosis of SI to residual colon [4]. Non-transplant autologous intestinal reconstruction surgeries, such as longitudinal intestinal lengthening and tailoring (LILT) and serial transverse enteroplasty (STEP), have been described in SBS, with the goals of increasing absorptive surface area and decreasing intestinal transit time. Several other surgical procedures have been proposed including tapering enteroplasty, construction of recirculating loops or intestinal valves, reversal of a short intestinal segment, and colonic interposition [4]. However, limited experience, precise patient selection, technical complexities, and suboptimal outcomes may preclude the use of such procedures [50].

Experience in intestinal transplantation (IT) has increased worldwide over time. The surgery has evolved through advancements in both organ procurement/preservation and multidisciplinary intensive care at dedicated centers. Three types of transplant surgeries include isolated IT, liver plus IT, and multivisceral transplantation including intestine, liver, stomach, duodenum, and pancreas. Surgical choice is based upon the presence of liver disease and extent of abdominal pathology. IT recipients require lifelong immunosuppression, the degree of which can predispose to several post-transplant complications including sepsis. Rejection, the most common cause of graft loss in IT recipients, reveals no biochemical markers [50]. Surgical management options in SBS have been described elsewhere [4, 51–53], and the details of IT are covered in a separate chapter of this book.

An approach to the management of SBS in Crohn's disease is presented in Fig. 11.1.

Conclusion and Future Directions

Despite recent developments in the management of SBS and IF, the conditions remain associated with limited treatment options. Nutritional and pharmacotherapeutic strategies vary broadly and must be individualized based on structural and functional intestinal anatomy, capacity for intestinal adaptation, clinical presentation, and response to therapy. Intestinal rehabilitation goals are to maximize absorptive potential of the remnant intestine and to reduce PN/IV requirements, with hopeful restoration of nutritional autonomy and enhancement in QOL [54]. Surgical interventions, particularly IT, are performed in a select SBS subset but remain costly options with substantial morbidity and mortality. Advancements in surgery and pharmacotherapy demonstrate promise in promoting intestinal rehabilitation and nutritional autonomy and provide growing areas of active research.

a) Determine SBS Etiology

- Prenatal

- Postnatal

- Post-Surgical

- Functional

b) Treat Inciting Conditions (if possible)

- Optimize medical therapy for Crohn's disease

c) Determine Remnant Anatomy

- Ileocolonic anastomosis*

- Jejunocolonic anastomosis⁰

- End-Jejunostomy, End-ileostomy

d) Anticipate Parenteral Nutrition, Fluid and Electrolyte Requirements

Small Intestinal Remnant Length	*Long-Term Nutritional and Fluid Support*
0-50 cm SI with colon-in-continuity:	PN
<100 cm SI with jejunostomy:	PN + IV fluids (saline +/- electrolytes)
	(85-100 cm SI may require IV fluid support only)
>50-100 cm SI with colon-in-continuity:	Oral or enteral nutrition
>100-150 cm SI with jejunostomy:	Oral or enteral nutrition + ORS
>150-200 cm SI with jejunostomy:	ORS

e) Determine Dietary, Hydration, and Nutrient Needs†

- *Macronutrients and oral fluid intake*

  • Promote hyperphagia with multiple meals throughout day

    - Proteins (1.0-1.5 g/kg/day); intact proteins +/- peptide-based formula

    - Carbohydrates (30-35 kcal/kg/day)

    - Fats (20-30% of daily energy intake); linoleic acid as 2-4% of total absorbed calories to prevent essential fatty acid deficiency

  • Colon present: ORS and/or hypotonic solution; restrict oxalate; complex carbohydrates/starches (metabolized to SCFAs in colon); soluble fiber for net secretors; medium- and long-chain triglycerides

  • Colon absent (jejunostomy/ileostomy): ORS; limit simple sugars; soluble fiber for net secretors; long-chain triglycerides

- *Micronutrients (fat- and water-soluble vitamins, minerals, and trace elements)*

  • Monitoring and repletion as needed

Fig. 11.1 Approach to the management of short bowel syndrome (SBS) in adults with Crohn's disease

f) Optimize Pharmacotherapy [†]

- Diarrhea: Anti-motility agents (diphenoxylate, loperamide, opiates); bile acid resins; octreotide
- Gastric acid hypersecretion (initial 6-months post-operatively): Proton pump inhibitors; histamine (H_2) receptor blockers
- Small intestinal bacterial overgrowth: Antibiotics
- Fat malabsorption: Pancreatic enzyme replacement
- Hormonal therapy for PN/IV dependence: r-hGH; GLP-2 analog

g) Consider Surgical Management (select SBS cases)

- LILT; STEP; Intestinal transplantation

h) Address Home PN and Catheter Care Needs

- Promote patient education in PN, catheter care, and aseptic technique
- Establish routine office visits and lab monitoring
- Cycle total PN at home
- Address patient awareness of common catheter-related complications, emergency contacts, and access to medical care
- Identify quality of life issues and ancillary support

i) Health Care Maintenance

- Follow patients over time based on SBS severity and clinical course
- Assess for bone health with DEXA scan; calcium and vitamin D supplementation
- Monitor vitamin, mineral, and trace element levels and replete as needed
- Encourage multidisciplinary care**

Fig. 11.1 (continued) Abbreviations: *DEXA* dual-energy X-ray absorptiometry, *GLP* glucagon-like peptide, *LILT* longitudinal intestinal lengthening and tailoring, *ORS* oral rehydration solution, *PN* parenteral nutrition, *r-hGH* recombinant human growth hormone, *SCFAs* short chain fatty acids, *SI* small intestine, *STEP* serial transverse enteroplasty. *Common with limited Crohn's disease resections. □Jejunoileal anastomosis is less common and infrequently associated with undernutrition; management is generally similar to patients with jejunocolic anastomosis. †Although general guidelines are provided, assessment and management approaches must be individualized. Close, frequent monitoring is recommended with appropriate modifications over time based on clinical response and progression. **Primary medical and specialist physicians; gastroenterologist; surgeon; psychiatrist; nutritionist; nurses and home health care workers; social workers; support groups, family/friends

References

1. Buchman AL, Scolapio J, Fryer J. AGA technical review on short bowel syndrome and intestinal transplantation. Gastroenterology. 2003;124(4):1111–34.
2. Shannon HE, Lutz EA. Comparison of the peripheral and central effects of the opioid agonists loperamide and morphine in the formalin test in rats. Neuropharmacology. 2002;42(2):253–61.
3. Kumpf VJ. Pharmacologic management of diarrhea in patients with short bowel syndrome. JPEN J Parenter Enteral Nutr. 2014;38(1 Suppl):38S–44.
4. Buchman A. Short bowel syndrome. In: Feldman M, Friedman LS, Brandt LJ, editors. Sleisenger and Fordtran's gastrointestinal and liver disease: pathophysiology, diagnosis, management. 9th ed. Philadelphia: Elsevier; 2010. p. 1779–95.
5. King RF, Norton T, Hill GL. A double-blind crossover study of the effect of loperamide hydrochloride and codeine phosphate on ileostomy output. Aust N Z J Surg. 1982;52(2):121–4.
6. Matarese LE. Nutrition and fluid optimization for patients with short bowel syndrome. JPEN J Parenter Enteral Nutr. 2013;37(2):161–70.
7. Fedorak RN, Bistritz L. Short bowel syndrome. In: Yamada T, editor. Textbook of gastroenterology. 5th ed. Oxford: Blackwell; 2009. p. 1295–321.
8. Windsor CW, Fejfar J, Woodward DA. Gastric secretion after massive small bowel resection. Gut. 1969;10(10):779–86.
9. Buxton B. Small bowel resection and gastric acid hypersecretion. Gut. 1974;15(3):229–38.
10. von Rosenvinge EC, Raufman JP. Gastrointestinal peptides and regulation of gastric acid secretion. Curr Opin Endocrinol Diabetes Obes. 2010;17(1):40–3.
11. Jeppesen PB, Staun M, Tjellesen L, Mortensen PB. Effect of intravenous ranitidine and omeprazole on intestinal absorption of water, sodium, and macronutrients in patients with intestinal resection. Gut. 1998;43(6):763–9.
12. Blandizzi C. Enteric alpha-2 adrenoceptors: pathophysiological implications in functional and inflammatory bowel disorders. Neurochem Int. 2007;51(5):282–8.
13. Buchman AL, Fryer J, Wallin A, Ahn CW, Polensky S, Zaremba K. Clonidine reduces diarrhea and sodium loss in patients with proximal jejunostomy: a controlled study. JPEN J Parenter Enteral Nutr. 2006;30(6):487–91.
14. McDoniel K, Taylor B, Huey W, Eiden K, Everett S, Fleshman J, et al. Use of clonidine to decrease intestinal fluid losses in patients with high-output short-bowel syndrome. JPEN J Parenter Enteral Nutr. 2004;28(4):265–8.
15. Nehra V, Camilleri M, Burton D, Oenning L, Kelly DG. An open trial of octreotide long-acting release in the management of short bowel syndrome. Am J Gastroenterol. 2001;96(5):1494–8.
16. Gomez-Herrera E, Farias-Llamas OA, Gutierrez-de la Rosa JL, Hermosillo-Sandoval JM. The role of long-acting release (LAR) depot octreotide as adjuvant management of short bowel disease. Cir Cir. 2004;72(5):379–86.
17. O'Keefe SJ, Peterson ME, Fleming CR. Octreotide as an adjunct to home parenteral nutrition in the management of permanent end-jejunostomy syndrome. JPEN J Parenter Enteral Nutr. 1994;18(1):26–34.
18. Bass BL, Fischer BA, Richardson C, Harmon JW. Somatostatin analogue treatment inhibits post-resectional adaptation of the small bowel in rats. Am J Surg. 1991;161(1):107–11; discussion 111–2.
19. Vanderhoof JA, Kollman KA. Lack of inhibitory effect of octreotide on intestinal adaptation in short bowel syndrome in the rat. J Pediatr Gastroenterol Nutr. 1998;26(3):241–4.
20. Hofmann AF, Mysels KJ. Bile acid solubility and precipitation in vitro and in vivo: the role of conjugation, pH, and Ca2+ ions. J Lipid Res. 1992;33(5):617–26.
21. Messing B, Crenn P, Beau P, Boutron-Ruault MC, Rambaud JC, Matuchansky C. Long-term survival and parenteral nutrition dependence in adult patients with the short bowel syndrome. Gastroenterology. 1999;117(5):1043–50.
22. Zorbtive® (somatropin [rNA origin]). Prescribing information. Rockland, MA: EMD Serono; 2003.

23. Byrne TA, Morrissey TB, Nattakom TV, Ziegler TR, Wilmore DW. Growth hormone, glutamine, and a modified diet enhance nutrient absorption in patients with severe short bowel syndrome. JPEN J Parenter Enteral Nutr. 1995;19(4):296–302.
24. Byrne TA, Persinger RL, Young LS, Ziegler TR, Wilmore DW. A new treatment for patients with short-bowel syndrome. Growth hormone, glutamine, and a modified diet. Ann Surg. 1995;222(3):243–54; discussion 254–5.
25. Byrne TA, Cox S, Karimbakas M, Veglia LM, Bennett HM, Lautz DB, et al. Bowel rehabilitation: an alternative to long-term parenteral nutrition and intestinal transplantation for some patients with short bowel syndrome. Transplant Proc. 2002;34(3):887–90.
26. Ellegard L, Bosaeus I, Nordgren S, Bengtsson BA. Low-dose recombinant human growth hormone increases body weight and lean body mass in patients with short bowel syndrome. Ann Surg. 1997;225(1):88–96.
27. Scolapio JS. Effect of growth hormone, glutamine, and diet on body composition in short bowel syndrome: a randomized, controlled study. JPEN J Parenter Enteral Nutr. 1999;23(6):309–12; discussion 312–3.
28. Seguy D, Vahedi K, Kapel N, Souberbielle JC, Messing B. Low-dose growth hormone in adult home parenteral nutrition-dependent short bowel syndrome patients: a positive study. Gastroenterology. 2003;124(2):293–302.
29. Szkudlarek J, Jeppesen PB, Mortensen PB. Effect of high dose growth hormone with glutamine and no change in diet on intestinal absorption in short bowel patients: a randomised, double blind, crossover, placebo controlled study. Gut. 2000;47(2):199–205.
30. Byrne TA, Wilmore DW, Iyer K, Dibaise J, Clancy K, Robinson MK, et al. Growth hormone, glutamine, and an optimal diet reduces parenteral nutrition in patients with short bowel syndrome: a prospective, randomized, placebo-controlled, double-blind clinical trial. Ann Surg. 2005; 242(5):655–61.
31. Parekh NR, Steiger E. Criteria for the use of recombinant human growth hormone in short bowel syndrome. Nutr Clin Pract. 2005;20(5):503–8.
32. Drucker DJ, Erlich P, Asa SL, Brubaker PL. Induction of intestinal epithelial proliferation by glucagon-like peptide 2. Proc Natl Acad Sci U S A. 1996;93(15):7911–6.
33. Tsai CH, Hill M, Asa SL, Brubaker PL, Drucker DJ. Intestinal growth-promoting properties of glucagon-like peptide-2 in mice. Am J Physiol. 1997;273(1 Pt 1):E77–84.
34. Brubaker PL, Izzo A, Hill M, Drucker DJ. Intestinal function in mice with small bowel growth induced by glucagon-like peptide-2. Am J Physiol. 1997;272(6 Pt 1):E1050–8.
35. Dube PE, Brubaker PL. Frontiers in glucagon-like peptide-2: multiple actions, multiple mediators. Am J Physiol Endocrinol Metab. 2007;293(2):E460–5.
36. Baldassano S, Liu S, Qu MH, Mule F, Wood JD. Glucagon-like peptide-2 modulates neurally evoked mucosal chloride secretion in guinea pig small intestine in vitro. Am J Physiol Gastrointest Liver Physiol. 2009;297(4):G800–5.
37. Wojdemann M, Wettergren A, Hartmann B, Holst JJ. Glucagon-like peptide-2 inhibits centrally induced antral motility in pigs. Scand J Gastroenterol. 1998;33(8):828–32.
38. Jeppesen PB, Hartmann B, Thulesen J, Graff J, Lohmann J, Hansen BS, et al. Glucagon-like peptide 2 improves nutrient absorption and nutritional status in short-bowel patients with no colon. Gastroenterology. 2001;120(4):806–15.
39. GATTEX® (teduglutide [rDNA origin]). Full prescribing information. Bedminster, NJ: NPS Pharmaceuticals; 2012.
40. Benjamin MA, McKay DM, Yang PC, Cameron H, Perdue MH. Glucagon-like peptide-2 enhances intestinal epithelial barrier function of both transcellular and paracellular pathways in the mouse. Gut. 2000;47(1):112–9.
41. Scott RB, Kirk D, MacNaughton WK, Meddings JB. GLP-2 augments the adaptive response to massive intestinal resection in rat. Am J Physiol. 1998;275(5 Pt 1):G911–21.
42. Jeppesen PB, Sanguinetti EL, Buchman A, Howard L, Scolapio JS, Ziegler TR, et al. Teduglutide (ALX-0600), a dipeptidyl peptidase IV resistant glucagon-like peptide 2 analogue, improves intestinal function in short bowel syndrome patients. Gut. 2005;54(9):1224–31.

43. Jeppesen PB, Gilroy R, Pertkiewicz M, Allard JP, Messing B, O'Keefe SJ. Randomised placebo-controlled trial of teduglutide in reducing parenteral nutrition and/or intravenous fluid requirements in patients with short bowel syndrome. Gut. 2011;60(7):902–14.
44. Tappenden KA, Edelman J, Joelsson B. Teduglutide enhances structural adaptation of the small intestinal mucosa in patients with short bowel syndrome. J Clin Gastroenterol. 2013; 47(7):602–7.
45. Jeppesen PB, Pertkiewicz M, Messing B, Iyer K, Seidner DL, O'keefe SJ, et al. Teduglutide reduces need for parenteral support among patients with short bowel syndrome with intestinal failure. Gastroenterology. 2012;143(6):1473–81. e3.
46. O'Keefe SJD, Jeppesen PB, Gilroy R, Pertkiewicz M, Allard JP, Messing B. Safety and efficacy of teduglutide after 52 weeks of treatment in patients with short bowel intestinal failure. Clin Gastroenterol Hepatol. 2013;11(7):815–23. e3.
47. Schwartz LK, O'Keefe SJ, Jeppesen PB, Pertkiewicz M, Youssef N, Fujioka K. Long-term safety and efficacy of teduglutide for the treatment of intestinal failure associated with short bowel syndrome: final results of the STEPS-2 study, a 2-year, multicenter, open-label clinical trial. Am J Gastroenterol. 2013;108:S101.
48. Iyer KR, Joelsson B, Heinze H, Jeppesen PB. Complete enteral autonomy and independence from parenteral nutrition/intravenous support in short bowel syndrome with intestinal failure-accruing experience with teduglutide. Gastroenterology. 2013;144:S–169.
49. Jeppesen PB. Pharmacologic options for intestinal rehabilitation in patients with short bowel syndrome. JPEN J Parenter Enteral Nutr. 2014;38(1 Suppl):45S–52.
50. American Gastroenterological Association. American Gastroenterological Association medical position statement: short bowel syndrome and intestinal transplantation. Gastroenterology. 2003;124(4):1105–10.
51. Abu-Elmagd K. The concept of gut rehabilitation and the future of visceral transplantation. Nat Rev Gastroenterol Hepatol. 2015;20.
52. Reyes JD. Intestinal transplantation: an unexpected journey. Robert E. Gross Lecture. J Pediatr Surg. 2014;49(1):13–8.
53. Frongia G, Kessler M, Weih S, Nickkholgh A, Mehrabi A, Holland-Cunz S. Comparison of LILT and STEP procedures in children with short bowel syndrome—a systematic review of the literature. J Pediatr Surg. 2013;48(8):1794–805.
54. Matarese LE, Jeppesen PB, O'Keefe SJ. Short bowel syndrome in adults: the need for an interdisciplinary approach and coordinated care. JPEN J Parenter Enteral Nutr. 2014;38(1 Suppl):60S–4.
55. http://www.fda.gov/downloads/Drugs/DrugSafety/MedicationErrors/UCM080654

Chapter 12
Small Bowel Transplantation

Philip J. Allan, Anil Vaidya, and Simon Lal

Abbreviations

CD	Crohn's disease
ECF	Enterocutaneous fistula
HPN	Home parenteral nutrition
IBD	Inflammatory bowel disease
IF	Intestinal failure
IFALD	IF associated liver disease
PSC	Primary sclerosing cholangitis
QoL	Quality of life
UC	Ulcerative colitis

P.J. Allan, M.B.B.S., B.Sc., D.P.H.I.L., M.R.C.P. (✉)
The Translational Gastroenterology Unit, Oxford University Hospitals NHS Trust, John Radcliffe Hospital, Headley Way, Oxford OX3 9DU, UK

The Oxford Transplant Centre, Oxford University Hospitals NHS Trust, Churchill Hospital, Oxford OX3 7LE, UK

The Intestinal Failure Unit, Salford Royal NHS Foundation Trust, Salford M6 8HD, UK
e-mail: philip.allan@ouh.nhs.uk

A. Vaidya, M.D.
The Oxford Transplant Centre, Oxford University Hospitals NHS Trust, Churchill Hospital, Oxford OX3 7LE, UK

S. Lal, M.B.B.S., Ph.D., F.R.C.P.
The Intestinal Failure Unit, Salford Royal NHS Foundation Trust, Salford M6 8HD, UK

© Springer International Publishing Switzerland 2016
A.N. Ananthakrishnan (ed.), *Nutritional Management of Inflammatory Bowel Diseases*, DOI 10.1007/978-3-319-26890-3_12

Introduction

Some conditions are more prone to developing intestinal failure (IF) than others; the risk of IF is inherent within inflammatory bowel disease (IBD), in particular in Crohn's disease (CD). In this chapter, we summarise the risk of developing IF in IBD, the history behind small bowel intestinal transplantation, the types of operations undertaken, the indications for having a transplant, and the risks and outcomes associated with transplantation.

Overview of IF

IF develops when a person's gut is unable to absorb sufficient water, electrolytes, macro- or micronutrients to maintain health. This typically occurs following gastrointestinal obstruction, resection, disease-related compromise of gut function, or dysmotility. Three IF types exist: Types 1, 2 and 3 [1, 2], where Type 1 is self-limiting and typically due to post-operative complications such as an ileus; Type 2 typically includes patients who develop sepsis and require a prolonged period on PN to provide nutritional stability prior to definitive reconstructive surgery; patients with Type 3 require long-term PN. It is this final category, type 3 that is the focus of the role of transplantation in patients with IBD in this chapter.

Risk of IF Development in IBD

The point prevalence of type 3 IF in IBD as a proportion of all IF cases is for Ulcerative Colitis (UC) 3 % and CD 29 % [3], but the overall incidence of patients with IBD developing IF is low. In UC, this is typically due to complications in those who were immunocompromised at the time of surgery, had a delayed timing of colectomy, required a reoperation or due to surgical complications following an unrelated event later in life [4]. In contrast, type 3 IF in CD results from three main reasons: recurrent uncomplicated operations removing bowel sequentially, complications following surgery for intra-abdominal sepsis or extensive disease in the small bowel uncontrolled by available therapy [4]. Following a first operation for CD, the risk of developing IF at 5, 10, 15 and 20 years is 0.8, 3.6, 6.1 and 8.5 % [5] and associations with developing IF are a younger age at diagnosis, stricturing disease at first operation or a family history of IBD [6, 7].

A Historical Perspective on Small Bowel Transplantation

Transplantation of tissue or organs has been part of modern medicine for the past 60 years. It was born out of the surgical and immunological knowledge at the time, but there were key medical developments that enabled it to become a reality.

The first key development was the ability to join blood vessels together, developed by a French surgeon Alexis Carrel in 1902. Following this, the first tissue transplant occurred in 1905 when Eduard Zirm transplanted a cornea in Moravia, modern day Czech Republic. Lastly, the regular use of blood transfusions during the First World War in 1918 brought an understanding of the requirement to match blood groups. However, it was not until 1954 when Joseph Murray transplanted a kidney as the first solid organ transplant in Boston, Massachusetts, and this was followed in 1963 by the first liver transplant by Thomas Starzl in Denver, Colorado. The first adult intestinal transplant reported was a combined liver and small bowel in 1988 by Grant and colleagues from London, Ontario, and the patient successfully survived over a year post-transplantation [8]. This had been preceded by paediatric experience [9, 10] and was followed in quick succession by others producing results of large series, especially from one of the most prolific centres, Pittsburg [11]. The advent of tacrolimus in 1989 brought improved immunosuppression and this, along with improved surgical techniques, led to an increase in the number of transplant performed each year until 2005, where it has remained stable [12]. In the UK, the number of intestinal transplants has risen from single figures (2000–2008) to 14–22 per annum (2011–2013) [13]. Outside North America and Europe, the number of transplant centres is increasing and with increasing activity. Of the worldwide transplants carried out between 2006 and 2011, 13 % were for patients with CD [12].

Types of Intestinal Transplantation

There are a number of different types of graft available, and the type transplanted is determined by the disease processes of the recipient. Some organs, such as the stomach and colon, may not be transplanted if during the preparatory operation in the recipient compromises are made during difficult dissection in a potentially hostile abdomen, in particular ensuring adequate access to the portal venous system and arterial blood supply. The donor organ quality and anatomical organisation may also impact on the final organs transplanted.

Small Bowel Transplant Alone

This is the simplest procedure as it requires insertion of jejunum and ileum attached to native duodenum, jejunum or stomach, and then the formation of distal ileostomy. If native colon remains in situ, then the option remains for a future return of intestinal continuity. In some instances, a donor ileum-native colon anastomosis will occur at transplantation and an access point or 'chimney' will be formed with ileum to facilitate access to the small bowel that can then be removed at a later date. Arterial supply is often via the abdominal aorta, mesenteric arteries or internal iliacs. Venous drainage may be either via the portal system (ideal) or via the inferior vena cava.

Modified Multivisceral

Extensive disease, in particular, affecting stomach, small bowel, colon, kidneys or pancreas would necessitate a modified multivisceral transplantation, incorporating multiple organs without the liver. Initially, it was thought that the colon proved problematic with increased risk of graft loss or recipient mortality [11]; however, it remains a very useful adjunct in salt and water management in the long run and is now being more commonly transplanted [14]. Arterial and venous supply would be dependent on the anatomy and required organs.

Multivisceral

This encompasses both combined liver with small bowel and full multivisceral including other organs such as stomach, colon, pancreas and kidneys. This is often reserved for those who have developed IF associated liver disease (IFALD) or, in the cases of patients with IBD, in those who have coexisting liver disease, such as primary sclerosing cholangitis (PSC). The advantage of a multivisceral is the provision of the organs en bloc with portal drainage already included, but this surgical advantage is tempered by patients who often have abdominal varices and a poorer physiological state at the outset that complicate the peri- and post-operative phase.

Abdominal Wall

In SBITx cases, the closure of the abdominal wall has frequently proved challenging, requiring plastic surgical techniques to assist in abdominal wall closure; in one study, 33 % of cases required plastic surgical techniques to provide satisfactory closure [15]. Patients who have suffered from complex CD, in particular those who have had multiple resections over a number of years or those who have complex fistulating disease requiring resection of significant abdominal surface area, are becoming better served through abdominal wall grafts, which were first reported in 2003 [16]. The lack of internal abdominal capacity could prevent sufficient closure of the abdominal wall at grafting. This would put the graft at risk, as arterial leakage, for example due to infection of the anastomosis, would result in graft loss and may be fatal. We have had good success with a number of patients requiring abdominal wall grafts [17] aided by the use of remote revascularisation of abdominal wall graft on the forearm whilst the intestinal graft is inserted to reduce cold ischaemia time during prolonged operations [18]. The presence of a sentinel skin flap on the forearm or the abdominal wall graft provides a visual checkpoint for patients to alert them to early signs of transplant rejection (see section 'Rejection') if a rash develops on the grafted skin but not on the body, or graft versus host disease (GVHD) (see section 'Graft Versus Host Disease') where the rash develops on the body but not on the graft.

IBD

For the majority of patients with IBD with type 3 IF, an isolated small bowel will suffice, unless there is evidence of other organ dysfunction, such as diabetes mellitus (where a pancreatic graft may be needed) or renal impairment due to conditions such as recurrent dehydration or oxalate nephropathy. In those with PSC or who have developed IFALD, then combined liver and small bowel would be required. In those with complex fistulating Crohn's disease or in those who have contraction of the abdominal cavity, abdominal grafts are proving a useful adjunct in their management.

Indications

The current choice between HPN and SBITx as the primary therapeutic options for patients with Type 3 IF is currently determined by predicted survival outcome. If a patient remains well and complication free, then HPN remains the superior long-term option; if complications develop or the patient has a high risk of death due to their underlying disease, then SBITx is the option of choice. Patients with IBD accounted 11 % of the SBITx in one centre [19], but account for 29 % of HPN cases in the UK [3]. The indications for transplantation are summarised in Table 12.1 and include both the American Gastroenterology Association and European guidelines for transplantation [20–23]. A recent joint publication between Oxford and Berlin has suggested a method to identify patients with CD for whom transplantation should be considered. The authors used a modified scoring system based on the American Gastroenterology Association SBITx referral guidelines. Each component of the scoring system was weighted according to the impact it might have on morbidity or lead to a poorer outcome post-SBITx (see Table 12.2): a score <2000 would not initiate a referral to a SBITx centre, a score 2000–5000 would initiate referral and a score >5000 would result in an urgent referral for SBITx [24]. In the authors' retrospective assessment of their combined 20 patients, the mean (standard deviation) score was 19350 (8397). As an example, any patient with CD on HPN who develops a single fungal central venous catheter (CVC) infection warrants a referral for consideration of transplantation.

Overall, among all groups undergoing SBITx, HPN failure accounts for 62 % cases, risk of dying due to underlying disease in 26 % of cases and low acceptance of HPN at 12 % [25]. A recent European 5-year multicentre study prospectively evaluated 545 patients with Type 3 IF assigned to two groups according to candidacy for SBITx based on the American Gastroenterology Association guidelines [25]. The authors found that only desmoids and IFALD were associated with increased risk of death on HPN and referral should be mandatory for patients with these conditions. However, recurrent CVC infections, venous thrombosis or ultrashort gut were not associated with an increased risk of death on HPN and so the authors concluded that patients with these conditions should only be considered for transplantation on a

Table 12.1 Indication for transplantation [20–23]

North American indications	European indications
1. Failure of home parenteral nutrition (HPN)	Irreversible, benign, chronic intestinal failure with no possibility of bowel rehabilitation associated with life-threatening complications of HPN
(a) Impending or overt liver failure	
(b) Central venous thrombosis of >2 central veins	Individual case-by-case decision for all patients
(c) Frequent and severe central venous catheter-related sepsis	
(d) Frequent episodes of severe dehydration despite intravenous fluids in addition to HPN	
2. High risk of death attributable to the underlying disease	
(a) Intra-abdominal invasive desmoid tumours	
(b) Congenital mucosal disorders	
(c) Ultrashort bowel syndrome	
3. Intestinal failure with high morbidity and low acceptance of HPN	
(a) Need for frequent hospitalisation, narcotic addiction or inability to function	
(b) Patient's unwillingness to accept long-term HPN	
	Non-indication
	High risk of death due to underlying disease
	Chronic dehydration
	Significantly impaired quality of life

Table 12.2 Scoring criteria for determining if patients with Crohn's disease warrant referral for SBITx [24]

Criteria	Points
HPN for irreversible intestinal failure	1000
Loss of catheter access	
Loss of 1 supracardiac catheter	500
Loss of ≥2 supracardiac catheters	5000
Catheter infection	
>1 Life-threatening catheter infection in 12 months	5000
1 fungal infection	5000
Impending or overt liver failure due to HPN	5000
Frequent dehydration leading to a decrease in eGFR by 20 mL/min at each episode	1000
Overt renal failure requiring renal replacement therapy	5000

(continued)

Table 12.2 (continued)

Criteria	Points
No ECF or stoma but <50 cm of good-quality bowel from duodenojejunal flexure (ultrashort gut)	2500
Proximal ECF or stoma and >100 cm of poor-quality distal bowel (strictured, matted, and obstructed and/or dilated)	5000
Persistence or recurrence of ECF after conservative management or attempted conventional surgical excision despite having optimal nutrition	5000
Prolonged hospital stay with organ dysfunction after last attempt at closure of ECF or any conventional surgical procedure to treat CD	5000
Presence of active CD	1000
Karnofsky performance status score >70 %	1000
Sensitisation status	
Unsensitised	1000
Sensitised	2500
Score analysis	
ITx not yet indicated: conventional surgical and medical management until score increases	<2000
ITx indicated: patient referral pathway should be considered and initiated	2000–5000
ITx definitely indicated: urgent referral should be made	>5000
ITx no longer indicated: transplantation does not represent a survival benefit	>30,000

case-by-case basis. Furthermore, no patient with poor quality of life or chronic dehydration died whilst remaining on HPN during the follow-up period of the study, leading the authors to suggest that such patients should not be considered for transplantation. Within the 545 patient cohort, only 22 underwent transplantation with a 54 % 5-year survival with all deaths occurring as a direct consequence of the transplant itself or immunosuppression. The wisdom of the subsequent position taken by the European Society of Parenteral and Enteral Nutrition to suggest restriction of SBITx to those indicated in Table 12.1 has been questioned by North American colleagues who have highlighted the worse survival rate in this European study compared to outcomes from larger series of patients ($n = 182$) with 75 % 5-year survival [26]. Whilst it is true that high volume centres may have better outcomes than low volume centres in SBITx, the same is the case for HPN care of Type 3 IF patients. At whatever stage of the patient journey, whether on HPN or awaiting SBITx, it is clearly important that care takes place in expert centres with good outcomes [20].

Outcomes of SBITx

In this section, we will review the complications associated with SBITx, survival, quality of life and risk of IBD recurrence. Any complication places the graft at risk of failure and the patient at risk of death. Graft failure will lead to patients resuming HPN and consideration of re-transplantation, even though the risk of success is less than the index transplant [27].

Complications

Rejection

Rejection is divided into acute rejection or chronic rejection. Acute rejection is further subdivided into hyperacute/accelerated acute, acute antibody mediated (humeral) rejection or acute cellular rejection. The interplay between innate and adaptive immune systems will be key to understanding the cause of rejection but also for directing therapy in the future.

Acute Rejection

Hyperacute and Accelerated Acute Rejection

In any transplant, the first principle is to ensure the recipient does not reject the graft. An initial hyperacute rejection is B-cell mediated and occurs within hours of transplantation, whilst an accelerated acute rejection occurs within days of transplantation. Clinical presentation involves marked vascular congestion, necrosis and inflammation of the graft. These rejections are caused by preformed antibodies from the recipient towards the donor; with good serological matching by tissue typing laboratories, such rejections are becoming less commonplace. In consideration of any candidate for transplantation, it is advisable to avoid the use of blood products if at all possible as this increases the exposure of the candidate to antigens that can contribute towards sensitisation.

Acute Antibody Mediated Rejection

A rising donor-specific antibody titre is important in diagnosing acute antibody mediated rejection. However, despite its name, T-cells may also be implicated in the underlying pathogenesis and may occur with or without acute cellular rejection. The antibodies initiate a cascade of inflammation associated with coagulation that results in intestinal injury.

Acute Cellular (T-Cell Mediated) Rejection

This is caused when effector immune T-cells overcome regulatory T-cells in both number and function. It is characterised by both superficial and deep inflammation and apoptosis of the mucosal surface. Acute rejection can occur at any point post-transplantation and has been reported to occur in 50–75 % (1990–2008) of intestinal transplants [28]. In patients transplanted with CD, acute rejection has been reported as the main reason for graft failure at 3 months (33 %) [19].

Chronic

In 15 % of cases, chronic rejection occurs [28], though in a report of patients transplanted with CD it occurred in 28 % [19]. It typically presents with increased stoma output or worsening nutritional status as the transplanted gut fails; it is the commonest cause of graft loss. Chronic rejection results in an insidious fibrosis that is mediated by the adaptive immune system that attacks the arterial blood supply to the graft. It is very challenging to diagnose and often goes undetected at the mucosal surface, in particular on histological assessment. Yet macroscopically on endoscopic assessment, it can cause villous flattening or loss; the whole graft becomes matted and thickened with widespread adhesions, irregular mucosal surface and intermittent ulcerations. The appropriate histological diagnosis is then made via a full thickness sample to assess the vasculature within the serosal surface and look for the pathognomonic signs: concentric intimal thickening of small to large-sized arteries with fibrous changes, medial hypertrophy of smooth muscle cells interspersed with foam cells and fibrosis in the adventitium [29]. Unfortunately, due to the fibrotic nature of chronic rejection, operating in such a hostile environment risks creating enterotomies or entero-cutaneous fistulae. Increasing immunosuppression can reduce some symptoms, but often the only course of action is to retransplant.

Infection

The risk of immunosuppressing a patient to control the risk of rejection is balanced by the risk of developing infections. These can be any pathogen, and often are commensal or ubiquitous pathogens. The risk of infection from one series [30] has been reported to be at a rate of 2.6 episodes per patient, with bacterial infections occurring in 61 % of infections and bacterial septicaemia in 15 %. Other infections include both fungal or parasites. Graft failure is caused by infections in 11 % in general series [28] and 18 % in a CD SBITx series [19].

Viral

Cytomegalovirus (CMV) and Epstein Barr Virus (EBV) are perhaps the two most important viruses in transplantation, mainly due to their almost ubiquitous nature within human communities.

CMV

CMV status is important in both the risk of developing de novo infection in a non-infected recipient from the donor or from another source, and through reactivation of a quiescent infection. As CMV is resident throughout the body, it can present in many ways including bone marrow suppression, CMV retinitis or CMV encephalitis and, perhaps most importantly, CMV enteritis. The presentation of a high output and fever should alert physicians to the risk of CMV enteritis. CMV prophylaxis using preparations such as oral ganciclovir is typically continued for 1-year post-transplantation. The risk associated with CMV is reducing with better immunosuppressive regimes, viral monitoring, prophylaxis and donor/recipient status matching [28, 31, 32].

EBV

EBV is associated with, but not exclusively the cause of, development of post-transplantation lymphoproliferative disorder (PTLD); where PTLD occurs, 97 % have a high EBV viral titre, but immunosuppression and splenectomy are the other main causes [28]. PTLD is treated with a mixture of reduction in immunosuppression to aid recovery of the recipient's immune surveillance strategies at keeping EBV under control and, in some cases, with chemotherapy, such as rituximab. The risk of developing PTLD is 50 %, but more recent larger series have shown a reduction in PTLD from 36 % at 5 years to 7 % [28]. It has also been associated with a high mortality risk where 29 % of those who contract it die (1990–1995) [28, 33, 34] but this again has not been reported in recent series where risk of death is related to age at diagnosis, 19 % if less than 5 years old, 0 % if over 10 years old [35].

Other Pathogens

Enteric

Patients are no less at risk of enteric infections. However, unusually high stoma outputs should alert health professionals to send stool samples for seasonal viral infections, such as adenovirus and norovirus, Clostridium difficile toxin and normal enteric infections, such as Salmonella, Shigella, Campylobacter among others.

Graft Versus Host Disease

As the intestine is resident to more white blood cells than any other non-lymphoid organ in the body, there is a fine line between acute rejection and GVHD. GVHD can affect a number of organs, but in particular seems to affect the skin, the liver (in non-liver transplants), the respiratory system and the bone marrow. GVHD has been reported in a large series (1994–2007, $n=241$) [36] to occur in 9 % of recipients, with children at greater risk than adults (12.4 % vs. 4.6 %, $p=0.05$), and isolated small bowel grafts at less risk than multivisceral grafts (4.4 % vs. 13.2 %, $p=0.05$). However, the mortality associated with contracting it is high with 18 % dying in one large series (1990–2008, $n=500$) [28]. There are no data looking at GVHD in patients with CD.

Renal Dysfunction

As already indicated, short bowel syndrome accounts for 65 % of SBITx indications [12], and renal impairment for patients on HPN is variably reported as occurring in 6–52 % [37, 38]. Whilst recurrent dehydration may be an indication for SBITx in North America, it is rare as a referral criteria [20]. Indeed, the risk of developing chronic renal failure is higher following SBITx than in patients remaining on HPN [37], which is most likely due to tacrolimus, though 80 % of adult SBITx patients experience an episode of acute kidney injury in the first year post-transplant [39]. In addition, in one centre, 9 % of surviving adults required renal replacement therapy during a median follow-up of 7.6 years with 50 % of these being dialysed and 50 % undergoing renal transplant [35].

Chylous Ascites

The lymphatic drainage is disrupted during explant and engraftment. In the first few days of commencing enteral nutrition, chylous ascites is not a common problem due to the use of medium chain triglycerides in polymeric feeds that are both absorbed through the lymphatics. However, delayed presentation can occur and should be treated by commencing a low fat diet.

Survival

As experience grows worldwide, there is an increased understanding of how best to manage these patients.

In contrast to graft failure rates reported in the North American Registry at 1-, 3- and 5-years of 26 %, 46 % and 48 %, respectively [40], graft loss at 1-, 3- and 5-years in CD patients is seen in 10 %, 35 % and 48 % for isolated small bowel grafts or 35 %, 43 % and 43 % in liver-intestinal grafts [19]. In large series in high workload centres (1990–2008, $n=453$ [28]; 1987–2009, $n=687$ [27]), 1-year patient survival is in excess of 80 %, 5 year of 51–61 % and 10 year 42 %. Patients with CD fair similarly, with one series (1987–2009, $n=86$) reporting 1 year 79 % and 5 year 43 % [19].

The survival benefits for those remaining on HPN is better; survival in those with short bowel syndrome on HPN at 1-, 5- and 10-years was 94 %, 70 % and 52 % determined from a large cohort ($n=268$) [41]. A smaller cohort ($n=40$ [42]) reported 1-, 3- and 5-year survival on HPN as 97 %, 82 % and 67 %. In both of these cohorts, malignancy as primary cause for IF had been excluded. This data is supported by a literature review of survival on HPN, which did include patients with cancer in 6/10 papers reported, where the 1-, 5- and 10-year survival was 91 %, 70 % and 55 % [43]. There is a perception that the comparison of patients who are on HPN to those who undergo SBITx is nonsensical as these are widely different groups; those undergoing SBITx have by definition developed complications from HPN. Alternatively, once the transplant outcomes improve to being close to HPN data then the question of timing of transplantation will be brought forward to making these equivalent options rather than merely being regarded as a life-saving option once HPN has failed or brought complications.

Quality of Life

The only study assessing some degree of quality of life (QoL) in CD patients pre- and post-SBITx used a modified Karnofsky performance status score and found that the mean pre-transplant score of 55.6 % rose to 74.4 % ($p < 0.001$) post-transplantation [24]. Previous understanding of QoL in patients with IBD undergoing SBITx had to rely on extrapolation of data from a study investigating pre- and post-SBITx in other conditions using the SF36 and an adapted HPN-QoL questionnaire [44]. In this study by Pironi and colleagues, SBITx patients faired better at ability to holiday/travel, fatigue, gastrointestinal symptoms, stoma management/bowel movements and global health/QoL but not significantly better for eating ability and had worse sleeping patterns, which may be related to the immunosuppression. Others have found that SBITx recipients have similar QoL to those who are stable on HPN but both are better than those with complicated IF on HPN [45]. Larger multicentre studies into those on HPN compared to those undergoing SBITx are needed to resolve the impact on QoL that SBITx has. Furthermore, specific large-scale studies on QoL for IBD patients are also required.

Risk of IBD Recurrence

There are case reports of 2 patients, transplanted in 1994, who develop recurrent CD, both clinical and histological evidence, at 7 months and 8 years post-SBITx [46, 47]. Yet others have reported 19 % [35] and 50 % [48] recurrence rates, though often this was histological recurrence but without clinical symptoms, which may be due to the underlying immunosuppression regimes.

Economic Impact

The cost of intestinal failure is high, and mainly through the forward costs of providing PN. Typically in the UK provision of PN for 5 days per week costs £35–40,000 if self-caring and £55,000 in those with nursing care [49]. In contrast, in the US may appear to be as high as $64,000 on HPN [50], and in Europe €9006 set up fee then €63,000 annually for HPN but €73,000 for initial SBITx and then €13,000 annually [51].

Whilst this is expensive for health care systems, and indirectly therefore to society, the personal cost varies. Unfortunately, heterogeneity in studies looking at QoL makes direct comparisons unclear. Yet having PN or a SBITx does affect an individual's ability to live a normal life, earn money and pay taxes. For example, employment on HPN can be anything from 0 to 52 % [52], 31 % of 151 adult SBITx patients in Pittsburgh were in work or education [28], and 35 % (41 patients) were in employment in a longer follow-up study from Pittsburgh [35]. The only comparative study looking at HPN and SBITx found that 56 % (6 % unemployed) of SBITx patients were in full- or part-time employment compared to 30 % (52 % unemployed) of HPN patients [44]. This may suggest that either patients who undergo SBITx are more motivated or do feel more able to undertake gainful employment than those who remain on HPN.

Conclusion

IBD is commonly associated with IF especially in CD. Most patients do well on HPN to maintain their physical, nutritional and personal well-being. Yet complications develop in some individuals, such as multiple CVC infections or venous thrombosis, or they have other complications—such as IFALD—that predispose them to require transplantation. The benefits of SBITx are improving year on year, and as expertise grows—both surgically and in better immunosuppression protocols—SBITx in time will be on a par with HPN. Encouragingly for patients with IBD, when required, transplantation is successful and patients often do well.

References

1. Lal S, Teubner A, Shaffer JL. Review article: intestinal failure. Aliment Pharmacol Ther. 2006;24:19–31.
2. Pironi L, Arends J, Baxter J, Bozzetti F, Pelaez RB, Cuerda C, Forbes A, Gabe S, Gillanders L, Holst M, Jeppesen PB, Joly F, Kelly D, Klek S, Oivind I, Olde Damink S, Panisic M, Rasmussen HH, Staun M, Szczepanek K, Van Gossum A, Wanten G, Schneider SM, Shaffer J, ESPEN endorsed recommendations. Definition and classification of intestinal failure in adults. Clin Nutr. 2015;34:171–80.
3. Smith T. Artificial nutrition support in the United Kingdom, 2000-2010, Vol. 2013. British Association of Parenteral and Enteral Nutrition Annual BANS Report; 2011.
4. Harrison E, Allan P, Ramu A, Vaidya A, Travis S, Lal S. Management of intestinal failure in inflammatory bowel disease: small intestinal transplantation or home parenteral nutrition? World J Gastroenterol. 2014;20:3153–63.
5. Watanabe K, Sasaki I, Fukushima K, Futami K, Ikeuchi H, Sugita A, Nezu R, Mizushima T, Kameoka S, Kusunoki M, Yoshioka K, Funayama Y, Watanabe T, Fujii H, Watanabe M. Long-term incidence and characteristics of intestinal failure in Crohn's disease: a multicenter study. J Gastroenterol. 2014;49:231–8.

6. Gearry RB, Kamm MA, Hart AL, Bassett P, Gabe SM, Nightingale JM. Predictors for developing intestinal failure in patients with Crohn's disease. J Gastroenterol Hepatol.
2013;28:801–7.
7. Nixon E, Allan P, Sidhu S, Abraham A, Teubner A, Carlson GL, Lal S. Development and
outcome of intestinal failure in Crohn's disease: 3 decades of experience from a national referral centre. Gut. 2014;63:A11.
8. Grant D, Wall W, Mimeault R, Zhong R, Ghent C, Garcia B, Stiller C, Duff J. Successful
small-bowel/liver transplantation. Lancet. 1990;335:181–4.
9. Starzl TE, Rowe MI, Todo S, Jaffe R, Tzakis A, Hoffman AL, Esquivel C, Porter KA,
Venkataramanan R, Makowka L, et al. Transplantation of multiple abdominal viscera. JAMA.
1989;261:1449–57.
10. Williams JW, Sankary HN, Foster PF, Loew JM, Goldman GM. Splanchnic transplantation.
An approach to the infant dependent on parenteral nutrition who develops irreversible liver
disease. JAMA. 1989;261:1458–62.
11. Todo S, Reyes J, Furukawa H, Abu-Elmagd K, Lee RG, Tzakis A, Rao AS, Starzl TE. Outcome
analysis of 71 clinical intestinal transplantations. Ann Surg. 1995;222:270–80; discussion 280–2.
12. Intestinal Transplant Registry Report. XII International small bowel transplant symposium.
Washington, DC: Intestinal Transplant Association; 2011.
13. NHS Blood and Transplant. Organ donation and transplantation activity report 2013, Vol.
2013. Hertfordshire: NHSBT; 2013. https://nhsbtmediaservices.blob.core.windows.net/organ-
donation-assets/pdfs/activity_report_2013_14.pdf.
14. Matsumoto CS, Kaufman SS, Fishbein TM. Inclusion of the colon in intestinal transplantation.
Curr Opin Organ Transplant. 2011;16:312–5.
15. Alexandrides IJ, Liu P, Marshall DM, Nery JR, Tzakis AG, Thaller SR. Abdominal wall closure after intestinal transplantation. Plast Reconstr Surg. 2000;106:805–12.
16. Levi DM, Tzakis AG, Kato T, Madariaga J, Mittal NK, Nery J, Nishida S, Ruiz P. Transplantation
of the abdominal wall. Lancet. 2003;361:2173–6.
17. Allin BS, Ceresa CD, Issa F, Casey G, Espinoza O, Reddy S, Sinha S, Giele H, Friend P,
Vaidya A. A single center experience of abdominal wall graft rejection after combined intestinal and abdominal wall transplantation. Am J Transplant. 2013;13:2211–5.
18. Giele H, Bendon C, Reddy S, Ramcharan R, Sinha S, Friend P, Vaidya A. Remote revascular-
ization of abdominal wall transplants using the forearm. Am J Transplant. 2014;14:1410–6.
19. Desai CS, Khan K, Gruessner A, Gruessner R. Outcome of intestinal transplants for patients
with Crohn's disease. Transplant Proc. 2013;45:3356–60.
20. Pironi L, Joly F, Forbes A, Colomb V, Lyszkowska M, Baxter J, Gabe S, Hebuterne X,
Gambarara M, Gottrand F, Cuerda C, Thul P, Messing B, Goulet O, Staun M, Van Gossum
A. Long-term follow-up of patients on home parenteral nutrition in Europe: implications for
intestinal transplantation. Gut. 2011;60:17–25.
21. Kaufman SS, Atkinson JB, Bianchi A, Goulet OJ, Grant D, Langnas AN, McDiarmid SV,
Mittal N, Reyes J, Tzakis AG. Indications for pediatric intestinal transplantation: a position
paper of the American Society of Transplantation. Pediatr Transplant. 2001;5:80–7.
22. Staun M, Pironi L, Bozzetti F, Baxter J, Forbes A, Joly F, Jeppesen P, Moreno J, Hebuterne X,
Pertkiewicz M, Muhlebach S, Shenkin A, Van Gossum A. ESPEN guidelines on parenteral
nutrition: home parenteral nutrition (HPN) in adult patients. Clin Nutr. 2009;28:467–79.
23. Buchman AL, Scolapio J, Fryer J. AGA technical review on short bowel syndrome and intestinal transplantation. Gastroenterology. 2003;124:1111–34.
24. Gerlach UA, Vrakas G, Reddy S, Baumgart DC, Neuhaus P, Friend PJ, Pascher A, Vaidya
A. Chronic intestinal failure after Crohn disease: when to perform transplantation. JAMA
Surg. 2014;149:1060–6.
25. Pironi L, Hebuterne X, Van Gossum A, Messing B, Lyszkowska M, Colomb V, Forbes A,
Micklewright A, Villares JM, Thul P, Bozzetti F, Goulet O, Staun M. Candidates for intestinal transplantation: a multicenter survey in Europe. Am J Gastroenterol. 2006;101:1633–43; quiz 1679.
26. Abu-Elmagd KM, Mazariegos G. Intestinal transplantation and the European implication:
impact of experience and study design. Gut. 2012;61:166; author reply 167.

27. Desai CS, Khan KM, Gruessner AC, Fishbein TM, Gruessner RW. Intestinal retransplantation: analysis of organ procurement and transplantation network database. Transplantation. 2012;93:120–5.
28. Abu-Elmagd KM, Costa G, Bond GJ, Soltys K, Sindhi R, Wu T, Koritsky DA, Schuster B, Martin L, Cruz RJ, Murase N, Zeevi A, Irish W, Ayyash MO, Matarese L, Humar A, Mazariegos G. Five hundred intestinal and multivisceral transplantations at a single center: major advances with new challenges. Ann Surg. 2009;250:567–81.
29. Swanson BJ, Talmon GA, Wisecarver JW, Grant WJ, Radio SJ. Histologic analysis of chronic rejection in small bowel transplantation: mucosal and vascular alterations. Transplantation. 2013;95:378–82.
30. Loinaz C, Kato T, Nishida S, Weppler D, Levi D, Dowdy L, Madariaga J, Nery JR, Vianna R, Mittal N, Tzakis A. Bacterial infections after intestine and multivisceral transplantation. Transplant Proc. 2003;35:1929–30.
31. Tzakis AG. Cytomegalovirus prophylaxis with ganciclovir and cytomegalovirus immune globulin in liver and intestinal transplantation. Transpl Infect Dis. 2001;3 Suppl 2:35–9.
32. Farmer DG, McDiarmid SV, Yersiz H, Cortina G, Restrepo GC, Amersi F, Vargas J, Gershman G, Ament M, Reyen L, Le H, Ghobrial RM, Chen P, Dawson S, Han S, Martin P, Goldstein L, Busuttil RW. Improved outcome after intestinal transplantation: an 8-year, single-center experience. Transplant Proc. 2000;32:1233–4.
33. Abu-Elmagd KM, Zak M, Stamos JM, Bond GJ, Jain A, Youk AO, Ezzelarab M, Costa G, Wu T, Nalesnik MA, Mazariegos GV, Sindhi RK, Marcos A, Demetris AJ, Fung JJ, Reyes JD. De novo malignancies after intestinal and multivisceral transplantation. Transplantation. 2004;77:1719–25.
34. Reyes J, Green M, Bueno J, Jabbour N, Nalesnik M, Yunis E, Kocoshis S, Kauffman M, Todo S, Starzl TE. Epstein Barr virus associated posttransplant lymphoproliferative disease after intestinal transplantation. Transplant Proc. 1996;28:2768–9.
35. Abu-Elmagd KM, Kosmach-Park B, Costa G, Zenati M, Martin L, Koritsky DA, Emerling M, Murase N, Bond GJ, Soltys K, Sogawa H, Lunz J, Al Samman M, Shaefer N, Sindhi R, Mazariegos GV. Long-term survival, nutritional autonomy, and quality of life after intestinal and multivisceral transplantation. Ann Surg. 2012;256:494–508.
36. Wu G, Selvaggi G, Nishida S, Moon J, Island E, Ruiz P, Tzakis AG. Graft-versus-host disease after intestinal and multivisceral transplantation. Transplantation. 2011;91:219–24.
37. Pironi L, Lauro A, Soverini V, Agostini F, Guidetti M, Pazzeschi C, Pinna A. Chronic renal failure in patients on long term home parenteral nutrition and in intestinal transplant recipients. In: International small bowel transplant symposium, Oxford; 2013.
38. Lauverjat M, Hadj Aissa A, Vanhems P, Bouletreau P, Fouque D, Chambrier C. Chronic dehydration may impair renal function in patients with chronic intestinal failure on long-term parenteral nutrition. Clin Nutr. 2006;25:75–81.
39. Suzuki M, Mujtaba MA, Sharfuddin AA, Yaqub MS, Mishler DP, Faiz S, Vianna RM, Mangus RS, Tector JA, Taber TE. Risk factors for native kidney dysfunction in patients with abdominal multivisceral/small bowel transplantation. Clin Transplant. 2012;26:E351–8.
40. OPTN/SRTR 2011 Annual data report, Vol. 2013. Department of Health and Human Services, Health Resources and Services Administration, Healthcare Systems Bureau, Division of Transplantation; 2012.
41. Amiot A, Messing B, Corcos O, Panis Y, Joly F. Determinants of home parenteral nutrition dependence and survival of 268 patients with non-malignant short bowel syndrome. Clin Nutr. 2013;32:368–74.
42. Pironi L, Paganelli F, Labate AM, Merli C, Guidetti C, Spinucci G, Miglioli M. Safety and efficacy of home parenteral nutrition for chronic intestinal failure: a 16-year experience at a single centre. Dig Liver Dis. 2003;35:314–24.
43. Pironi L, Goulet O, Buchman A, Messing B, Gabe S, Candusso M, Bond G, Gupte G, Pertkiewicz M, Steiger E, Forbes A, Van Gossum A, Pinna AD. Outcome on home parenteral nutrition for benign intestinal failure: a review of the literature and benchmarking with the European prospective survey of ESPEN. Clin Nutr. 2012;31:831–45.

44. Pironi L, Baxter JP, Lauro A, Guidetti M, Agostini F, Zanfi C, Pinna AD. Assessment of quality of life on home parenteral nutrition and after intestinal transplantation using treatment-specific questionnaires. Am J Transplant. 2012;12 Suppl 4:S60–6.
45. Cameron EA, Binnie JA, Jamieson NV, Pollard S, Middleton SJ. Quality of life in adults following small bowel transplantation. Transplant Proc. 2002;34:965–6.
46. Sustento-Reodica N, Ruiz P, Rogers A, Viciana AL, Conn HO, Tzakis AG. Recurrent Crohn's disease in transplanted bowel. Lancet. 1997;349:688–91.
47. Kaila B, Grant D, Pettigrew N, Greenberg H, Bernstein CN. Crohn's disease recurrence in a small bowel transplant. Am J Gastroenterol. 2004;99:158–62.
48. Harpaz N, Schiano T, Ruf AE, Shukla D, Tao Y, Fishbein TM, Sauter BV, Gondolesi GE. Early and frequent histological recurrence of Crohn's disease in small intestinal allografts. Transplantation. 2005;80:1667–70.
49. Specialised intestinal failure and home parenteral nutrition services (adult)—definition no. 12. Specialised Services National Definitions Set, Vol. 2013. Specialised Services National Health Service; 2010.
50. Piamjariyakul U, Ross VM, Yadrich DM, Williams AR, Howard L, Smith CE. Complex home care: part I—utilization and costs to families for health care services each year. Nurs Econ. 2010;28:255–63.
51. Roskott A, Groe H, Krabbe P, Rings E, Serlie M, Wanten G, Dijkstra G. Cost-effectiveness of intestinal transplantation (ITx) for adult patients with permanent intestinal failure (IF) depending on home parenteral nutrition. In: International small bowel transplant symposium, Oxford; 2013.
52. Baxter JP, Fayers PM, McKinlay AW. A review of the quality of life of adult patients treated with long-term parenteral nutrition. Clin Nutr. 2006;25:543–53.

Index

A

AhR. *See* Aryl hydrocarbon receptor (AhR)
Air embolism, 160
Anemia
  IBD, 54
  iron deficiency, 53
  vegetarians/children, 54
Antibacterial activity, vitamin D, 36
Aryl hydrocarbon receptor (AhR)
  cruciferous vegetables, 9
  DHNA administration, 9
  environmental substances, detoxification, 9
  microbial metabolites/dietary
     factors, 9
Autophagy and vitamin D, 36

B

Bifidobacteria-fermented milk (BFM), 137
Biotin (Vitamin B7), 84
Bowel resection, 184
Bowel rest, 120–121

C

Calcium, 89–90
Cardiovascular disease, 208
Catheter related bloodstream infection
    (CRBSI), 161
Chromium, 94
Clostridium difficile infection, 43, 204
Colon cancer and vitamin D, 44
Colorectal cancer (CRC), 80
Copper, 93–94
CRC. *See* Colorectal cancer (CRC)

Crohn's disease (CD), 66, 216, 221
  pediatric and adult studies, 6
Cyanocobalamin (Vitamin B12)
  amino acid and fatty acid metabolism, 80
  anemia, 81
  CD patients, 81
  Cochrane meta-analysis, 81
  Crohn's disease, 80
  diagnosis, 81
  ileoanal pouch anastomosis, 81
  methylmalonic acid and homocysteine
     levels, 81
  micronutrients, 70–71, 80
  neurologic and skeletal changes, 80
  neuronal myelin formation, 80
  oral/sublingual, 81
  physiological processes, 80
  red meats and marine sources, 80
  terminal ileal resections, 81

D

Dendritic cells and vitamin D, 37
Diarrhea, 201, 202
  fat malabsorption, 203
  gastric acid hypersecretion
    clonidine, 202
    fluid and electrolyte, 202
    intestinal resection, 202
    octreotide, 202
    opium tincture, 201
    peptic ulcer disease, 202
    transdermal/oral, 202
  rapid intestinal transit, 200
  small intestinal bacterial overgrowth, 203

© Springer International Publishing Switzerland 2016
A.N. Ananthakrishnan (ed.), *Nutritional Management of Inflammatory Bowel Diseases*, DOI 10.1007/978-3-319-26890-3

Printed in the United States
By Bookmasters